RETT SYNDROME:
THERAPEUTIC INTERVENTIONS

DISABILITY STUDIES

JOAV MERRICK - SERIES EDITOR –
NATIONAL INSTITUTE OF CHILD HEALTH
AND HUMAN DEVELOPMENT,
MINISTRY OF SOCIAL AFFAIRS, JERUSALEM

Contemporary Issues in Intellectual Disabilities
V.P. Prasher (Editor)
2010. ISBN: 978-1-61668-023-7

Disability from a Humanistic Perspective: Towards a Better Quality of Life
Shunit Reiter (Editor)
2011. ISBN: 978-1-60456-412-9

Pain Management Yearbook 2009
Joav Merrick (Editor)
2011. ISBN: 978-1-61209-666-7

Pain. Brain Stimulation in the Treatment of Pain
Helena Knotkova and Ricardo Cruciani Joav Merrick (Editors)
2011. ISBN: 978-1-60876-690-1

Cancer in Children and Adults with Intellectual Disabilities: Current Research Aspects
Daniel Satgé and Joav Merrick (Editors)
2011. ISBN: 978-1-61761-856-7

Pain Management Yearbook 2010
Joav Merrick (Editor)
2011. ISBN: 978-1-61209-972-9

Neural Plasticity in Chronic Pain
Helena Knotkova, Ricardo A. Cruciani and Joav Merrick (Editors)
2011. ISBN: 978-1-61324-657-3

Rett Syndrome: Therapeutic Interventions
Meir Lotan and Joav Merrick (Editors)
2011. ISBN: 978-1-61728-080-1 (Softcover)

Rett Syndrome: Therapeutic Interventions
Meir Lotan and Joav Merrick (Editors)
2011. ISBN: 978-1-61728-614-8 (Hardcover)

DISABILITY STUDIES

RETT SYNDROME:
THERAPEUTIC INTERVENTIONS

MEIR LOTAN
AND
JOAV MERRICK
EDITORS

For permission to use material from this book please contact us:
Telephone 631-231-7269; Fax 631-231-8175
Web Site: http://www.novapublishers.com

NOTICE TO THE READER

The Publisher has taken reasonable care in the preparation of this book, but makes no expressed or implied warranty of any kind and assumes no responsibility for any errors or omissions. No liability is assumed for incidental or consequential damages in connection with or arising out of information contained in this book. The Publisher shall not be liable for any special, consequential, or exemplary damages resulting, in whole or in part, from the readers' use of, or reliance upon, this material. Any parts of this book based on government reports are so indicated and copyright is claimed for those parts to the extent applicable to compilations of such works.

Independent verification should be sought for any data, advice or recommendations contained in this book. In addition, no responsibility is assumed by the publisher for any injury and/or damage to persons or property arising from any methods, products, instructions, ideas or otherwise contained in this publication.

This publication is designed to provide accurate and authoritative information with regard to the subject matter covered herein. It is sold with the clear understanding that the Publisher is not engaged in rendering legal or any other professional services. If legal or any other expert assistance is required, the services of a competent person should be sought. FROM A DECLARATION OF PARTICIPANTS JOINTLY ADOPTED BY A COMMITTEE OF THE AMERICAN BAR ASSOCIATION AND A COMMITTEE OF PUBLISHERS.

Additional color graphics may be available in the e-book version of this book.

LIBRARY OF CONGRESS CATALOGING-IN-PUBLICATION DATA

Rett syndrome : therapeutic interventions / editors, Meir Lotan, Joav Merrick.
    p. ; cm.
  Includes bibliographical references and index.
  ISBN 978-1-61728-080-1 (Softcover)
  1. Rett syndrome--Treatment. I. Lotan, Meir. II. Merrick, Joav, 1950-
  [DNLM: 1. Rett Syndrome--therapy. WM 300]
  RJ506.R47.R485 2010
  618.92'8588--dc22
                        2010027262

Published by Nova Science Publishers, Inc. † *New York*

Contents

Foreword

The time for intensive therapeutic efforts for individuals with Rett syndrome (RS) is NOW. The word "Rett" means "right" in Danish and Norwegian and we believe that it certainly is the right syndrome to study. I (ML) was completely taken by these amazing girls, since the first time I met them in 1992 and began to try to unveil the riddle called Rett syndrome. This fascination drove me deeper and deeper into "Rett land" and the present book is the result of that journey.

According to a Rett legend during 1960s, a young Swedish physician and pediatric neurologist by the name of Bengt Hagberg in Uppsala had seen his first undiagnosed patient (a 4 year old girl in the emergency room) with Rett syndrome. The girl was showing peculiar intriguing signs and a very unusual progression of her condition. She was born after a normal pregnancy and delivery, developed normally until she suddenly and dramatically regressed. He kept her file and slowly encountered more and more clients showing similar features and in Manchester in 1981 at a pediatric neurology conference presented his first 16 cases. At this meeting other physicians approached him and told him about other cases. Professor Jean Aicardi, child neurologist from Paris and Karin Dias from Lissabon started to work together on a scientif paper describing their cases.

Together they presented their finding at a conference in Toronto in 1981 and when their presentation was finished another physician ran up to them "Ich bin Rett, ich bin Rett und will jetzt mit Ihnen sprechen" (I am Rett, I am Rett and want to talk to you now) [1]. This was Andreas Rett (1924-1997) a child neurologist from Austria, who was designated to become the health ministrer in the goverment of Bruno Kreisky and had already published his first cases in 1966 in the German language [2]. He had observed two young patients who were waiting to see him in his clinic. Both were sitting on their parents laps waving their hands in a similar manner. After going through his files he found a collection of more of these patients and wrote about his discovery in a German medical journal [2], but the publication had not received wide recognition. He at once invited the other three child neurologists to Vienna and in April 1992 they all came to visit the clinic of Andreas Rett. It turned out that Rett was in the position that once had belonged to Sigmund Freud and here in the same location many girls and adolescents were waiting to be examined by the four physicians. That afternoon it was decided to call the syndrome Rett syndrome and their findings of 35 cases were described soon afterwards in Annals of Neurology [3].

Another player in the Rett syndrome puzzle is the Howard Hughes Medical Institute investigator Huda Zoghbi, who in 1983 as a neurology fellow encountered her first RS patient and because of that encounter decided to enter research to search for the genetic cause. Zoghbi's group at Baylor College of Medicine worked in collaboration with researchers led by Uta Francke, an Howard Hughes Medical Institute investigator at Stanford University School of Medicine. Zoghbi and Francke, along with members of their laboratories, narrowed the search down for the RS gene by analyzing shared and unshared DNA sequences in a small number of Rett families. By 1998, the search was narrowed to about 200 candidate genes. Israeli postdoctoral fellow Ruthie Amir of Zoghbi's laboratory followed the advice of Igna Van den Veyver, a member of Zoghbi's lab, that MECP2 would be an excellent candidate gene. Amir found mutations in MECP2 that were similar in about 30 percent of their RS patients. The researchers reported their discovery in the October 1999 issue of the journal Nature Genetics [4].

These events and our long lasting work with RS patients have initiated our interest in writing the present book. But the most significant event that drove us to collect paraprofessionals for this project was the reversal of Rett syndrome signs in a mouse model in the laboratory of Adrian Bird [5]. Due to the rapid progression of gene therapy and the vast interest of the global scientific community, it is our belief that within a matter of years a cure can be found for individuals with Rett syndrome.

Until such time arise we would like to share our clinical experiences with other clinicians, so individuals with RS across the globe will receive the best health related intervention and support. It is our firm belief that intensively adapted intervention could prevent some of the secondary deteriorating signs that lead to what is now known as "the fourth stage of RS" [6].

We hope that keeping this specific group of clients at their best functional status and optimal medical condition would become the aim of other devoted health-related professions enabling them to maximize the gain of recovery. This book is the collected experience of an extremely devoted group of people that have spent major part of their professional lives working with individuals with RS, trying to unveil and overcome this debilitating syndrome.

We hope that the knowledge presented in this book would give the readers some tools that will assist health care professional to better assist Rett syndrome clients and their families in dealing with this condition.

Senior Lecturer Meir Lotan, BPT, MScPT, PhD
Department of Physical Therapy, Ariel University Center of Samaria, Ariel, Israel. E-mail: ml_pt_rs@netvision.net.il

Professor Joav Merrick, MD, MMedSci, DMSc
Ministry of Social Affairs and National Institute of Child Health and Human Development, Jerusalem and Kentucky Children's Hospital, University of Kentucky, Lexington, United States. E-mail: jmerrick@zahav.net.il

References

[1]   Lagerkvist B. [Rett hade rätt men tolkade snett.] Läkartidningen 2007;104(1-2):61-3. [Swedish]

[2]   Rett A. On an unusual brain atrophy syndrome with hyperammonemia in childhood. Wein Med Wochenschr 1966;116(37):723–6. [German].

[3]   Hagberg B, Aicardi J, Dias K, Ramos O. A Progressive syndrome of autism, dementia, ataxia, and loss of purposeful hand use in girls: Rett syndrome: Report of 35 cases. Ann Neurol 1983;14(4):471–9.

[4]   Amir RE, Van Den Veyver IB, Wan M, Tran CQ, Franke U, Zoghbi H. Rett syndrome is caused by mutations in X-linked MECP2, encoding methyl CpG binding protein 2. Nat. Genet 1999;23:185–8.

[5]   Guy J, Gan J, Selfridge J, Cobb S, Bird A. Reversal of Neurological Defects in a Mouse Model of Rett Syndrome. Science 2007;315(5815):1143-7.

[6]   Hagberg B. Rett syndrome: Clinical and biological aspects. London: Mac Keith, 1993.

In: Rett Syndrome: Therapeutic Interventions
Editors: Meir Lotan and Joav Merrick

ISBN: 978-1-61728-080-1
©2011 Nova Science Publishers, Inc.

Chapter I

Rett Syndrome: An Introduction with Emphasis on Clinical Characteristics and Intervention

Meir Lotan, BPT, MScPT, PhD[*]

Israeli Rett Syndrome Association, National Evaluation Team and National Rett Syndrome Clinic, Chaim Sheba Medical Center, Ramat-Gan, and Department of Physical Therapy, Ariel University Center of Samaria, Ariel, Israel

Rett syndrome (RS) is a genetic disorder affecting mainly females. It is caused in the majority of cases by a mutation in MECP2, an X-linked gene, and considered the most common genetic disorder in females after Down syndrome, resulting in multiple disabilities. This chapter is an introduction to RS. It presents a basic understanding of the common characteristics of the disorder, and the variants from the classical expression of the syndrome. It will review the current literature on RS, focusing particularly on the clinical features of the disorder. The intention of the chapter is to provide a clear and up-to-date picture of the disorder to assist the clinician in working with this population.

Introduction

Rett syndrome (RS) was first described as a clinical entity in the German literature by Andreas Rett in 1966 [1]. During the period 1966-69, Rett (1924-1997) reported on further 22 cases of females with this disorder and regularly lectured on this topic throughout Austria and Germany [2]. In 1982 he published a second article on the effectiveness of music in the management of individuals with this disorder, again in the German language [3]. Bengt Hagberg and his associates from Sweden were responsible for bringing awareness of this

---

[*] Correspondence: Meir Lotan, BPT, MScPT, PhD, Department of Physical Therapy, Ariel University Center of Samaria, IL-40700 Ariel, Israel. E-mail: ml_pt_rs@netvision.net.il

disorder to the English speaking medical community in 1983 with a description of 35 individuals with strikingly similar clinical features of: "progressive autism, loss of purposeful hand movements, ataxia, and acquired microcephaly" [4]. Since then it has been observed that RS affects mainly females and is found in a variety of racial and ethnic groups worldwide with a variable clinical phenotype [5]. The estimated incidence of RS is 10-15 per 100,000 females [6], although a higher incidence rate has been reported by some researchers [7-9]. It is considered to be the second most common cause of multiple disabilities in females resulting from a genetic disorder, after Down's syndrome [10,11].

RS is a severe neuro-developmental disorder characterized by losses in the areas of intellectual functioning, fine and gross motor skills and communicative ability. Other features include deceleration of head growth and the development of stereotypic hand movements, occurring after a period of apparently normal development. Individuals with RS often develop seizures, disturbed breathing patterns, characterized by hyperventilation and periodic apnoea, (among other abnormalities), scoliosis, growth retardation, and gait apraxia [12]. The main diagnostic indicators will be outlined in the next section.

Diagnosis RS results from an X-linked dominant mutation in MECP2 gene [13,14]. To date mutations in this gene can be found in about 90% of females presenting with the classical phenotype of this disorder [15]. Despite the high specificity and sensitivity regarding genetic diagnosis, clinicians still rely primarily on a clinical diagnosis. This is characterized by a specific developmental profile and certain clinical diagnostic criteria being met [16,17]. The diagnostic criteria for classical and variant RS as outlined by Hagberg et al [17] are as follows :

Classical RS inclusion criteria

- Apparently normal prenatal and perinatal history
- Psychomotor development normal during the first 6 months (may be delayed from birth)
- Normal head circumference at birth
- Postnatal deceleration of head growth (most individuals)
- Loss of purposeful hand skills between 0.5–2.5 years
- Stereotypic hand movements
- Evolving social withdrawal, communication dysfunction, loss of acquired speech, cognitive impairment
- Impaired or deteriorating locomotion

The first three clinical criteria may not be applicable to severely affected females; other criteria will not apply to those who are mildly affected and are only identified due to positive findings of mutations in MECP2.

Supportive criteria

- Breathing disturbances while awake
- Bruxism
- Impaired sleeping pattern from early infancy
- Abnormal muscle tone accompanied by muscle wasting and dystonia

- Peripheral vasomotor disturbances
- Progressive scoliosis or kyphosis
- Growth retardation
- Hypotrophic small and cold feet and/or hands

Exclusion criteria

- Organomegaly or other evidence of a storage disorder
- Retinopathy, cataract, or optic atrophy
- History of perinatal or postnatal brain damage
- Identifiable inborn error of metabolism
- Neurodegenerative disorder
- Acquired neurological disorder due to severe infection or head trauma

Genetic diagnosis

In 1999 mutations in the MECP2 gene were found in patients with a clinical diagnosis of Rett syndrome (RS) and these aberrations were considered the main cause for this disorder [13,14]. Rett syndrome is inherited in an X-linked dominant manner. Approximately 99.5% of cases are sporadic single occurrences in a family, resulting from a de novo mutation in the embryo with RS. 0.5% of the cases are inherited either by a mutation carrier mother or by gametic mosaicism (that can occur in both parents). In most familial cases the carrier mother has favorably skewed X-chromosome inactivation that results in her being unaffected or only slightly affected [18].

In case of a carrier mother the recurrence risk is 50%. If a mutation is not identified in leukocytes of the mother [19], the risk to siblings of the proband is below 0.5% (since germline mosaicism in either parent cannot be excluded). Because of this fact, it is advisable to offer prenatal screening to couples who have had a child with RS or mental retardation due to a MECP2 mutation whether or not the disease-causing mutation has been identified in the mother, since it is not possible for the father to carry pathogenic mutation without phenotypic expression of RS [20].

Stages of rett syndrome

The prenatal and perinatal period appears to be normal in individuals with RS. There is also apparently normal developmental progress for the first 5–6 months of life. Head circumference at birth is within the normal range, with subsequent deceleration of head growth, and microcephaly emerging at around four months post-natally [21,22]. At this stage minor developmental abnormalities are evident in the majority of these children such as mild hypotonia, poor suck, a weak cry and a calm disposition. Such minor signs are difficult to detect even by experts in developmental disabilities [23,24]. Despite close evaluation by experts in the field of spontaneous movements in the early month of the child with RS were development is smilingly normal and despite findings of abnormal movement in these children. No specific abnormal movements could be related to small babies with RS that might be used as markers for early detection and diagnosis [24, 25]. The development of RS is usually described in four stages [12, 26]:

Stage I - early onset stage

Between three months and three years there is reduction or loss of acquired skills such as purposeful hand function, vocalization, and communication skills. A short period of developmental stagnation then commences. This stage is not always clear to diagnose as it is very short and overlaps with stage two.

Stage II - rapid destructive stage

The second stage occurs when the child is between the ages of approximately 1 and 4 years. This stage is usually short, often with a duration of weeks to several months. It is often characterized by rapid regression in language and motor skills. For some girls the characteristics of this stage may be extreme screaming and crying episodes by 18-24 months of age [27]. Additional characteristics include autistic like behaviors, panic-like attacks, bruxism, episodic apnea and/or hyperpnea, seizures, gait ataxia and apraxia and tremors. The emergence of stereotypical hand mannerisms is the prominent feature of this stage. Intermittent esotropia is common, and vasomotor changes are often noted, especially in the lower limbs, as well as deceleration in head growth. After this period of rapid deterioration, RS becomes relatively stable.

Stage III - plateau stage

The third stage is usually apparent from preschool age to adulthood. Apraxia and other motor problems are more prominent during this long stage. The individual with RS will usually show less irritability, and enhanced awareness of her surroundings. This stage can last for decades and as a result may enable the person to make gains in various skills.

Stage IV - late motor deterioration stage

This stage is characterized by reduced mobility. Hagberg suggests individuals losing their walking ability will be defined as stage IVA while those who have never been ambulant move directly from Stage II to IV at age 10 and are regarded as stage IVB [12]. Despite motor deterioration at this stage, there is no decline in cognition communication or hand skills. At this stage individuals with RS may develop dystonia and foot and hand deformities as they grow older.

Clinical characteristics of RS

The principal clinical characteristics of RS and their developmental pattern suggests abnormal development of the cortex in and dysfunction of sub-cortical regulator systems, brain stem, basal forebrain nuclei, and basal ganglia.

Functional disturbances in RS such as breathing, cardiac rate, swallowing, peripheral vasomotor disturbances, sleep, bowel motility, and salivation indicate that there is significant brain stem involvement [28,29]. The cardiac and breathing abnormalities are related to dys-regulation of autonomic tone with failure to regulate vagal (parasympathetic) tone and respiratory rhythm [30].

The key distinguishing feature of RS is the intense, and almost continuous, stereotypic hand movements [31], which develop after a period of purposeful hand use at infancy. These hand mannerisms include hand wringing, hand washing, clapping, patting, or other hand automatisms and occur only during waking hours [12]. A jerky truncal ataxia and an ataxic gait pattern are other prominent features. Other features include breathing dysfunction, EEG abnormalities, spasticity, peripheral vasomotor disturbance, scoliosis and growth retardation. RS may also occur in the presence of other disorders [32 33] in which case appropriate diagnosis can be delayed.

Variant phenotypes of rett syndrome

Many variants of the disorder have been described, which may display different clinical profiles than that presented by the individual with classical RS [34]. Broad clinical variability may be observed among individuals leading to what is termed "atypical forms". These variations may be milder or more severe than the classic RS phenotypes [10,35].

Inclusion criteria

- At least 3 of the 6 main criteria mentioned above for classic RS
- At least 5 of the 11 supportive criteria mentioned above
- Absence of or deterioration in hand skills
- Deterioration in or loss of speech (including babble)
- Hand stereotypes
- Reduction or loss of communication skills
- Deceleration of head growth from early childhood
- Regression in social interactions followed by recovery

Supportive criteria

- Breathing irregularities including air swallowing or abdominal bloating
- Bruxism
- Abnormal locomotion
- Scoliosis or kyphosis
- Lower limb amyotrophy

- Cold, discolored feet, usually hypotrophic
- Sleep disturbances, including night time screaming
- Inexplicable episodes of laughing or screaming
- Apparently diminished pain sensitivity
- Intense eye contact and/or eye pointing

A variant form of RS might present as a more severe or a milder form of the classic disorder. In the severe variants there is no normal developmental period. Individuals with milder variants experience less dramatic or late regression and a milder expression of the characteristics of RS [36]. In this group one might find the "Forme fruste" (FF) [37] or the preserved speech variant (PSV). Although initially thought to be a disorder exclusively affecting females, males with a Rett-like phenotype have been reported occasionally with various phenotypes including severe neonatal encephalopathy [38,39]. As MECP2 mutations and their particular effects are better understood with time and research, characterization of the various phenotypes associated with mutations of this gene should be possible. The different types of RS are further discussed below.

Early epileptic varinat is a severe variant with no period of normal early development. Early features include congenital hypotonia, poorly acquired developmental milestones and infantile epileptic encephalopathy that can include infantile spasms and hypsarrhytmic EEG or other intractable seizure forms, [19,40]. The girl (rarely boy) may later develop a severe manifestation of RS or a classical one [12,41] a significant number of these cases were found to have mutations in a different X-linked gene, CDKL5, its product is involved in phosphorylation of MECP2. In a second variant the early "normal development" is completely absent making diagnosis difficult. This type is referred to as "congenital RS", early seizures are not consistent in this form and head circumference maybe small from birth [11]. Recently several cases with congenital RS were found to have mutations in an autosomal gene FOXG1 on chromosome 14 [42]. So far hardly any MECP2 mutations have been diagnosed in those exhibiting early epileptic form.

Forme fruste (FF)

A known variant of RS with milder clinical features. In this form of RS the clinical signs appear at an older age (around age 2-3 years or older), after the child has already developed expressive language. It is not always easy to connect this regression to the classical appearance of RS but usually with the passing years more and more features of RS are apparent [10]. Individuals with Forme Fruste RS usually present milder reduction in head circumference, better functional hand use, and sometimes the hand mannerisms are more subtle [37].

Preserved speech variant (PSV)

Lately suggested as Zappela RS variant). These children experience a gradual regression that begins after the third year. They do lose part of their purposeful hand use and can develop seizures, although they retain the ability to walk [48]. In this form of RS some language is preserved. However, expressive language is seldom fully coherent. Most of these individuals also show a milder expression of other symptoms of RS some showing more autistic features [43,44].

Mildly affected females

MECP2 mutations have been identified in females with a RS variant, mild learning disability, and even in a few women with no apparent symptoms who demonstrate extreme skewed X-chromosome inactivation [14,45].

Angelman-like RS

These individuals show Angelman-like dysmorphism and behavioral characteristics. They exhibit refined hand function, usually observed in manual stereotypies and manipulate objects in an autistic manner. They usually exhibit superior ability in the area of mobility but demonstrate less social skills and involvement than most individuals with RS [46].

Males with RS

There were several case reports on males with Rett syndrome phenotype even before the discovery of the relation of RTT to the MECP2 gene [47-49], but none of them have presented with the full clinical characteristics of the disorder. An 47,XXY karyotype [50,51] and postzygotic MECP2 mutations resulting in somatic mosaicism have been associated with males meeting the clinical criteria for Rett syndrome [52,53]. Males with a 46,XY karyotype, however, can also be affected by mutations in MECP2. In later publications several males have been positively identified as carriers of the RS mutated gene [38,54-56]. It seems that like females with RS, males with MECP2 mutations show a wide phenotypic spectrum ranging from mild mental retardation through classic Rett -like picture to severe neonatal encephalopathy [57]. They might die at an early age or leave to become adults with intellectual and developmental disability [54,55].The severity of the clinical picture relates to the location and type and mutation. Males with mutations described in females usually have a much worse and severe picture while the ones which are relatively mildly affected and hardly show any Rett like features carry mutations which were not reported to be harmful in females.

Genotype-phenotype correlations

Despite some findings showing some correlation between genotype and phenotype by some, other researchers like Cheadle et al [58] and Huppke et al [59] reported several patients with the same mutation but different phenotypes, the findings suggesting that factors other than mutation type influence disease severity. One such factor is the pattern of X-chromosome inactivation (XCI). Females who have a mutation but have favorably skewed XCI may have milder symptoms or none at all [14]. These conflicting findings are due, in part, to different criteria for determining severity and classifying mutations of the examined participants. Evolution of the phenotype with age and variable expressivity arising from individual variability in X-chromosome inactivation patterns are among other reasons the findings varied [60]. Therefore the below reported findings should be interpreted cautiously with the knowledge that individuals with RS tend to present extreme individual versatility.

Table I-1. Genotype-phenotype correlations summation of investigation

#	The evaluated mutations	Findings	N	Article
1	R133C	Less severe phenotype expression Preserved speech, Better hand movements Usually walking Normocephaly.	24	[61]
2	Truncating mutations	Positive correlation to breathing abnormalities,	78	[14]
	Missense mutations	Scoliosis more common		
3	Missense mutations	Milder features of RS than clients with truncating mutations	44	[58]
	Late truncating mutations	Milder phenotypes than early truncating mutations		
4	Late truncating mutations	less typical presentation than cases with missense and early truncating mutations	116	[62]
	Early truncating mutations	More severe outcome than cases with missense and late truncating mutations.		
5	Missense mutations such as A140V	significant mental retardation in males mild cognitive impairment in females	-----	[54]
6	R294X and R306C	Reduced risk for scoliosis	554	[63]
7	Nonsense mutations	more severe phenotype	---	[64]
	p.R168X	Most severe impairment		
8	genotype-phenotype correlation has not been established		142	[65]
9	Genotype/phenotype correlation studies, in particular in groups of patients with the same mutation, did not offer definitive and interesting data.		64	[66]

Differential diagnosis

In 1997 Leonard investigated the primary diagnosis of 82 girls later positively diagnosed with RS [6]. Despite the fact that more than 50% of individuals with RS presented with clear characteristics of stage II of RS before the age of 15 months [67], only 11 (13%) were diagnosed initially with RS. This is despite the fact that the research population in Leonard's inquiry had visited the physician at the relatively advanced average age of 17 months. Diagnoses given to the remaining cases (N=71) included developmental delay or 'cognitive impairment' (N=42; 60%), hypotonic C.P. (N=14; 19%), autism (N=9; 12%) and 'maternal anxiety' (N=6) [6]. In a present on-going investigation to detect undiagnosed adults with RS living in residential setting across Israel, more than 100 new cases were detected. These individuals were found to be diagnosed (some with overlapping diagnosis) with: Mental Retardation (85%) Cerebral Palsy (33%) and Autism (12%) (Unpublished data). These findings generally correspond with Leonard's report. Therefore to emphasize the distinction between these groups of patients we present some features which might assist in making a differential diagnosis.

Rett syndrome

- Normal development to 6-18 months
- Progressive loss of skills with loss of speech and hand function
- Profound mental retardation in all intellectual domains according to conventional intellectual testing
- Acquired microcephaly, growth retardation, and poor weight gain
- Stereotyped hand-clasping, hand-wringing, or hand washing movements are present in every case; tooth-grinding and breath-holding are also common
- Gait deteriorates and is characteristically straight kneed, wide based and ataxic; some girls may become non-ambulatory
- Language is mostly absent
- Eye contact is present
- Most children have very poor hand function
- Seizures develop in 75% -80% of the population usually appearing for the first time between ages 1 and 3 years
- Behavior modification techniques do not significantly impact target problem behaviors, yet many parents report this form of intervention was beneficial for their daughter with RS.
- The syndrome occurs almost exclusively in females.

Early infantile autism

- Onset before 30 months of age, and often from early infancy
- Loss of previously acquired skills does not occur; generally slower rate of development
- Level of cognitive functioning is varied; 40% are reported to have IQs < 50 and 30% have IQs > 70; additionally, there is subtest scatter in intellectual assessment, with more efficient performance in manipulative or visual spatial skills and immediate memory, while verbal abilities and abstract thinking are found to be more impaired
- Physical development is usually normal
- Stereotyped behavior is more varied, ranging from self stimulatory behaviors to object manipulation
- Gross motor skills are mostly and sometimes impressively superior
- Language may be absent; if speech is present, peculiar speech patterns such as immediate and delayed echolalia and pronominal reversal are often observed
- Eye contact with others may be avoided
- Ritualistic behavior may involve manipulation of objects in an odd and stereotypical way. Other obsessive behaviors may also be present
- Seizures develop in 25% of the population in adolescence and early adulthood

- Children have been found to respond well to behavior modification techniques
- The disorder occurs more in males than females, with a 3:1 ratio.

Cerebral palsy (CP)

- Onset from birth, unless the result of a specific postnatal insult, occurring up to the age of first year.
- Delayed acquisition of normal developmental milestones and skills; physical handicap interferes with motor development
- Level of functioning is varied; IQ in CP may range from below normal to above average and varies according to several intervening factors. Educational attainment often depends on the person's health and access to appropriate education
- Physical development may be influenced by the extent of motor involvement and as a result of additional medical complications
- Stereotyped behavior is not typically a characteristic of this diagnosis
- Gross motor development is delayed or abnormal; ambulatory status is related to the type and severity of cerebral palsy
- Receptive language is generally much better than expressive; expressive language ability is related to the extent of motor interference
- Eye contact is present
- Ability to manipulate objects is influenced by the extent of motor impairment
- Seizures are present in 86% of individuals with spastic quadriparetic cerebral palsy and 12% of those with athetoid cerebral palsy
- Behavior modification interventions may be appropriate for specific situations
- The disorder occurs slightly more frequently in boys than girls.

Pathogenesis in rett syndrome

When considering the vast clinical/neurological signs displayed by individuals with RS, there are relatively few pathological findings within the neural system of individuals with RS [68]. The brain in individuals with RS are usually small and densely packed with neurons. The fact that the brain weight of individuals with RS is 60%-80% of expected weight in age matched females without RS [69] may explain the microcephaly observed in this population. Decreased dendritic spines and arbors have been noted [70]. The densely packed cells at the cortex, thalamus, basal ganglia, amygdala, and hippocampal areas resemble the brain of a young infant [71]. In individuals with RS entering their second decade of life, mild loss of neurons and moderate non-specific gliosis is observed [71]. Most of the basal ganglia structures seem relatively normal, yet the severe movement disturbances observed in RS can be attributed to abnormality in the Substantia Nigra [69 72].

MECP2 expression in postmitotic neurons is critical for brain function, and a delicate balance of MeCP2 is required for proper neuronal maturation in the postnatal period [73]. MeCP2 was believed to be expressed ubiquitously in all tissues and stages of development, but it is now accepted that its highest expression is in mature neurons and its lowest expression is in glia. Expression in spinal cord and hindbrain, which are early developing systems, precede expression in the hippocampus and cerebral cortex [74,75]. The gene expression develops progressively from deep cortical to superficial layers following cortical laminar development (''inside-out''). This is consistent with the role of MeCP2 in postmigrational neuronal development and synaptogenesis, making it a marker of mature neurons in the postnatal brain [76]. The gradual increased expression of MeCP2 in human brain continues during childhood [77]. It is becoming clear that, MeCP2 has no significant role in early embryonic stages and is not involved significantly in cell fate decisions. Gross brain tissue in girls with RS appears to be relatively normal. Microcephaly is related to the decreased size of neuronal cell bodies, whereas higher packing density is related to reduced pyramidal neurons, dendritic spines, and arborization. These changes are most prominent in layers 2/3 projection neurons of prefrontal, postfrontal, and anterior temporal regions and less prominent in the occipital regions, as has been shown in autism [78-80].

Using immunoblotting techniques, the RS brain shows reduction in all dendritic proteins, but mainly in microtubule-associated protein (MAP)-5 (early dendritic differentiation marker) and MAP-2 (associated with dendritic branching) [81,82]. Minicolumn structures are arranged more tightly, similar to autism brain [83], because of decreased MAP-2 cytoskeleton protein in the subplate neurons [81]. Synaptic development is impaired [84]. Abnormal levels of neurotrophic proteins, neurotransmitters, and their receptors were described in several studies [85]. Presently, researchers are looking for downstream targets for MECP2 regulation. General gene expression profile analysis reported that less than 5% of genes are significantly altered, and, more commonly, are up-regulated [86,87].

Brain-derived neurotrophic factor (BDNF) was found to be a major target for MeCP2 by two separate laboratories. BDNF is a neurotrophin that is essential for adult neuronal plasticity, learning, and memory. MeCP2 is associated with methylated CpG sequences which upstream the BDNF promoter. Dissociation from the promoter, which is phosphorylation dependant, results in a switch to a transcriptionally permissive chromatin state. Up-to-date findings are consistent with reduced expression of BDNF in RS while, basically, BDNF expression should be up-regulated. A disrupted response to activation related to higher BDNF basal levels in Mecp2-deficient mice might explain this paradox. Otherwise, low or absent BDNF levels and abnormally high levels produce aberrant maturation and reduced dendritic arborization [88-90].

Recently, McGill and colleagues [91] demonstrated MeCP2 binding to methyl CpG dinucleotides on the corticotrophin (CRH) gene promoter. CRH is overexpressed in Mecp2308 mutant mice, resulting in elevation of corticotropin and adrenal steroids causing increased anxiety-like behaviors and abnormal stress response. Frequently encountered anxiety-like behaviors in patients who have RS and increased urinary cortisol secretion are consistent with this mechanism of function. Repeated corticosteroid exposures and elevated CRH can affect dendritic branching and synaptic plasticity and cause memory impairment, making CRH regulation even more significant.

Clinical characteristics of rett syndrome

Individuals with RS display a wide variety of clinical abnormalities most of which are listed below.

- Ambulation (crawling & walking). Most children with RS begin to crawl later than normally expected and usually display abnormal forms of crawling. Most of them will not show customary reciprocal crawling, some of them compensate by scooting, bunny hopping, or rolling [92]. Walking is achieved in 50%-85% of children with RS [12,93] . Those who do achieve walking ability, usually do so after the age of 19 months. There have been anecdotal reports by parents regarding initiation of walking by their daughters as late as at 16 years of age. The regular walking pattern of individuals with RS is a wide based, straight kneed ataxic gait. Many of them start toe walking at later stages which necessitates intense physical therapy or orthopedic intervention. At the second or third decade of life, 33%-85% of those who have achieved the ability to walk might lose the ability to do so [12, 94].

- Apraxia is a broad term relating to situations in which one is having difficulties in performing a motor act on demand or in learning a new motor function. It is derived from a deficit in sensory (tactile, proprioceptive, vestibular) information processing, causing a skewed body schema disabling the child's ability to engage in motor planning [95]. This difficulty affects the child in all functional areas (feeding, movement, speech, hand function). Given the immense functional impact of apraxia in RS, it is recommended that the child with RS should be treated in accordance with the 'Guidelines on intervention with children with apraxia' [2,96,97].

- Breathing abnormalities. Most (84%) individuals with RS present with some form of breathing abnormality such as apnea, hyperventilation, breath holding, as well as deep breathing and apneustic breathing and bloating, usually from stage III on in the disorder [98,99]. These abnormalities are apparent during walking hours alone [100], and are probably due to defects in neurochemical signaling resulting from abnormal patterns of neurotransmitter and neuromodulatorexpression. It is believed that Breathing dysregulation in RS results from disturbances in mechanisms that modulate the respiratory rhythm, acting either alone or in combination with more subtle disturbances in rhythm and pattern generation [99]. It is important to note that breathing irregularities during sleep are a sign of a respiratory problem not associated with Rett Syndrome and these should be examined by a physician since they may be indicative of an acquired illness [92]. According to Julu, and his associates [101], individuals with RS show 13 types of breathing irregularities divided into four main categories. Some of these respiratory irregularities respond to medication, others do not. An expert in the field of RS should be consulted with regard to the child's breathing pattern and the proper care advised [102]. The breathing categories identified by Julu et al., are the following: breath holding, forced expiration, Feeble/Shallow breathing and Valsalva breathing.

- Feeble/shallow breathing. Individuals with this type of breathing display low PO_2 and raised PCO_2 which can lead to repeated episodes of exaggerated simultaneous increases in cardiac sensitivity to baroreflex, cardiac vagal tone, and blood pressure. During such incidents the functional indices of the whole brain stem are simultaneously and momentarily increased, a situation referred to by the authors as "brain stem storms." Such sudden large increases in vagal tone combined with poor ventilation, raised carbon dioxide, and hypoxia carry a risk of cardiac arrest [101]. Individuals with RS presenting this type of breathing are more susceptible than other individuals with RS to a phenomenon termed "Brain stem shutdown" (characterized by a drop in arterial blood pressure). In severe cases the brain stops controlling the heart rate and the pacing of the heart is transferred to the internal pacer. At this point the child can look lifeless, therefore proper diagnosis and treatment is essential. Researchers are suggesting clinical intervention when respiratory abnormalities of the child with RS are prominent. Treatment with ampakine CX546 in mice with RS for 3 days was found to restore normal respiratory frequency and ventilation [103].

- Balance and coordination. When walking, the person with RS has to manage her unreliable sensory processes (apraxia), her fear of movement, her fluctuating muscle tone, and poor muscular control attributed to ataxia. The combination of such challenges inflicts severe functional limitations upon the individual with RS. Therefore, many of these girls will find it hard to handle tasks such as ascending or descending staircases, walking on uneven surfaces, running and more. On the other hand some children with RS have been known to be able to use a trampoline, ride a bicycle, ski, or use roller blades. A daily low intensity, short term treadmill program has been found to improve functional ability in children with developmental disabilities [104] including four girls with RS [105]. These reports, and the assumption that the fourth stage of RS might be prevented in some cases, if intervention is appropriate and focused enough [106], support the case for early intervention and intense programs for this population.

- Body schema. Due to the problem of sensory imbalance of children with RS and immaturity in cerebral functioning it is probable that the concept of body schema is incomplete. This could be concluded from the apraxia shown by many of the persons with RS and from the skewed midline [107-109] presented by some. Their fear of movement is probably caused by this same problem. Experiencing such sensory uncertainty on a continuous basis could cause a sense of fear and insecurity leading to reluctance to engage in movement. To reduce some of the anxiety associated with movement in the individual with RS the application of a daily program which would provide an experience of intense proprioceptive input (deep pressure), in order to help the individual with RS in building up a sense of orientation in space is recommended [2,109].

- Bruxism (teeth grinding). Teeth grinding during waking hours is evident in 53%-95% of individuals with RS. It is usually more intense in the younger age groups and generally disappears in adults [110]. Bruxism is typical in periods of excitement or anxiety. Teeth grinding may cause damage mainly to incisors and canines, but molars can be damaged as well [111].

- Cognitive abilities. Individuals with RS display functional abilities corresponding with a severe to profound level of intellectual disability. Nevertheless, conventional intelligence tests require the use of hand function and expressive linguistic ability on the part of the person being tested. These skills are almost entirely absent in individuals with RS, thereby questioning the appropriateness of these instruments for this specific population. Regardless of the findings using conventional intellectual assessment tools, it is apparent that these individuals possess learning ability [112-115] and that learning skills can be enhanced when these girls are sufficiently motivated. Findings also show that learning is maintained after a 'washout' period [114]. It is also apparent that learning, including literacy skills [115], is possible in this population throughout adulthood [110].

- Communication. The initial normal-like development of the child with RS leads to the belief that their communicative attunement and intentionality are preserved and therefore could later be used to successfully implement alternative communication [116]. Individuals with RS indicate an emotional and social need to communicate, yet this need is masked by their disabilities [117], making their efforts to communicate hard for others to interpret. Nevertheless, when motivation levels are sufficiently high in a person with RS and those attending to her are attentive, she will be able to convey her needs and wants, greatly improving her quality of life [118,119]. Some individuals with RS use pictures, body language, and gestures [110] to assist them in communication. The use of AAC (Alternative and Augmentative Communication) can compensate for the severe communication difficulties experienced by these girls [120], and is therefore highly recommended for individuals with RS. It is recommended that every individual with RS should be evaluated with regard to assistance in the area of communication skills (preferably by an expert in the field of AAC and RS) and the most appropriate communication approach chosen according to the child's skills and personality [113].

- Digestive system. Many (74%) individuals with RS experience gastrointestinal problems [114]. Intestinal problems detected in individuals with RS include gastro-esophageal reflux (GER), bowel dysmotility, constipation, and functional megacolon. GER is more common in non-ambulant girls and will present with regurgitation of food, vomiting, dysphagia related to esophagitis, chronic cough and recurrent aspirations. Evaluating the gastro-esophageal junction's function by milk scans and pH probe is suggested in the more severe cases. Treatment is usually effective and includes anti-reflux agents, antacids, smaller and thickened feedings, and proper positioning .When these interventions fail, surgery in the form of funduplication and gastrostomy might be suggested. One of the most common problems for individuals with RS is constipation. Severe and recurring constipation can cruelly impede quality of life. In extreme cases, fecal impaction, volvulus, and intussusceptions occur [122]. A diet including a high fluid and fiber intake with occasional use of stool softeners can help prevent acute intestinal crises and prevent or minimize the occurrence of constipation [2]. When those measures are ineffective in controlling constipation, Miralax (polyethylene glycol) has been found highly effective and is tolerated better than milk of magnesia. Recent observations regarding a large number of girls with RS have detected significant gallbladder dysfunction, notably in girls under the age of 20 years. The findings included both gallbladder dysfunction and gallstones. These findings present a significant problem in RS. The frequency seems to be far greater than expected in a normal population of children [46]. In the event of otherwise unexplained distress in girls with RS, a medical evaluation should give specific consideration to the possibility of gallbladder dysfunction.

- EEG findings. Certain EEG findings common to the disorder are not unique to Rett syndrome. However, they are relatively specific and include the slowing of the occipital dominant background activity with very frequent spike or sharp wave discharges mainly in central regions accentuated during sleep early in the course of the syndrome (usually during the regression stage). There is also loss of non-rapid eye movement (NREM) sleep characteristics. Later in the course of the disorder (end of stage 3–stage 4) there is evidence of slowing of background with decreased epileptiform activity. Video/EEG monitoring reveals frequent episodes of apnea and hyperventilation, laughing, screaming, and vacant staring spells with no consistent EEG correlates [123].

- Emotional responses. The child with RS usually develops from birth experiencing common parental affection as any other child, in a manner that supports the development of normal emotional responses [124]. At the beginning of stage II of RS the child might experience extreme disorientation [110] and her physical deterioration might lead to frustration, anger, sadness, fear and surprise and a sense of loss. This loss of control over her body and mind is incomprehensible to the child and can cause her to burst in to anger and rage or to give in to an emotional withdrawal and apathy. At the end of that turbulent stage, the end of functional deterioration, the child usually regains some of her emotional balance which can be observed by calmer disposition. Nevertheless the person with RS will be dependent on others for most of her daily needs and their responses to her will affect her behavior and her emotional expression for better or for worse [125]. Negative emotional expressions are common especially in two phases in individuals with RS. During stage two behaviors such as screaming, hair pulling, biting, hitting, pacing, anxiety, inattentiveness and hyperactivity can be observed, while the adolescent with RS (10-20 years of age) might present behaviors such as: moodiness, sleeplessness, poor appetite, loss of weight, loss of interest in activities they enjoyed previously, unexplained crying and signs resembling depression. These behaviors have been attributed to constipation, hyperventilation, bowel pain, a noisy environment, excessive stimulation and temperature changes. These changes can shift from laughter to dissatisfaction and back again within seconds. An emotional state can last for a few minutes or up to several hours. The fact that the individual with RS has a full range of emotional states [124] has to be understood and addressed by her caregivers. Her difficulty in communicating clearly mean that it is the responsibility of the caregiver to get to know the child well, to decipher the cause of her discomfort and to try and resolve the problem, thereby addressing her emotional well-being as well. A current hypothesis suggests that the reduced catecholamines in the brain of individuals with RS are associated with abnormal synaptic function responsible for the changes in mood and behavior of girls with Rett syndrome. According to this assumption behavioral changes can be modified by medications that increase serotonin and norepinephrine at central synaptic sites. An on going research is now being conducted as to the efficiency of such medication (such as: Venlafaxine, Citalopram or Celexa) on behavior of children with RS. Yet the author believes that even in the case were these drugs be found effective, it is recommended to try conservative emotional approaches and use such drugs only in severe cases where the child's behavior is completely unexplained and uncontrolled and is extremely harming the person with RS and her interactions with her surroundings.

- Epilepsy. Seizures have been reported in 30%-90% of individuals with RS [11,12,123]. Seizures occur more frequently once the disorder stabilizes (at the end of stage II - usually between 2-5y of age), However, an early epileptic variant with neonatal seizures or hypsarrhythmia, followed by classical Rett clinical picture is well delineated [126,127]. Epilepsy is easier to control in individuals showing late onset epilepsy than early onset epilepsy with seizures appearing after the age of 5 more likely to be well controlled [128]. RS severity was found to correlate with more severe epilepsy, while parameters associated with milder phenotypic expression (preserved speech, normal head circumference, preserved ambulation) were inversely related [129, 130]. Epilepsy in RS might be difficult to treat, with recent findings suggest 34.4% having intractable epilepsy [128].

All kinds of epileptic seizures are present in individuals with RS [131] with generalized tonic-clonic seizures and partial complex seizures most common [132], yet one should be aware of a high rate of nonepileptic paroxysmal events [12, 126, 127, 133]. Such episodes mimicking epileptic events might actually be related to motor activity such as twitching, jerking, and trembling, or a cardiac arrhythmia associated with a prolonged QT interval [131]. These events are not correlated with epileptiform activity on EEG. On the other hand, clinical events accompanying EEG epileptiform activities, such as absence episodes or flexor spasms, are not always recognized as seizures by the parents [131]. Recently we have identified two girls in which stereotypes were actually accompanied by epileptiform activity on the EEG, suggesting that if movements are very rhythmic and mainly unilateral a video EEG should be performed (Unpublished data).

Therefore the use of E.E.G video-telemetry is advised to reveal the fact that "observed attacks\mannerisms" are in actuality events of breath holding and in this case should not be controlled with anti-convulsant medication [123]. Use of video EEG for further defining these episodes or at least discussing them with an expert in the field of RS will prevent the inappropriate use of anti-epileptic drugs. Evidence shows that epileptic activity in RS is reduced and is mostly easily controlled in individuals reaching adolescence [131]. In many cases seizures are easily controlled by medications. However, in others they can be intractable. Common pharmacological interventions with this population include valproic acid, lamotrigine, topiramate, carbamazepine and recently keppra. The use of phenol-barbitone, and to a lesser extent benzodiazepines, can severely impact on the level of alertness and responsiveness of the client with RS to the point of sudden pseudo-motor deterioration. Their use should be avoided as much as possible

- Feeding. Individuals with RS usually enjoy eating, and present a developed sense of taste with obvious food preference [110]. It was established that frequent small meals during the day with added carbohydrate foods can support growth as well as weight gain in individuals with RS [92]. Due to functional limitations meal times are usually prolonged. Individuals with RS are usually very slim averaging at 17.5 BMI. The normal Body Mass Index for their peer group is 21-26 [121]. This lower BMI appears to be due to altered energy balance [134] Furthermore, it has been found that many children with RS suffer from mild to moderate malnutrition [92], as their caloric intake is 70% of the norm due to their feeding difficulties [135]. Feeding problems are common in RS [121,136]. Some of the difficulties experienced at meal times include spitting, immature chewing patterns, exaggerated gag reflex, reflux, swallowing difficulties, and intestinal problems [137]. In order to increase pleasure associated with the experience of eating, the physical and human environment should be individually assessed and adapted as necessary [2]. In a situation where the addition of nutritional supplements does not address the problem of insufficient caloric intake, a gastro-intestinal tube might need to be considered. After such surgical interventions individuals with RS have been found to gain weight, demonstrate an improved growth rate, present less agitation and irritability and had better energy levels as were evidenced by an ability to function at higher activity levels [138,139].
- Growth failure. Most individuals with RS show a decrease in growth and weight gain presented in average BMI measures at 17.5 [121]. Growth failure is detected in 85%-90% of individuals with RS and the situation appears to worsen with age [11,92,138,140]. If not addressed, girls with RS can become dangerously malnourished. Such a situation might arise despite a healthy appetite, and meals of lengthy duration, which may create the illusion that the child has a high caloric intake. It is postulated that this poor growth rates are the result of poor coordination of both the oropharyngeal and gastroesophageal processes, which leads to poor caloric intake and high energy expenditure [134-137]. As a result of this it is essential that persons with RS should have a fat and carbohydrates enriched diet, with vitamins and minerals supplemented. Regular supervision by a dietitian with expertise in RS is highly recommended. In some cases where nutrient uptake is low and conventional food supplements are not enhancing the child's development sufficiently, a gastrointestinal tube is recommended. Anecdotally, the information available to date suggests that all parents, who agreed to this operation were very pleased with the results.
- Head circumference. At birth, head circumference is usually found to be within the lower normal percentile [59]. Between 2-4 or 5-12 months post delivery [21,22] head growth has been found to gradually decrease, resulting in true or relative microcephaly [141]. Steinbom and his associates [142] reported a correlation between head circumference and functional abilities of children with RS at one year of age but those findings were preliminary and were not supported by other research groups.
- Hearing. Due to communication limitations of individuals with RS it is a complex task to perform a conventional hearing test. Nevertheless, it has been widely observed that the sense of sound appears to be extremely well developed in individuals with RS. It is common knowledge that they love music [143-146], they have been found to remember special sounds and have the ability to connect them to

specific events. They love the sound of children singing and the whisper of adults [110] and music has been established as a key motivator for learning in this population [112,113]. In a single report, a slight to moderate loss of hearing loss was found in 17.3% of the participants. Hearing loss was mainly found in adults participants in this study and was attributed to lengthy use of anti-convulsant medication [147].

- Hyperkinetic movement. Hyperkinetic movement is characteristic of those individuals with RS who are able to walk. It is believed that the child with RS can identify her goal and direction of movement but that this movement is interfered with by ataxia and apraxia. Consequently, gross motor movements in girls with RS may be perceived by the external observer as senseless or aimless roaming [92].

- Limited hand use. Most children with RS acquire some form of hand function in their first year. Such hand function might include gripping objects, self feeding, and some parents even report the ability of their children to finger dial on a phone, or to flip pages of a book at a very young age. From about 8 months up to approximately 4 years of age these children gradually lose hand function. It was found that 33.6% of children with RS have a left hand preference, 40.7% show right handedness, and 25.7% show no preference in hand use [148]. Children with left handedness usually show dominance transference to the right at age 7-8 years [110]. The assumption is that poor functional abilities of individuals with RS are not derived from lack of ability rather from the combination of apraxia and lack of opportunity to engage this ability [149]. Despite the deterioration of functional hand use individuals with RS can and should be taught hand skills and how to regain those which have been lost, as there is evidence to show that this ability improves with such intervention[150].

- Language. The development of language in infants with RS is extremely rare. In infancy, vocalisations as well as proto-speech, are slower to develop and are usually poorer than would be expected of babies without RS. In our experience some girls retain the ability to express a few words, this ability is usually expressed in situations of stress ("afraid", "Mammy") or when highly excited ("cookie", "dog"). It is believed that most individuals with RS have good verbal comprehension, understanding the meaning of many words. They also enjoy listening to children and adults speaking and are extremely fond of stories. When given the chance many individuals with RS can acquire literacy to the level of a couple of dozen of words. The preserved speech variant (PSV) comprises 1-4% of all individuals with RS [43,151,152]. These individuals have the ability to speak, usually with an odd and sparse vocabulary.

- Life expectancy. Due to the rarity of RS, and its relative novelty in the scientific world [4], very little is known about long term prognosis and life expectancy. While there are a few women in their 40's and 50's with a diagnosis of RS, there have been too few women studied to make reliable estimates beyond age 40. Many women with RS can now be expected to live into their 40s and beyond, assuming that they have no undue medical complications [153]. In fact in a present on-going investigation to detect undiagnosed adults with RS living in residential setting across Israel, 29 women were found over the age of 60 years (Unpublished data). Females with RS typically survive into adulthood, but the incidence of sudden, unexplained death is significantly higher than in other adults of similar age [154]. These sudden deaths may be due, in part, to the higher incidence of longer QT intervals, T-wave abnormalities, and reduced heart rate variability in RS [155,156]. It might also be related to SUDEP (Sudden death due to epilepsy) [157] or other 'Complications of Rett syndrome' [158] such as breathing abnormalities [101].

- Muscle shortening. Muscle shortening is common in individuals with RS presenting with high muscle tone. It should be observed, however, that in the case of girls exhibiting low muscle tone in the early years, they may gradually experience increased muscle tone with age [94]. The first muscle influenced by hypertonia is usually the gastrocnemius. Toe-walking is usually observed as a result. In severe cases the person with RS can lose her ability to walk. This phenomenon can be addressed by the physical therapist through a daily standing program, or by using specially designed active splints, or through serial casting [2]. In severe cases the orthopedic surgeon might suggest botulinum toxin (botox) treatment or surgery. Other muscles tending to shorten are the hip adductors, and in wheelchair bound individuals, the hip flexors. Another group of muscles in danger of shortening are the anterior muscles of the shoulder girdle. This happens due to rarity of hand function in this population and the constant hand mannerisms usually performed at the midline at chest level [159]. Girls with RS should be routinely examined for evidence of muscle shortening by the physical therapist, and the orthopedic surgeon. An appropriate intervention program should be implemented if required.

- Muscle tone. Individuals with RS present with abnormal muscle tone. Most children with RS show a gradual change from very low muscle tone or even severe hypotonia at birth and during the first stage of RS. Gradually some (about 40%) will develop high muscle tone including spasticity and/or rigidity that will initiate from the shin muscles. About 30% will remain hypotonic and the rest will show fluctuating/dystonic muscle tone [94]. Individuals with RS who show the least muscle tone (hypotonia) as infants appear to become the most rigid or hypertonic in adulthood [93]. Such unbalanced muscle tone accompanying ataxia and apraxia will severely affect the child's posture and stability thus severely harming her ability to move or function in any way. These difficulties require intensive physical therapy or other health related intervention programs (such as hydrotherapy, hyppotherapy, or occupational therapy) aimed at reducing muscle tone and enhancing functional capacities.

- Orthopedic problems. Over the years with the progression of RS some of the following orthopedic problems can arise.

  o   Scoliosis. It has be found that 83% of children with RS experience scoliosis to a severe degree, while a deviation of at least 10 degrees may be detected in the spine in all other persons with RS [12]. According to Kerr [94] 90% will develop scoliosis and in 60% it could be defined as severe. Scoliosis in RS becomes apparent between the ages of 3 and 18 years. The median age at onset of scoliosis was found at 9.8 years, with the likelihood of scoliosis development increasing with advancing age. By 6 years of age, 25% of individuals with RS were diagnosed with scoliosis, and 75% of this group of clients is diagnosed with scoliosis by 13 years of age [160].

       When the spinal curve exceeds 50 degrees surgery is generally advised by an orthopedic surgeon to alleviate difficulties in walking, spinal mobility and respiratory function. An early diagnosis followed by an intensive physical therapy program was found useful in reversing the spinal deformity in a child with RS [161], and prevented the need to perform surgery in several others [137]. Intensive physical therapy is recommended in this situation by all experts in the field of RS [105, 109, 162-165]. Bracing has not been found to be an efficient means of preventing or improving the progression of scoliosis [166], but it can provide support and improve function since it can help the very hypotonic\flaccid individual maintain an erect posture. When the condition of the child during the pre-surgery period was found as severe, most parents have agreed that surgery was the right option after the procedure has completed [167].

o   Kyphosis. Kyphosis is more frequent in mobile individuals with RS. In most cases it is not significant enough to require intervention. However due to a constant forward posture involving the shoulder girdle associated with stereotypical hand movements, it is advisable to check for kyphosis during routine visits to the orthopedic surgeon and physical therapist. In the case of muscle shortening at the anterior aspect of the chest's musculature, intervention will be required, either by the physical therapist or the orthopedic surgeon [2].

o   Hip instability. This orthopedic problem is not extremely common in individuals with RS. It presents more commonly in those who do not walk. [168]. Hip dislocation may be avoided through the use of preventive measures such as daily standing program, manual exercises to keep full range of motion in the joint, serial casting, the use of hydrotherapy to strengthen the muscle around the joint, or by using botolinum toxin at specific injection sites [2].

o   Feet deformities. This is represented by a deviation from the normal alignment of the feet, which is caused by asymmetry in muscle activation. It is common among wheelchair users and severely affected individuals with RS [168].

- Osteoporosis/osteopenia occurs frequently in females with RS and decreased bone mineral density has been reported in very young girls as well as adults in comparison to controls [169]. It is assumed that this phenomenon results from poor bone formation. As a result of osteoporosis pathological fractures can occur [170]. As might be expected, fractures are more common in non-ambulatory children highlighting again the importance of preserving walking ability [171]. Anti-epileptic drugs are also known to have a negative effect on Vitamin D absorption and therefore are seen as playing a contributory role in osteoporosis [172]. Recent findings suggest that the first and only non CNS Gene influenced by MECP2 is related to bone osteoblastic-osteoclastic balance and its elevation because of mutated MECP2 brings to increased bone absorption and early osteoporosis[173]. These findings support the need for routine checking of bone density from childhood, and commencement of physical programs such as intensive standing and walking [165] Nutritional supplements as well as medical interventions if required, as preventive measures.

- Pain sensation. Decreased sensitivity to pain has been reported a number of times in this population by researchers [12,27,92,110]. Other neuro-chemical findings in this population support the possibility of a decreased reaction to pain. Kalmanchey [174] found reduced conduction velocity in peripheral neural pathways in individuals with RS. Witt-Engerstrom, & Hagberg, [175] found a reduction in the number of dorsal root ganglia that serve as ascending pathways to painful stimuli towards brain pain centers. Budden, Myer, & Butler [176] reported high values of Beta-endorphins in the spinal fluids of individuals with RS. Moreover, low levels of P-substance (a neurotransmitter involved in relaying pain sensation), were also found in the neural systems of individuals with RS [177]. The accumulating evidence supports the notion that pain sensation is reduced in individuals with RS. Due to these findings and since verbal communication in individuals with RS is lacking, manual treatments should be performed with caution and persons with RS should be carefully checked for possible tissue damage with any unexplained change in mood or behavior.

- Pregnancy (of the mother) and perinatal period (of the client with RS). No common complications have been documented during these periods. A study by Huppke et al [59] found that head circumference, although smaller than expected, is within the normal range at delivery. Birth weight is also low but again within the normal range. This research also found that in 30 out of the 70 (42%) cases investigated, minor pregnancy complications were reported. However, these findings are not specific to RS.

- Prolonged reaction time. It is common knowledge that individuals with RS display prolonged reaction time [110,115,117,178-181]. Researchers in the field report responses occurring 30 seconds and even longer after a request was presented to the participants [115]. The fact that the child might be intensely occupied with breathing irregularities and appears to be gazing vaguely at the object to be manipulated might be wrongly interpreted as the child misunderstanding the request or losing interest in the task. All these behaviors are the child's way of preparing for appropriate action. Individuals with RS should be allowed the amount of time they need to succeed in accomplishing a task. Provided with appropriate motivators, reaction time can be reduced considerably [114].

- Sensory system. The sensory system of individuals with RS has never been thoroughly investigated. Nevertheless accumulating reports suggest that the sensory system does not function normally in this population. Lindberg observed [110] that individuals with RS show difficulties in receiving, deciphering and processing of external stimuli. This observation has been supported by anecdotal reports from parents. In the turbulent second stage of RS many individuals show extreme agitation with regard to external stimuli through various sensory modalities. Management of these sensory difficulties requires reduced stimulation and a quiet and a relaxing atmosphere. [182,183]. The tactile system has been reported as overly sensitive especially around the mouth and face. This can be observed in sensitivity to tooth brushing, and resistance to different food textures. In our experience some children react negatively (i.e. crying, face frowning, hand pulling) to proprioceptive input involving the arms. Taste and olfactory senses on the other hand, seem not to be affected [92], despite occasional reports to the contrary [184]. The auditory and visual systems are considered the most functional with regard to sensory input in this population [30,92]. Many individuals with RS rely on the visual system as their main communication system and use eye gaze to indicate choices. Eye gaze can be used to interact with concrete objects or communication symbols. This system has been found to be preserved and function at a reasonable level even amongst the most highly affected individuals, and into late adulthood [12], except for a few cases where girls were found to exhibit problems with their eyesight such as myopia (shortsightedness), and hyperopia (farsightedness) [92].

  o   The auditory system is also a very active sensory pathway enabling the individual with RS to enjoy the sounds of music and human voices which have been found to be particularly stimulating for them. Somato-sensory and auditory abilities have been tested several times in individuals with RS and have been found to be within the norm or slightly deviated from different control groups [185-187].

○   Vision. Despite the fact that the eyes are a major channel of communication in individuals with RS, 50%-100% of them display slight visual problems [110,188], as well as unusual ways of using the eyes. They tend to look at an object peripherally before focusing on it. This phenomenon was defined by Barbo Lindberg [110] as "Eyes who can see without looking" (p. 25). About 80% of individuals with RS show a slight strabismus (crossing of the eyes) at a young age (during the first decade of life). This slight strabismus disappears as the girls get older [2].

- Sleep patterns. Individuals with RS show significant sleep problems especially during stages II-III of the disorder. Some individuals find it difficult to fall asleep. Some might do so only when extremely exhausted and might need the use of medication [189-191]. In some instances children can wake up during the night with idiopathic crying or laughing spells. As a result of night-time wakening, during which they can be fully alert and active, they are subsequently very tired the following day. These spells usually occur in clusters of several days to weeks and subside spontaneously [192,193]. Nocturnal seizures, gastroesophageal reflux, and constipation are possible causes of disturbed sleep and it is important to assess for the presence of these and treat accordingly. Children with RS were reported to sleep more than their peers and this tendency increases with age [192,193]. In contrast to control groups, individuals with RS have been found by some researchers to continuously experience repeated short cycles of deep and REM (Rapid Eye Movements) sleep. It is hypothesized that this pattern is a result of a Dopaminergic/Serotonergic system abnormality [190,191]. Various solutions have been found useful in helping the individual with RS and her family achieve an improved night's sleep. These include medications [189] such as melatonin, barbiturates, benzodiazepines and other sedatives. Other more traditional methods might include cooling or warming of the room (according to each individual's preference), deep massage, a white noise machine, a water bed, a car ride, soft music, hot bath before sleep time, maintaining high activity levels throughout the day, and more [92:123].

- Stereotypical hand movements. Hand mannerisms are apparent in all individuals diagnosed with RS. They appear simultaneously with loss of hand function and are typically performed at the body midline, at chest level. These vigorous movements are apparent in 30%-72% of the individual's waking hours [31]. These movements intensify when the person with RS is exited/hungry/tired and they stop only when she is asleep. The movements are not symmetrical [194] and can be performed as hand-clasping, hand-wringing, or hand washing sometimes touching the mouth and tongue. Usually, the individuals who exhibit more intense hand stereotypical movements also display better manual functional abilities. These movements are involuntary and do not usually include the use of objects (except in the case of Angelman type RS). Neither are they used for protection or as a response to a sensorial need [31]. Voluntarily stopping the hand movement is usually very difficult for the individual with RS, although some can withdraw from those continuous movements, for a short period on demand. It is speculated that the stereotypical movements are a result of a neuro-chemical imbalance in the dopaminergic, monoaminergic and cholinergic systems [195,196]. Despite the fact that in late stages of RS the stereotypical movements subside they can still be observed [87].

Management

As of today there is no known medical intervention that will cure a person with RS. Yet, medical interventions can offer symptomatic relief. The aim of interventions in RS is to provide support and comfort to the individual with RS and her family. A multidisciplinary team approach is advised [11,197, 198] and should aim to maximize abilities and facilitate any emerging skills. Psychosocial support for the families, development of an appropriate rehabilitation/education plan, and assessment of available community resources should also be provided. Parent support groups are a vital aspect in providing support for families of individuals with RS [198].

Pharmaceutical intervention

A number of pharmacological treatments for RS have been suggested and investigated with regard to alleviating symptoms of this disorder:

- L-carnitine has been tested in a double-blind trial as a possible therapeutic agent. Despite caregiver's reports on improvements in patients' general well-being, significant functional improvements were not observed by the researchers [199].
- Naltrexone, an oral opiate antagonist was investigated due to the fact that elevated opioids had been observed in the Cerebro-Spinal Fluid (CSF) of individuals with RS. Although it decreased breathing dysrhythmias and had some sedating properties, its efficacy is controversial due to reports on deterioration in the course of the disorder due to use of this drug [200].
- Risperidone or selective serotonin uptake inhibitors and other medications such as chloral hydrate, hydroxyzine, or diphenhydramine along with melatonin have been somewhat successful in treating agitation in a group of children with PDD[201].
- Carbidopa/levodopa has been tried for reducing rigidity in populations other than RS [202].
- Magnesium has been introduced for individuals with RS in an attempt to reduce episodes of hyperventilation [203].
- Melatonin has been found to possess some beneficial effects on sleep disturbances [189].
- A trial involving dietary supplementation with folate and betaine based on the assumption that some alleles of the affected genes could be altered by dietary methyl supplementation did not show any significant benefits for individuals with RS [46].
- Folinic acid was found to normalize 5-MHTF and 5-HIAA levels in the CSF of four patients with RS in a study by Raemakers and his associates thereby leading to partial clinical improvements in those patients. Therefore the researchers suggested

that folinic acid should be used to increase folate metabolites in the CSF of individuals with RS [204]. However, these finding were not replicated in a further study by Neuel and his associates [205].

- An on-going study is being conducted by Naidu and her associates to test the efficacy of Dextromethorphan as a glutaminergic blocker. Preliminary results show some benefits in epilepsy control and general well-being for the participants.
- Recent reports demonstrate that BDNF over-expression in brain tissue of individuals with RS was related to a slower disease progression. Therefore Tsai [206] suggests a manipulation of BDNF expression in the brain through the use of lithium and other antidepressants. AS of today, since as an increase in central BDNF levels or signaling in human as well as animal studies [206] was not found, no clinical trial was performed yet to assert this hypothesis. Based on the finding of abnormal adreneragic activity in brainstem as a contributor to respiratory dysfunction and on positive response of mutant mice to Desipramine (an adrenalin reuptake blocking agent) on their breathing dysfunction and longevity a current study on the effect of desipramine on breathing is being carried now in France [207]
- IGF-1 (insulin growth factor-1) was found to be influenced by MECP2 and increasing its level in a mouse model was related to increased longevity, better locomotion and improvement in breathing abnormalities. Based on these findings a clinical study is currently taking place in Boston Children's Hospital [208].

Medications to be avoided in persons with rett syndrome

Prolonged heart rate corrected QT values have been reported in association with RS [155,199]. In order to prevent electrocardiogram QT abnormalities and cardiac arrhythmias certain drugs should not be administered to individuals with RS. These include prokinetic agents (i.e. cisapride), antipsychotics (i.e. thioridazine), antiarrhythmics (i.e. quinidine, sotolol, amiodarione), anaesthetic agents (i.e. thiopental, succinylcholine), and certain antibiotics (i.e. erythromycin, ketoconazole) [209].

Allied health professional intervention

Occupational and physical therapy are crucial in maintaining function and preventing deterioration while improving well-being for the individual with RS and her family. Augmentative communication is essential for enhancing the child's control over her environment. Music is a key element which can be used to great effect in conjunction with other therapeutic interventions. Music therapy has been found to be most beneficial as well as therapeutic horseback riding and therapeutic swimming [122]. The above mentioned interventions are most effective if there is ongoing therapeutic dialog between the different professionals involved and a 'multi-disciplinary milieu' maintained [198]. Lately it has been reported that environmental enrichment in the mouse model by adding play objects, adding sound and light stimuli to the cages has a positive effect on these mice locomotion, breathing and longevity possibly through elevation of BDNF levels.This finding was replicated in several labs and extrapolating these results to individuals with RS suggests the importance of non pharmacological interventions especially enrichment of their environment by cognitive and sensory situations [210]. These results support earlier findings of the effectiveness of a daily treadmill training program in enhancing functional abilities of four girls with RS [105].

Physical therapy

The clinical characteristics of RS include the expression of several challenging physical disabilities. Scoliosis is found in approximately 65-85% of girls with RS [12,122]. Physical therapy intervention has been found to reduce the progression of scoliosis [161]. Some girls require bracing, while others require surgical intervention [122,163]. Increased tone in the Achilles tendon is one of the earliest manifestations of onset of rigidity, usually followed by toe walking. It is important to maintain ambulation, and conventional physical therapy intervention methods can keep the Achilles tendons stretched [2,107,122,165]. Bilateral ankle foot orthosis (AFO) might be considered as a measure to prevent foot deformities, maintain foot alignment, and keep the heel cords lengthened. Botolinum toxin injections are also useful in this situation [167,168]. More information regarding this topic can be found in the chapter on physical therapy.

Occupational therapy

Many common difficulties can be addressed by an occupational therapist knowledgeable in the area of RS. Such problems can include the sensory abnormalities presented by individuals with RS, low motivation levels, stereotypical hand movements, poor hand function, and short attention span. Regulating sensory imbalance in these individuals can be assisted using the Snoezelen approach [183,212] or the sensory integration approach [213]. Low motivation levels can result from the enormous challenges every action presents to the apraxic, dystonic, and ataxic individual with RS. Enabling the individual to engage with the environment by using switches to operate daily appliances and continuous training in managing challenging situations can help the child overcome some of her barriers [2]. Overcoming the repetitive hand mannerisms and improving hand function can be accomplished using different approaches. Some therapists favor hand restraints in order to inhibit the repetitive purposeless hand movements. The use of soft splints is occasionally helpful in training in specific hand skills such as self feeding and communication. Splinting has been found to be helpful in decreasing agitation and self injurious behaviors in some individuals with RS [122]. Due to individual differences in the presentation of RS the effect of splinting should be individually evaluated for each client. Attention span can be increased by the use of quiet environments when individual interventions are taking place. Active involvement in various activities such as eating, operating musical instruments and the use of computer programs are all recommended and can be supported by the involvement of an OT. (More information regarding this topic could be found in the chapter on occupational therapy in this book)

Speech therapy

Research and information about the cognitive and communicative potential of females with RS is scarce and sometimes produces contradictory and indefinite outcomes [117,180, 181,214].

It has been reported that people with RS can communicate with the use of gestures, vocalizations and body positioning [27], and by establishing positive contact with people's faces/eyes, using smiles when they wish to answer in the affirmative [215]. The loss of expressive language in the majority of individuals with RS requires the intervention of a speech pathologist experienced in the use of Assistive and Augmentative Communicative (AAC) devices. Such aids are used for making choices which empower the person with RS and facilitate environmental control. Alternative forms of communication include communication boards, technical devices, eye pointing, body language, and hand pointing. Each child's abilities need to be recognized and encouraged by those who are involved in her care [114]. More information regarding this topic could be found in the chapter on communication.

Music therapy

Females with RS have been observed to be very responsive to music [144]. When music has been used therapeutically by trained practitioners, interventions have been shown to promote and motivate desire to interact and communicate with surroundings, as well as developing cognitive, affective, sensory-motor and physical skills [110,144-146,216-222]. Current knowledge of the value of music therapy with the person with RS, suggests that it can stimulate many aspects of development. It can assist in promoting choice making, enhancing vocalization, hand use and function, and improving eye contact. It also opens channels for emotional and communicative expression [145,146,162,215-218,220,223] and assists learning [114]. More information regarding this topic could be found in the chapter on music therapy.

Hydrotherapy

Individuals with RS face difficulties that affect them in many daily situations. Hydrotherapy can be a very useful medium in which to conduct physical therapy exercises. Warm water helps reduce spasticity and softens rigid tissues. In addition to supporting the client's unbalanced posture, water provides the individual with RS with massive physical stimulation. It can help to calm someone who is afraid of motion. In the water the individual with RS is able to move more slowly, with more ease and freedom, and without the fear of falling or hurting her self [224].

The aims of aquatic therapy for the individual with RS are similar to other general therapeutic goals such as enhancing relaxation [183, 224]; improving hand function; maintaining and improving transitioning skills [85,86,107-109,225]; regulating breathing patterns; preventing potential orthopedic problems and treating existing ones [139,164, 189,190,224]; re-assembling the "midline" [84,108,109]; improving equilibrium, coordination and communication; regulation of the sensory system; improvement of social skills; and general support of physical activity [189,190,224]. More information regarding this topic could be found in the chapter on hydrotherapy.

Hippotherapy

Hippotherapy is part of a range of experiences known as "equine assisted activities". Hippotherapy refers to the use of the movement of the horse by a skilled and licensed professional to address impairments, functional limitations, and disabilities in persons with nerve, muscular, skeletal, vestibular and/or behavioral problems, as part of an integrated treatment approach aimed at improving physical function.

The experience of equine-assisted movement provides the participant with a variety of sensory-motor experiences through changes of position on the horse. These changes produce active mobilization of the pelvis, lumbar spine and hip joints; develop body symmetry and awareness; equilibrium reactions leading to improved posture, balance, coordination, motor-planning, strength and/or endurance, timing and rhythm [192,226]. Resent findings suggest that a hippotherapy program specifically adapted for girls with RS can improve stability, improve equilibrium reduce the scoliotic curve [227]. More information regarding this topic could be found in the chapter on hippotherapy.

Summary

In this review an outline of the clinical features of Rett Syndrome has been introduced. The intention was to provide an update with reference to recent developments on the syndrome to the reader who has some familiarity with the condition and to introduce this syndrome to individuals taking their first clinical steps in "Rettland". We hope that this chapter together with other chapters in the book will add to the reader's existing knowledge and advance the quality of care and management received today by individuals with RS around the world.

References

[1]   Rett A. Uber ein eigartiges hirnatrophisches Syndrom bei Hyperammoniamie in Kindesalter. Wien Med Wochenschr 1966;116:723–38.

[2]   Lotan M. The management of individuals with Rett syndrome. Tel-Aviv: Isr Rett Syndr Assoc, 2006. [Hebrew]

[3]   Rett A. Grundlagen der Musiktherapie und Music-Psychologie. Stuttgart: Harrer, 1982. [German]

[4]   Hagberg B, Aicardi J, Dias K, Ramos O. Progressive syndrome of autism, dementia, ataxia and loss of purposeful hand use in girls: Rett's syndrome: Report of 35 cases. Ann Neurol 1983;14:471–9.

[5]   Hagberg B, Hagberg G. Rett syndrome: epidemiology and geographical variability. Eur Child Adolesc Psych 1997;1:5–7.

[6]   Leonard H, Bower C, English D. The prevalence and incidence of Rett syndrome in Australia. Eur Child Adolesc Psych 1997;1:8–10.

[7]   Fombonne E, Simmons H, Ford T, Meltzer H, Goodman R. Prevalence of pervasive developmental disorders in the British nationwide survey of child mental health. Int Rev Psychiat 2003;15(1-2):158-65.

[8]   Skesedel OH, Von-Tetzchner S, Aspelund F, Herder GA, Lofterld B. Rett Syndrome: Geographic variation in prevalence in Norway. Brain. Dev 1997;19:258-61.

[9]   Pini G, Milan M, Loppella M. Rett Syndrome in northern Tuscany (Italy): Family tree studies. Clin Genet 1996;50:486-90.

[10]   Hagberg B. Rett syndrome: clinical peculiarities and biological mysteries. Acta. Paediatr 1995;84:971–6.

[11]   Ellaway C, Christodoulou J. Rett syndrome: Clinical characteristics and recent genetic advances. Disabil Rehabil 2001;23:98-106.

[12]   Hagberg B. Rett syndrome: Clinical and biological aspects. London: Mac Keith, 1993.

[13]   Amir RE, Van Den Veyver IB, Wan M, Tran CQ, Franke U, Zoghbi H. Rett syndrome is caused by mutations in X-linked MECP2, encoding methyl CpG binding protein 2. Nat Genet 1999;23:185–8.

[14]   Amir RE, Van den Veyver IB, Schultz R, Malicki DM, Tran CQ, Dahle EI, et al. Influence of mutation type and X chromosome inactivation on Rett syndrome phenotypes. Ann Neurol 2000;47:670–9.

[15]   Neul JL, Zoghbi HY. Rett syndrome: a prototypical neurodevelopmental disorder. Neuroscientist 2004;10(2):118-28.

[16]   Trevethan E, Moser H. Diagnostic criteria for Rett syndrome. The Rett Syndrome Diagnostic Criteria Work Group. Ann. Neurol 1998;23:425–8.

[17]   Hagberg B, Hanefield F, Percy A, Skjeldal O. An update on clinically applicable diagnostic criteria in Rett syndrome. Comments to Rett Syndrome Clinical Criteria Consensus Panel Satellite to European Paediatric Neurology Society Meeting, Baden Baden, Germany, 11 September 2001. Eur J Paediatr Neurol 2001;6:293–7.

[18]   Kerr AM, Belichenko P, Woodcock T, Woodcock M. Mind and brain in Rett disorder. Brain Dev 2001;23(Suppl 1):S44-9.

[19]   Mari F, Azimonti S, Bertani I, Bolognese F, Colombo E, Caselli R, et al. CDKL5 belongs to the same molecular pathway of MeCP2 and it is responsible for the early-onset seizure variant of Rett syndrome. Hum Mol Genet 2005;15(14):1935-46.

[20]   Young JI, Zoghbi HY. X-Chromosome inactivation patterns are unbalanced and affect the phenotypic outcome in a mouse model of Rett syndrome. Am J Hum Genet 2004;74(3):511–20.

[21]   Schults RR, Glaze DG, Motil KJ, Armstrong DD, Del-Junco DJ, Hubbard CR, et al. Rett syndrome in a boy with a 47,XXY karyotype confirmed by a rare mutation in the MECP2 gene. Neuropediatrics 2001;32:162-4.

[22]   Naidu S. Research findings on Rett syndrome. IRSA annual conference; may; Las-Vegas, Nevada. Tape RS 9, 2000.

[23]   Burford B. Identifying early signs of Rett disorder and their implications for development. A lecture presented at the international course on Rett syndrome. June 16-18, Ostersund, Sweden, 2003.

[24]   Einspieler C. Signs of Rett disorder in the first six month of life. A lecture presented at the international course on Rett syndrome. 16-18 June, Ostersund, Sweden, 2003.

[25]   Einspieler C, Kerr AM, Prechtl HFR. Is the Early Development of Girls with Rett Disorder Really Normal? Pediatr Res 2005;57(5 Part 1):696-700.

[26]   International Rett Syndrome Association web site. FAQ: What are the stages of Rett syndrome? http://www.rettsyndrome.org/main/adults-intro.htm Accessed May 29. 2006.

[27]   Coleman M, Brubaker J, Hunter K, Smith G. Rett Syndrome: A survey of North American patients. J Ment Def Res 1988;32:117-24.

[28]   Julu. PO. Autonomic dysfunction and aspects of pharmacological treatment. A lecture presented at the international course on Rett syndrome. 16-18 June: Ostersund, Sweden, 2003.

[29]   Julu PO, Witt Engerstrom I. Assessment of the maturity-related brainstem functions reveals the heterogeneous phenotypes and facilitates clinical management of Rett syndrome. Brain. Dev 2005;27(Suppl 1):S43-53.

[30]   Kerr AM, Witt Engerstrom I. The clinical background to the Rett disorder. In: Kerr AM, Witt-Engerstrom I, eds. Rett disorder and the developing brain. Oxford: Oxford Univ Press,2001:1-26.

[31]   Lotan M. Roth D. The effect of hand vibrators on the hand stereotypes and function in Rett syndrome. Two case studies. Isr Physiother Quart 1996;52:23-6. [Hebrew].

[32]   Leonard H, Weaving L, Eastaugh P, Smith L, Delatycki M, Witt Engerstrom I, Christodoulou J. Trisomy 21 and Rett syndrome: a double burden. J Paediatr Child Health 2004;40:406–9.

[33]   Ellaway CJ, Badawi N, Raffaele L, Christodoulou J, Leonard H. A case of multiple congenital anomalies in association with Rett syndrome confirmed by MECP2 mutation screening. Clin Dysmorph 2001;10:185–8.

[34]   Hagberg B, Gillberg C. Rett variants—rettoid phenotypes. In: Hagberg B, Anvret M, Wahlstrom J, eds. Rett syndrome. Clinical and biological aspects. London: MacKeith Press, 1993:40-60.

[35]   Hanfield F, Hagberg B, Percy AK. Molecular and neurobiology aspect of Rett Syndrome. Neuropediatrics 1995;26:60-1.

[36]   Hagberg BA. Rett syndrome: clinical peculiarities, diagnostic approach, and possible cause. Pediatr Neurol 1989;5(2):75-83.

[37]   Hagberg B, Rasmussen P. "Forme fruste" of Rett syndrome-a case report. Am J Med Genet 1986;1(1Supp):175-81.

[38]   Ben-Zeev B, Yaron Y, Schanen NC, Wolf H, Brandt N, Ginot N, Shomrat R, Or R Urtreger A. Rett syndrome: clinical manifestations in males with MECP2 mutations. J Child Neurol 2002;17(1):20-4.

[39]   Moog U, Smeets EE, van Roozendaal KE, Schoenmakers S, Herbergs J, Schoonbrood-Lenssen AM, Schrander-Stumpel CT. Neurodevelopmental disorders in males related to the gene causing Rett syndrome in females (MECP2). Eur J Paediatr Neurol 2003;7(1):5-12.

[40]   Scala E, Ariani F, Mari F, Caselli R, Pescucci C, Longo I, et al. DKL5/STK9 is mutated in Rett syndrome variant with infantile spasms. J Med Genet 2005;42(2):103-7.

[41]   Lin MY, Wang PJ, Lin LH, Shen YZ. The Rett Syndrome and Rett-like Syndrome: A board concept. Brain Dev 1991;13:228-31.

[42]   Ariani H, Hayek G, Rondinella D, Artuso R, Mencarelli MA, Spanhol-Rosseto A, et al. FOXG1 is responsible for the congenital variant of Rett syndrome. Am J Hum Genet 2008;(1):89-93.

[43]   Zappella M, Mari F, Renieri A. Should a syndrome be called by its correct name? The example of the preserved speech variant of Rett syndrome. Eur J Pediatr 2005;164(11):710-2.

[44]   Yamashita Y, Kondo I, Fukuda T, Morishima R, Kusaga A, Iwanaga R, Matsuishi T. Mutation analysis of the methyl-CpG-binding protein 2 gene (MECP2) in Rett patients with preserved speech. Brain Dev 2001;23(Suppl 1):S157-60.

[45]   Wan M, Lee SS, Zhang X, Houwink-Manville I, Song HR, Amir RE, et al. Rett syndrome and beyond: recurrent spontaneous and familial MECP2 mutations at CpG hotspots. Am J Hum Genet 1999;65:1520-9.

[46]   Percy AK, Lane JB. Rett syndrome: model of neurodevelopmental disorders. J Child Neurol 2005;20(9):718-21.

[47]   Percy AK. International research review. Paper presented at the IRSA 12th annual conference; May 24-27; Boston, MA; Tape 622-15, 1996.

[48]   Schanen NC. A severely affected male born into a RS kinderred supports x-lined. Am J Hum Genet 1998;63:267-9.

[49]   Schanen NC, Kurczynsk TW, Brunelle D, Woodcock MM, Dune LS, Percy AK. Neonatal encephalopathy in two boys in families with recurrent Rett Syndrome. J Child Neurol 1998;13:229-31.

[50]   Leonard H, Silberstein J, Falk R, Houwink-Manville I, Ellaway C, Raffaele LS, Engerstrom IW, Schanen C. Occurrence of Rett syndrome in boys. J Child Neurol 2001;6:333-8.

[51]   Schwartzman JS, Bernardino A, Nishimura A, Gomes RR, Zatz M. Rett syndrome in a boy with a 47,XXY karyotype confirmed by a rare mutation in the MECP2 gene. Neuropediatrics 2001;32(3):162-4.

[52]   Clayton-Smith J, Watson P, Ramsden S, Black GC. Somatic mutation in MECP2 as a non-fatal neurodevelopmental disorder in males. Lancet 2000;356:830-2.

[53]   Topcu M, Akyerli C, Sayi A, Toruner GA, Kocoglu SR, Cimbis M, Ozcelik T. Somatic mosaicism for a MECP2 mutation associated with classic Rett syndrome in a boy. Eur J Hum Genet 2002;10:77–81.

[54]   Dotti MT, Orrico A, De Stefano N, Battisti C, Sicurelli F, Severi S, et al. A Rett syndrome MECP2 mutation that causes mental retardation in men. Neurol 2002;58:226–30.

[55]   Hoffbuhr K. Testing for the gene. IRSA annual conference; May 18-21: Las-Vegas, Nevada. Tape RS 5, 2000.

[56]   Villard L, Kpebe A, Cardoso C, Chelly PJ, Tardieu PM, Fontes, M. Two affected boys in a Rett syndrome family: clinical and molecular findings. Neurology 2000; 55(8):1188-93.

[57]   Marcu S, Nissenkorn A, Lerman-Sagie T, Menascu S, Landau D, Shorer Z, et al. MECP2 Gene rearrangement in five males in the Rett Israeli Cohort, 24 Feb, 2009. presented at the international conference of the Asian Society for Child Neurology, 2010.

[58]   Cheadle JP, Gill H, Fleming N, Maynard J, Kerr A, Leonard H, et al. Long-read sequence analysis of the MECP2 gene in Rett syndrome patients: correlation of disease severity with mutation type and location. Hum Mol Genet 2000;9:1119-29.

[59]   Huppke P, Laccone F, Kramer N, Engel W, Hanefeld F. Rett syndrome: analysis of MECP2 and clinical characterization of 31 patients. Hum Mol Genet 2000;9:1369-75.

[60]   Ham AL, Kumar A, Deeter R, Schanen NC Does genotype predict phenotype in Rett syndrome? J Child Neurol. 2005 Sep;20(9):768-78.

[61]   Leonard H, Colvin L, Christodoulou J, Schiavello T, Williamson S, Davis M, et al. Patients with the R133C mutation: is their phenotype different from patients with Rett syndrome with other mutations? J Med Genet 2003;40:e52.

[62]   Charman T, Neilson TC, Mash V, Archer H, Gardiner MT, Knudsen GP, et al. Derepression of BDNF transcription involves calcium-dependent phosphorylation of MeCP2. Science 2003;302(5646):885-9.

[63]   Percy AK, Lee HS, Neul JL, Lane JB, Skinner SA, Geerts SP, et al. Profiling scoliosis in Rett Syndrome. Pediatr Res, in press.

[64]   Li MR, Pan H, Bao XH, Zhu XW, Cao GN, Zhang YZ, Wu XR. Correlation between MECP2 genotype and phenotype in Chinese patients with Rett syndrome Zhonghua Er Ke Za Zhi 2009;47(2):124-8.[Chinese]

[65]   Kondo I, Yamagata H. [Mutation spectrum and genotype-phenotype correlation of MECP2 in patients with Rett syndrome] No To Hattatsu 2002;34(3):219-23. [Japanese].

[66]   Giunti L, Pelagatti S, Lazzerini V, Guarducci S, Lapi E, Coviello S, et al. Spectrum and distribution of MECP2 mutations in 64 Italian Rett syndrome girls: tentative genotype/phenotype correlation. Brain Dev 2001;23(Suppl 1):S242-5.

[67]   Witt-Engerstrom I. Rett Syndrome in Sweden. Neurodevelopment disability- pathophysiology. Goteborg University: Goteborg, Sweden, 1990.

[68]   Bauman ML, Kemper TL, Arin DM. Microscopic observations of the brain in Rett Syndrome. Neuropediatrics 1995;26:105-8.

[69]   Percy AD. The pattern of growth failure in Rett syndrome. Am J Disabl Child 1993;147:633-7.

[70]   Armstrong DD. Neuropathology of Rett syndrome. Ment Retard Dev Disabil Res Rev 2002;8:72-6.

[71]   Jellinger KA. Rett Syndrome - an update. J Neural Transm 2003;110(6):681-701.

[72]   Kitt CA, Wilcox BJ. Preliminary evidence for neurodegenerative changes in the substantia nigra of Rett Syndrome. Neuropediatrics 1995;26:114-8.

[73]   LaSalle JM, Hogart A, Thatcher N. Rett syndrome: a Rosetta stone for understanding the molecular pathogenesis of autism. Int Rev Neurobiol 2005;7:131–65.

[74]   Reichwald K, These J, Winches T, Wiehe T, Weitzel J, Strätling WH, et al. Comparative sequence analysis of the MECP2 locus in human and mouse reveals new transcribed regions. Mamm Genome 2000;11:182–90.

[75]   Shahbazian MD, Antalffy B, Armstrong D, Zoghbi HY. Insights into Rett syndrome: MeCP2 levels display tissue and cell specific differences and correlate with neuronal maturation. Hum Mol Genet 2002;11:115–24.

[76]   Kishi N, Macklis JD. MECP2 is progressively expressed in post-migratory neurons and is involved in neuronal maturation rather than cell fate decisions. Mol Cell Neurosci 2004;27:306–21.

[77]   Neul JL, Zoghbi HY. Rett syndrome: a prototypical neurodevelopmental disorder. Neuroscientist 2004;10(2):118–28.

[78]   Subramaniam B, Naidu S, Reiss AL. Neuroanatomy in Rett syndrome: cerebral cortex and posterior fossa. Neurology 1997;48:399–407.

[79]   Armstrong D, Dunn JK, Antalffy B, Trivedl R. Selective dendritic alterations in the cortex of Rett syndrome. J Neuropathol Exp Neurol 1995;54:195–201.

[80]   Kishi N, Macklis JD. Dissecting MECP2 function in the central nervous system. J Child Neurol 2005;20:753–9.

[81]   Kaufmann WE, Naidu S, Budden S. Abnormal expression of microtubule associated protein 2 in the neo-cortex of Rett syndrome. Neuropediatrics 1995;26:109–13.

[82]   Kaufmann WE, Worley PF, Taylor CV, Bremer M, Isakson PC. Cyclo-oxygenase 2 expression during rat neocortical development and in Rett syndrome. Brain Dev 1997;19:25–34.

[83]   Casanova MF, Buxhocveden DP, Switala A, Roy E. Rett syndrome as a minicolumnopathy. Clin Neuropathol 2003;22:163–8.

[84]   Kauffman WE. Cortical development in Rett syndrome: molecular, neurochemical and anatomical aspects. In: Kerr AM, Engerstrom W, editors. Rett disorder and the developing brain. England: Oxford Univ Press, 2001:85-110.

[85]   Armstrong DD. Neuropathology of Rett syndrome. Ment Retard Dev Disabil Res Rev 2002;8:72–6.

[86]   Clanton C, Jean OH, Hyder K, Chenchik A, Khimani AH, Narayanan V, et al. Gene expression profiling in post-mortem Rett syndrome brains: differential gene expression and patient classification. Neurobiol Dis 2001;8:847–65.

[87]   Tudor M, Akbarian S, Chen RZ, et al. Transcriptional profiling of a mouse model for Rett syndrome reveals subtle transcriptional changes in the brain. Proc Natl Acad Sci USA 2002;99:15536–41.

[88]   Chen WG, Chang Q, Lin Y. Depression of BDNF transcription involves calcium dependant phosphorylation of MeCP2. Science 2003;202:885–9.

[89]   Martinowich K, Hattori D, Wu H. DNA methylation related chromatin remodeling in activity dependant BDNF gene regulation. Science 2003;202:890–3.

[90]   Kaufmann WE, Johnston MV, Blue ME. MeCP2 expression and function during brain development: implications for Rett syndrome's pathogenesis and clinical evolution. Brain Dev 2005;27:S77–87.

[91]   91.   McGill BE, Bundle SF, Yayalaoglu MB, Carson JP, Thaller C, Zoghby H. Enhanced anxiety and stress induced corticosterone release are   associated   with   increased   CRH expression in a mouse model of Rett syndrome. Proc Natl Acad Sci USA 2006;103:18267–72.

[92]   Hunter K. The Rett Syndrome handbook. Washington, DC: Int Rett Syndr Assoc, 1999.

[93]   Witt-Engerstrom I, Hagberg B. The Rett syndrome: gross motor disability and neural impairment in adults. Brain Dev 1990;12(1):23-6.

[94]   Kerr AM. The future for Rett syndrome girls. Int Rett Syndr Assoc Newsletter 1992;13-14.

[95]   Ayres AJ. Sensory integration and the child, 5th ed. Los Angeles, CA: Western Psychol Serv, 1982.

[96]   Fisher AG, Murray EA, Bundy AC. Sensory integration theory and practice. Philadelphia, PA: FA Davis, 1991.

[97]   Ayres AJ. Sensory integration and learning disorders. Los Angeles, CA: Western Psychol Serv, 1972.

[98]   Mount RH, Hastings RP, Reilly S, Cass H, Charman T. Behavioral and emotional features in Rett syndrome. Disabil Rehabil 2001;23:129-38.

[99]   Katz DM, Dutschmann M, Ramirez JM, Hilaire G. Breathing disorders in Rett syndrome: progressive neurochemical dysfunction in the respiratory network after birth. Respir Physiol Neurobiol. 2009;168(1-2):101-8.

[100]   Elian M, Rudolf ND. EEG and respiration in Rett Syndrome. Acta Neurol Scand 1991;83:123-8.

[101]   Julu PO, Kerr AM, Apartopoulos F, Al-Rawas S, Witt Engerström I Engerström. L, Gamal AJ, Hansen S. Characterization of breathing and associated central autonomic dysfunction in the Rett disorder. Arch Dis Child 2001;85:29-37.

[102]   Witt-Engerstrom IW. Autonomic monitoring in Rett syndrome at the Swedish Rett Center, Froson. A handout received at the annual conference, Washington, DC, 2001.

[103]   Ogier M, Wang H, Hong E, Wang Q, Greenberg ME, Katz DM. Brain Derived Neurotrophic Factor and respiratory function improve after ampakine treatment in a mouse model of Rett Syndrome. J Neurosci 2007;27:10912–17.

[104]   Lotan M, Isakov E, Kessel S, Merrick J. Physical fitness and functional ability of children with intellectual disability: Effects of a short-term daily treadmill intervention. ScientificWorldJournal 2004;(4):449-57.

[105]   Lotan M, Isakov E, Merrick J. Improving functional skills and physical fitness in children with Rett syndrome. J Intell Disabil Res 2004;48(8):730-5.

[106]   Ben –Zeev B. Lessons from Rett syndrome and the MECP2 gene as a model for a neuro-developmental disorder. Ann Conf Rare Dis, Sheba Med Center, Ramat-Gan, Israel, 2004 Dec 09.

[107]   Hanks SB. Motor disabilities in the Rett syndrome and physical therapy strategies. Brain Dev 1990;12:157–61.

[108]   Hanks SB. Physical therapy strategies. Paper presented at the IRSA 12th Annual Conference: May 24-27, Boston, MA. Tape 622-08, 1996.

[109]   Hanks SB. Why physical therapy? Rett Gazette 2001;1-2,6-8

[110]   Lindberg B. Understanding Rett Syndrome: A practice guide for parents, teachers and therapists. Toronto: Hognefe Huber, 1991.

[111]   Peak J, Eveson JW, Scully C. Oral manifestation of Rett's Syndrome. Br Den J 1992;172:248-9.

[112]   Elefant C. Speechless yet communicative: Revealing the person behind the disability of Rett syndrome through clinical research on songs in music therapy. In: Aldridge D, di Franco G, Ruud E, Wigram T, eds. Music therapy in Europe. Rome: ISMEZ, 2001.

[113]   Elefant C. Music, choice making and communication in Rett syndrome. A lecture presented at the international course on Rett syndrome. 16-18 June, Ostersund, Sweden, 2003.

[114]   Elefant C, Wigram T. Learning ability in children with Rett syndrome. Brain Dev 2005;27(Suppl 1):S97-S101.

[115]   Koppenhaver D, Erickson KA, Harris B, McLellan J, Skotko BG, Newton RA. Storybook-based communication intervention for girls with Rett syndrome and their mothers. Disabil Rehabil 2001;23(3/4):149-59.

[116]   Sigafoos J, Woodyatt G. Educational implications of Rett syndrome. Eur J Ment Disabil 1996;3(11):19-28.

[117]   Sigafoos J, Woodyatt G, Tucker M, Roberts-Pennell D, Pittendreigh N. Assessment of potential communication acts in three individuals with Rett syndrome. J Dev Phys Disabil 1999;12(3):203-16.

[118]   Sigafoos J. Communication development and aberrant behavior in children with developmental disabilities. Edu Train Ment Retard Dev Disabil 2000;35(2):168-76.

[119]   Sigafoos J, Woodyatt G, Keen D, Tait K, Tucker M, Roberts-Pennell D, Pittendreigh N. Identifying potential communicative acts in children with developmental and physical disabilities. Commun Disord Quart 2000;21(2):77-86.

[120]   Beukelman DR, Mirenda P. Augmentative and alternative communication; Management of severe communication disorders in children and adults. 2nd edition, Baltimore, MD: Paul H Brooks, 1998.

[121]   Leonard S. The Australian Rett syndrome study inaugural report. Western Australia: Telethon Inst Child Health Res, 2002.

[122]   Budden SS. Rett syndrome: habilitation and management reviewed. Eur Child Adolesc Psychiatr 1997;6(1Suppl):103-7.

[123]   Glaze D. Epilepsy. Paper presented at the IRSA 12th Annual Conference. May 24-27, Boston, MA, Tape 622-18, 1996.

[124]   Elefant C. Emotional/musical communication of children with RS. A lecture at an annual conference on RS. Sheba hospital, Ramat-Gan, Israel, 2005.

[125]   Sansom D, Krishnen UH, Corbett J, Kerr A. Emotional and behavioral aspects of Rett Syndrome. Dev Med Child Neurol 1993;35:340-5.

[126]   Ben Zeev Ghidoni B. Rett syndrome. Child Adolesc Psychiatric Clin North Am 2007;16:723-43.

[127]   Steffenburg U, Hagberg B. Epilepsy in a representative series of Rett syndrome. Acta Paediatr 2001;90:34-9

[128]   Nissenkorn A, Gak E, Vecksler M, Reznik H, Menascu S, Ben-Zeev, B. Epilepsy in Rett syndrome. The experience of a National Rett Center. Epilepsia, in press.

[129]   Jian L, Nagarajan L, De Klerk N, Ravine D, Bower c, Anderson A, Williamson S, Christodoulou J, Leonard H. Predictors of seizure onset in Rett syndrome. J Pediatr 2006;149:542-7.

[130]   Jian L, Nagarajan L, De Klerk N, Ravine D, Christodoulou J, Leonard H. Seizures in Rett syndrome: an overview from a one-year calendar study. Eur J Paediatr Neurol 2007;11:310-7.

[131]   Glaze DG, Schultz RJ, Frost JD. Rett syndrome: characterization of seizures versus non-seizures. Electroencephalogr Clin Neurophysiol 1998;106:79-83.

[132]   Witt-Engerstrom I. Age-related occurrence of signs and symptoms in the Rett syndrome. Brain Dev 1992;14:S11-20.

[133]   Cooper RA, Kerr AM, Amos PA. Rett syndrome: clinical examination of clinical features, serial EEG and video-monitoring in understanding and management. Eur J Pediatr Neurol 1998;2:127-135.

[134]   Motil KJ, Schultz R, Brown B, Glaze DG, Percy A.K. Altered energy balance may account for growth failure in Rett Syndrome. J Child Neurol 1994;9:315-9.

[135]   Thommessen M, Kase BF, Heiberg A. Growth and nutrition in ten girls with Rett Syndrome. Acta Pediatrica 1992;81:686-9.

[136]   Motil KJ, Schultz RJ, Browning K, Trautwein L, Glaze DG. Oropharyngeal dysfunction and gastroesophageal dysmotility are present in girls and women with Rett syndrome. J Pediatr Gastroenterol Nutr 1999;29(1):31-7.

[137]   Budden SS. Management of Rett syndrome: a ten year experience. Neuropediatr 1995;26:75–7.

[138]   Motil KJ, Schultz RJ, Wong WW, Glaze DG. Increased energy expenditure associated with repetitive involuntary movement does not contribute to growth failure in girls with Rett syndrome. J Pediatr 1998;132(2):228-33.

[139]   Motil K. Nutrition and weight management. Paper presented at the IRSA 12th annual conference; May 24-27; Boston, MA; Tape 622-11, 1996.

[140]   Reilly S, Cass H. Growth and nutrition in Rett syndrome. Disabil Rehabil 2001;23:118-28.

[141]   De Bona C, Zappella M, Hayek G, Meloni I, Vitelli F, Bruttini M, et al. Preserved speech variant is allelic of classic Rett syndrome. Eur J Hum Genet 2000;8(5):325-30.

[142]   Stenbom Y, Engerstron IW, Hagberg B. Gross motor disability and head growth in Rett syndrome. Neuropediatrics 1995;26:85-6.

[143]   Bergstrom-Isacsson M. Ways to resolve agitation. A lecture presented at the international course on Rett syndrome. June 16-18, Ostersund, Sweden, 2003.

[144]   Merker B, Bergstrom-Isacsson M, Witt Engerstrom I. Music and the Rett disorder: The Swedish Rett center survey. Nord J Music Ther 2001;10(1):42-53.

[145]   Wigram T. Assessment and treatment of a girl with Rett syndrome. In: Bruscia K, ed. Case studies in music therapy. Gilsum, NH: Barcelona Publ, 1991.

[146]   Wigram T. A model of assessment and differential diagnosis of handicap in children through the medium of music therapy. In: Wigram T, Saperston B, West R, eds. The art and science of music therapy: A handbook. Chur, Switzerland: Harwood Acad, 1995.

[147]   Pillion JP, Rawool VW, Bibat G, Naidu S. Prevalence of hearing loss in Rett syndrome. Dev Med Child Neurol 2003;45(5):338-43.

[148]   Umansky R, Watson JS, Colvin L, Fyfe S, Leonard S, de Klerk N, Leonard H. Hand preference, extent of laterality, and functional hand use in Rett syndrome. J Child Neurol 2003;18(7):481-7.

[149]   Jacobsen K, Viken A, Von Tetchner S. Rett syndrome and aging: A case study. Disabil Rehabil 2001;23(3/4):160-6.

[150]   Piazza CC, Nederson C, Fisher W. Teaching self-feeding skills to patients with Rett Syndrome. Dev Med Child Neurol 1993;35:991-6.

[151]   Zappella M, Gillberg C, Ehlers S. The preserved speech variant: a subgroup of the Rett complex: a clinical report of 30 cases. J Autism Dev Disord 1998;28:519-26.

[152]   Zappella M. The preserved speech variant of the Rett complex: a report of 8 cases. Eur Child Adolesc Psychiatry 1997;6(Suppl 1):23-5.

[153]   Smeets EE, Chenault M, Curfs LM, Schrander-Stampel CT, Frijns JP. Rett syndrome and long-term disorder profile. Am J Med Genet A 2009;149A(2):199-205.

[154]   Kerr AM, Julu PO. Recent insights into hyperventilation from the study of Rett syndrome. Arch Dis Child 1999;80:384-7.

[155]   Sekul EA, Moak JP, Schultz RJ, Glaze DG, Dunn JK, Percy AK. Electrocardiographic findings in Rett syndrome: An explanation for sudden death? J Pediatr 1994;125:80-2.

[156]   Guideri F, Acampa M, Hayek G, Zappella M, Di Perri T. Reduced heart rate variability in patients affected with Rett syndrome. A possible explanation for sudden death. Neuropediatrics 1999;30:146-8.

[157]   Annegers JF, Coan SP. SUDEP: overview of definitions and review of incidence data. Seizure 1999;8(6):347-52.

[158]   Byard RW. Forensic issues and possible mechanisms of sudden death in Rett syndrome. J Clin Forensic Med 2006;13(2):96-9.

[159]   Elian M, De M, Rudolf N. Observations on hand movement in Rett Syndrome: A Pilot Study. Acta Neurol Scand 1996;94:212-4.

[160]   Ager S, Fyfe S, Christodoulou J, Jacoby P, Schmitt L, Leonard H, Predictors of scoliosis in Rett syndrome. J Child Neurol 2006;21(9):809-13.

[161]   Lotan M, Merrick J, Carmeli E. Scoliosis management in Rett syndrome. A case study. ScientificWorldJournal 2005;5:264-73.

[162]   Lotan M, Elefant C. Physiotherapy and music therapy for a girl with Rett syndrome – a dual treatment approach. Fysioterapeuten 2006;13(2):15-20.

[163]   Rossin L. Effectiveness of therapeutic and surgical intervention in the treatment of scoliosis in Rett syndrome. A seminar work. Pittsburgh, PA: Univ Duquesne, 1997:1-19.

[164]   McClure MK, Battaglia C, McClure RJ. The relationship of cumulative motor asymmetries to scoliosis in Rett Syndrome. Am J Occup Ther 1998;52:196-204.

[165]   Weeks L. Rett Syndrome. A lecture given at Sydney Australia; February, 1997.

[166]   Haung TS, Lubicky SP, Hammerberg KW. Scoliosis in Rett syndrome. Orthoped Rev 1994;23:931-7.

[167]   Sponseller P. Orthopedic update in Rett syndrome. Rett Gazette 2001; Spring:1,4-5.

[168]   Tsurel S. Orthopedic aspects of Rett's syndrome, Harefuah 2000;139(7-8):104-5. [Hebrew]

[169]   Haas RH, Dixon SD, Sartoris DJ, Hennessy MJ. Osteopenia in Rett syndrome. J Pediatr 1997;131(5):771-4.

[170]   Budden SS, Gunness ME. Bone histomorphometry in three females with Rett syndrome. Brain Dev 2001;23:S133-7.

[171]   Cepollaro C, Gonnelli S, Bruni D, Pacini S, Martini S, Franci MB, et al. Dual X-ray absorptiometry and bone ultrasonography in patients with Rett syndrome. Calcif Tissue Int 2001;69:259-62.

[172]   Gough H, Goggin T, Bissessar A, Baker M, Crowley M, Callaghan N. A comparative study of the relative influence of different anticonvulsant drugs, UV exposure and diet on vitamin D and calcium metabolism in out-patients with epilepsy. Q J Med 1986;59(230):569-77.

[173]   Xiao P, Chen Y, Jiang H, Liu YZ, Pan F, Yang TL, et al. In vivo genome-wide expression study on human circulating B cells suggests a novel ESR1 and MAPK3 network for postmenopausal osteoporosis. J Bone Miner Res 2008;23(5):644-54.

[174]   Kalmanchey R. Evoked potentials in the Rett syndrome. Brain Dev 1990;12(1): 73-6.

[175]   Witt- Engerstrom I., Hagberg B. The Rett Syndrome: Gross motor disability and neural impairment in adults. Brain Dev 1990;12(1):23-6.

[176]   Budden SS, Myer ED, Butler IJ. Cerebrospinal fluid studies in Rett syndrome: Biogenic amines and B-Endorphins. Brain Dev 1990;12(1):81-4.

[177]   Armstrong DD, Kinney H. The neuropathology of the Rett disorder. In: Kerr AM, Witt-Engerstrom I, eds. Rett disorder and the developing brain. Oxford: Oxford Univ Press, 2001:57-84.

[178]   Sigafoos J, Laurie S, Pennell D. Preliminary assessment of choice making among children with Rett syndrome. J Assoc Pers Severe Handicaps 1995;20:175-84.

[179]   Sigafoos J, Laurie S, Pennell D. Teaching children with Rett syndrome to request preferred objects using aided communication: Two preliminary studies. Augment Altern Commun 1996;12:88-96.

[180]   Woodyatt G, Ozanne A. Communication abilities and Rett syndrome. J Autism Dev Disord 1992;22:155-73.

[181]   Woodyatt G, Ozanne A. Intentionality and communication in four children with Rett syndrome. Aust NZ J Dev Disabil 1994;19:173-83.

[182]   Kaufmann WE, Johnston MV, Blue ME. MeCP2 expression and function during brain development: implications for Rett syndrome's pathogenesis and clinical evolution. Brain Dev 2005;27(Suppl 1):S77-S87.

[183]   Lotan M, Shapiro M. Management of young children with Rett syndrome in the multi-sensory environment. Brain Dev 2005;27(Suppl 1):S88-S94.

[184]   Ronnett GV, Leopold D, Cai X, Hoffbuhr KC, Moses L, Hoffman EP, Naidu S. Olfactory biopsies demonstrate a defect in neuronal development in Rett's syndrome. Ann Neurol 2003;54(2):206-18.

[185]   Percy AK, Zoghbi H, Riccardi VM. Rett syndrome: initial experience with an emerging clinical entity. Brain Dev 1985;7(3):300-4.

[186]   Bader GG, Witt-Engerstrom I, Hagberg B. Neurophysiological findings in the Rett syndrome, II: Visual and auditory brainstem, middle and late evoked responses. Brain Dev 1989;11(2):110-4.

[187]   Bader GG, Witt-Engerstrom I, Hagberg B. Neurophysiological findings in the Rett syndrome, I: EMG, conduction velocity, EEG and somatosensory-evoked potential. Brain Dev 1989;11(2):102-9.

[188]   Saunders KJ, McCulloch DL, Kerr AM. Visual function in Rett Syndrome. Dev Med Child Neurol 1995;37:496-504.

[189]   McArthur AJ, Budden SS. Sleep dysfunction in Rett syndrome: a trial of exogenous melatonin treatment. Dev Med Child Neurol 1998;40:186–92.

[190]   Nomura Y. Sleep in relation to other behaviors in Rett syndrome. A lecture presented at the international course on Rett syndrome; 16-18 June; Ostersund, Sweden, 2003.

[191]   Nomura Y. Early behavior characteristics and sleep disturbance in Rett syndrome. Brain. Dev 2005;27(Suppl 1):S35-S42.

[192]   Piazza CC, Fisher W, Kiesewetter BS, Bowman L, Moser H. Aberrant sleep patterns in children with Rett Syndrome. Brain Dev 1990;2:488-93.

[193]   Piazza CC, Fisher W, Moser H. Behavioral treatment of sleep dysfunction in patients with Rett Syndrome. Brain. Dev 1991;13:232-7.

[194]   Weiss M. Intervention and assessment of hand behavior. Paper Presented at the IRSA 12th. Annual Conference. 24-27 May, Boston, MA. Tape: 622-07, 1996.

[195]   Nomura Y, Segawa M. Motor symptoms of the Rett syndrome: abnormal muscle tone, posture, locomotion and stereotyped movement. Brain Dev 1992;14 (Suppl):S21-8.

[196]   Matsuishi T, Yamashita Y, Kusaga A. Neurobiology and neurochemistry of Rett syndrome. Brain. Dev 2001;23(Suppl 1):S58-61.

[197]   Cass H, Reilly S, Owen L, Wisbeach A, Weekes L, Slonims V, Wigram T, Charman T. Findings from a multidisciplinary clinical case series of females with Rett syndrome. Dev Med Child Neurol 2003;45(5):325-37.

[198]   Lotan M, Wein J, Elefant C, Sharf A, Yoshei Y. The Rett syndrome evaluation center in Israel. A play based assessment model. A poster presented at the annual Israeli Physical therapy association conference, Dead sea, Israel, 2005.

[199]   Ellaway C, Williams K, Leonard H, Higgins G, Wilcken B, Christodoulou J. Rett syndrome: randomized controlled trial of L-carnitine. J Child Neurol 1999;14:162 –7.

[200]   Percy AK, Glaze DG, Schultz RJ, Zoghbi HY, Williamson D, Frost JD Jr, et al. Rett syndrome: controlled study of an oral opiate antagonist, naltrexone. Ann Neurol 1994;35:464-70.

[201]   Shea S, Turgay A, Carroll A, Schulz M, Orlik H Smith I, Dunbar F. Risperidone in the treatment of disruptive behavioral symptoms in children with autistic and other pervasive developmental disorders. Pediatrics 2003;114(5):634-41.

[202]   Scheife RT, Schumock GT, Burstein A, Gottwald MD, Luer MS. Impact of Parkinson's disease and its pharmacologic treatment on quality of life and economic outcomes. Am J Health Syst Pharm 2000;57(10):953-62.

[203]   Egger J, Hofacker N, Schiel W, Holthausen H. Magnesium for hyperventilation in Rett's syndrome. Lancet 1992;340:621–2.

[204]   Ramaekers VT, Hansen SI, Holm J, Opladen T, Senderek J, Hausler M, et al. Reduced folate transport to the CNS in female Rett patients. Neurology 2003;61(4):506-15.

[205]   Neul JL, Maricich SM, Islam M, Barrish J, Smith EO, Bottiglieri T, et al. Spinal fluid 5-methyltetrahydro-folate levels are normal in Rett syndrome. Neurology 2005;64(12):2151-2.

[206]   Tsai SJ. Lithium and antidepressants: Potential agents for the treatment of Rett syndrome. Med Hypotheses 2006;67(3):626-9.

[207]   Roux JC, Dura E, Moncla A, Mancini J, Villard L. Treatment with desipramine improves breathing and survival in a mouse model for Rett syndrome. Eur J Neurosci. 2007;25(7):1915-22.

[208]   Tropea D, Giacometti E, Wilson NR, Beard C, McCurry C, Fu DD, et al. Partial reversal of Rett Syndrome-like symptoms in MeCP2 mutant mice, PNAS 2009;106(6):2029-34.

[209]   Weaving LS, Ellaway CJ, Gécz J, Christodoulou J. Rett syndrome: clinical review and genetic update. Med Genet 2005;42:1-7.

[210]   Kondo M, Gray LJ, Pelka GJ, Christodoulou J, Tam PP, Hannan AJ. Environmental enrichment ameliorates a motor coordination deficit in a mouse model of Rett syndrome – Mecp2 gene dosage effects and BDNF expression. Eur J Neurosci 2008;27(12):3342-50.

[211]   Ellaway CJ, Sholler G, Leonard H, Christodoulou J. Prolonged QT interval in Rett syndrome. Arch Dis Child 1999;80:470–2.

[212]   Lotan M, Merrick J. Rett syndrome management with Snoezelen or controlled multi-sensory environment. A review. Int J Adolesc Med Health 2004;16(1):5-12.

[213]   Schmidt J. What to look for in a sensory integration evaluation, especially when complex issues are involved. Rett Gazette 2003 Spring:2-4.

[214]   Van Acker R. Using computers to promote communication and adaptive Hand use in girls with Rett syndrome. Paper presented at the International Rett syndrome 12th annual conference. May; Boston, MA, 1996.

[215]   Burford B, Trevarthen C. Evoking communication in Rett syndrome: Comparisons with conversations and games in mother-infant interaction. Eur Child Adolesc Psychiatr 1997;6(suppl 1):1-5.

[216]   Coleman KA. Music therapy in Rett syndrome. Educational and therapeutic intervention in Rett syndrome. Clinton, MD: IRSA, 1987:93-110.

[217]   Elefant C, Lotan M. Rett syndrome: Dual intervention – music and physical therapy. Nord J Music Ther 2004;13(2):172-82.

[218]   Hill SA. The relevance and value of music therapy for children with Rett syndrome. Br J Spec Educ 1997;24(3):124-8.

[219]   Wigram T, Cass H. Music therapy within the assessment process for a therapy clinic for people with Rett syndrome. Paper presented at the Rett Syndrome World Conference in Sweden, 1996.

[220]   Wesecky A. Music therapy for children with Rett syndrome. Am J Hum Genet 1986;24(suppl 1):253-7.

[221]   Montague J. Music therapy in the treatment of Rett syndrome. Glasgow: Rett Syndrome Assoc, 1998.

[222]   Takehisa K, Takehisa-Silvestri G. Intermediate results of music therapy in interdisciplinary work with Rett syndrome in institut Haus der barmherzigkeit, Vienna. Institut Haus der Barmherzigkeit, Vienna, Austria, not dated.

[223]   Hadsell NA, Coleman KA. Rett syndrome: A Challenge for music therapists. Music Ther Perspect 1988;5:52-5.

[224]   Lotan M, Hadar-Frumer M. Aquatic Rehabilitation for Individuals with Rett syndrome. Aquatic Phys Ther 2004;12(1):6-16.

[225]   Beuchel K. Physical therapy and gross motor skills in Rett syndrome. A handout received at the IRSA annual conference, May, Washington, 2001.

[226]   Graffman K. Hippotherapy: never heard of it. Rett Gazette 2002;Winter:3-5.

[227]   Maciques Rodríguez E, Lotan M. Therapeutic horseback riding (hippotherapy) for individuals with Rett syndrome: A review with a case study. Int J Child Health Human Dev 2008;1(1):39-53.

In: Rett Syndrome: Therapeutic Interventions
Editors: Meir Lotan and Joav Merrick

ISBN: 978-1-61728-080-1
©2011 Nova Science Publishers, Inc.

Chapter II

Rett Syndrome: Reflections on the Constraints and Opportunities in Therapy

Alison M Kerr, MB, ChB, DCH, FRCP, FRCP&CH, MD, OBE[*]

Section of Psychological Medicine, Division of Community Based Sciences, Academic
Centre, Gartnavel Royal Hospital, Glasgow, United Kingdom

More than twenty years of clinical and research experience with affected people in the British Isles has provided insight into particular challenges for therapists, educators or parents wishing to facilitate learning and to support the development of skills in people with Rett syndrome. This chapter considers the challenges in two groups - those due to constraints imposed by the disabilities associated with the disorder and those stemming from the opportunities, often masked by the disorder, allowing the development of skills that depend on less affected areas of the brain. Because the disorder interferes with the synaptic links between neurones, those functions of the brain that are most dependent on complex neural networks are the most affected. These functions include speech, memory, learning, general planning of fine movements especially those of the hands. Emotional and hormonal responses appear relatively intact. Whereas the physical limitations of the disease leads to frustration, a good understanding of the better preserved areas of control can encourage progress in learning, the building of satisfying relationships and a better quality of life.

Introduction

The Rett disorder is due to mutation of the gene MECP2 at the tip of the X chromosome [1,2] and responsible for at least 80-90% of cases presenting with "classic" Rett syndrome [3]. The classic picture was first described in young girls, when the condition was thought to be degenerative and confined to females [4-6]. The occurrence of a developmental regression at around one year of age led to the initial assumption that the child was born healthy and then suffered inevitable deterioration, but it has since become clear that the disease is not progressive [7]. It is recognized in many adults and in a few boys [8] and it is evident that although the earliest signs are subtle and frequently missed the disease affects the development and function of the brain even before birth [9,10]. It is also appreciated that there is a very wide range in severity [11] the most severe and the mildest cases, as might be expected, showing the cardinal signs to a greater or lesser degree than the "classic" case [11]. This variation in severity is due in part to the fact that all female cells have two X chromosomes, but use only one. The variable extent to which the neurones are dependent on the X chromosome with the faulty gene therefore influences the severity of the condition in that person. The exact position of the mutation in the gene MECP2 and other factors determining the expression of the gene also affect severity. Experience in the United Kingdom (UK) suggests that a remarkably consistent group of clinical problems is to be found in affected cases, however mild or severe they may be. It is the constraints and opportunities associated with this highly characteristic Rett disorder profile that will be explored here.

Collaborations

The development of the Rett Syndrome Support organisations in 1985 in Scotland (RSA Scotland) and England (RSAUK) made possible a working relationship with the author through which the organisations funded a medical advisory service for families and their professional advisers. This included teaching sessions and clinics at which people with Rett could be examined at the request of their families. The wealth of resulting clinical experience laid the foundation for further clinical, epidemiological and neurophysiological research and a nation-wide survey recording the health of each reported person, the British Isles Survey (BIS or BIRS), based until 2005 in Glasgow, now transferred to the University of Wales Institute of Medical Genetics in Cardiff, Wales. Reliable data from all sources are entered on a database [12]. Key items are recorded at five-year intervals from birth and throughout life. A simple BIS scoring system for severity has been validated against later severity and survival [13]. The score includes muscle tone disturbance, locomotion, scoliosis, occurrence of epilepsy and feeding difficulty. The early score has been shown to rise until 15-20 years of age and then to stabilise [13]. A separate BIS health score is based on the items: persistent epilepsy, episodes of respiratory or other illness, body weight and the parent's opinion of health [14]. It is through these activities that reports and observations have been gathered indicating practical problems and successes in therapy.

---

* Correspondence: Alison M Kerr, MB, ChB, DCH, FRCP, FRCP&CH, MD, OBE, 29 Fountain Road, Bridge of Allan, Stirling FK9 4AT E-mail: amk5m@clinmed.gla.ac.uk

Why is the clinical profile of the Rett disorder so specific?

In Rett disorder the fault in the gene MECP2 leads to failure of production of its active protein MeCP2 that is important for the normal development and function of the brain [15,16]. It also influences the expression of several other genes that are important for brain growth and function. MeCP2 normally plays a part in the brain stem regulation of heart rate and breathing and is of great importance in the cerebral cortex [17]. As the brain grows and matures throughout infancy and childhood the affected neurones fail to make adequate connections with each other. That failure profoundly disturbs the functions that are most dependent on multiple neuronal connections - the "neural networks". Most severely affected are therefore finely controlled movement, speech, thought, memory and imagination, while many functions that rely less on complex neuronal interactions are relatively spared. This pervasive but selective pattern of abnormality in the brain leads to the distinct pattern of disability - the 'disease profile' - that is characteristic for the disorder. It is important to note that this profile is remarkably consistent regardless of the level of severity [18]. For example hand use and speech are always impoverished, even in the least affected people who may speak and write [18]. Posture and balance are always measurably disturbed even in those who can walk and run. Peripheral reception of sight and sound appears normal while central processing of these signals is defective and this is true of both severe and mild cases [19]. Control of heart rate, blood pressure and respiratory rhythm appears to be disturbed in everyone although to a variable extent [20].

Constraints and hidden opportunities

While progress in research provides the hope that it will become possible to prevent or rectify the defects in the brain, much can now be achieved in reduction of the impact of these on function and quality of life for the person with Rett and the family.

The primary need for assessment

As for any person with disabilities, accurate diagnosis and a thorough functional assessment are the foundation for therapy and such assessments should be repeated at intervals throughout life to ensure that the individual's needs are met and possibilities recognised [21]. Such assessments benefit from the expertise of a range of therapists. In the United Kingdom we call on the services of physiotherapist, occupational therapist, music therapist and other communication therapists, dietician, optometrist and audiometrician. When such expertise is not available the careful observations of the family or carer may still provide a valuable guide to care and provision. Families and carers are quick to learn from the professionals and their observations should always be recorded as part of a formal assessment. The aim of the assessment is to discover and minimise the impact of disabilities and to discover and support competences.

Posture and locomotion

Posture is invariably disturbed in Rett, There appears to be reduced appreciation of the position of the body in space (proprioception). There is also disturbance of the tension in muscles (muscle tone) required to support the body and to allow smooth and accurate movement. That area of function is dependent upon continuous monitoring and adjustment by the complex neural networks in the brain that are specifically disabled in Rett. In the youngest children the defect is manifest as reduced muscle tension (hypotonia) – "floppiness", most marked in the most severe. This reduced muscle tone is usually superceded by an abnormal increase in tone (hypertonia or dystonia) usually first evident at the ankles (the calf muscles) finally affecting most areas. The most severely affected children cannot stand or walk without support and many within this group of clients hold the tendency for contractures to develop at the joints. Acute dystonic episodes are common and involuntary movements may affect muscles in the face, limbs and spine. The increased muscle tension commonly affects some muscle groups more than others and one side of the body more than the other. In the spine this probably contributes to the almost invariable development of scoliosis, requiring surgical correction in about half [22]. Early detection of these evolving problems gives the best opportunity for the provision of appropriate support. The therapist must understand and accommodate these disabilities in any plans.

At least as important for the individual is encouragement and opportunity to be active, using the whole body as fully as possible. It is in such activity that the hidden movement skills of people with Rett usually become apparent. The families' observations are of particular value. It will be seen that although planned movements are poor, spontaneous movements and postural adjustments can be surprisingly fluent and appropriate in such activities as managing a swing, swimming, horse riding and dancing. Such skills clearly give satisfaction to the individual and may improve with practice, benefiting body and mind. Triggers for such useful spontaneous actions appear to include a strong level of motivation combined with low demand and a relaxed environment. Since music appeals to almost everyone with Rett it has become one of the most highly valued of the therapies and may be combined with other physical therapies to relax and to motivate the individual as well as holding a major place in communication therapy [23]. Water at a comfortable temperature in a pleasant, supported environment is also an excellent facilitator for many people with Rett and physiotherapy may be most successful in such a pool.

Involuntary movements

The extraordinary stereotyped movements and the failure of useful hand activity characteristic in Rett reflect the inability of the brain to organise finely controlled hand movements and the release of more primitive alternating patterns [24]. Research studies indicate that the individual has very little control of these repetitive rhythms. The movements increase with agitation and abate with relaxation and so may mislead the therapist into believing that they constitute a form of intentional communication. On the contrary, useful communication is sometimes assisted when these movements are interrupted. As with the unexpected postural and locomotor skills the best use of the hands tends to be seen when the individual is well motivated, not stressed by demands and allowed plenty of time to act in a relaxed atmosphere [25].

Feeding and nutrition

Feeding difficulties are common in all but the mildest cases. These include positioning difficulties, inadequate mouth closure, interruption of feeding by involuntary movements, erratic respiratory rhythm, inability to chew and move food around the mouth, aspiration of food or fluids into the lungs, reflux of acid material from the stomach leading to reflux oesophagitis and ingestion of air with sometimes painful bloating [26]. When severe these difficulties necessitate specialist assessment and in some cases direct percutaneous nutrition. A good nutritional state is essential for everyone and without it existing skills are likely to be lost and other problems exacerbated. Although expert support may be necessary it should also be kept in mind that simple strategies such as withdrawal from a noisy dining room with extra time for assistance may reduce the most severe difficulties at meal times.

Control of cardiac and respiratory rhythm

The involuntary abnormal breathing patterns in Rett also require understanding and accommodation by the therapist. Breathing becomes irregular when even the least affected people become agitated and a variety of abnormal rhythms are commonly present whenever the individual is awake and alert. These may include breath holding, deep breathing and inadequate ventilation [27]. These disturbances may cause further agitation so that a vicious cycle is produced. Severely disturbed respiratory rhythm stresses the already defective control of blood pressure and heart rate leading to several types of non-epileptic "vacant spell" [27,28]. Interestingly such attacks very rarely culminate in an epileptic seizure. True epilepsy, associated with disturbance of the electrical discharges in the cortex also occurs in about half of all cases and when severe should be treated with anticonvulsant medication. However non-epileptic vacant spells are much more common than epilepsy and major difficulties arise when these are mistakenly medicated as intractable epilepsy. When in doubt, brain stem and electroencephalographic monitoring are recommended [27]. Any such interruption of awareness seriously interferes with performance and the therapist has to make allowance for such events.

Mood

Sudden mood swings are especially common in children during the early infancy regression period but occur also in older children and adults with Rett disorder. During regression the levels of the excitatory neurotransmitter glutamate are known to be abnormally high [29] and this may result in agitation and pain. A quiet situation with soft music, favoured by the individual, may allow relaxation and permits the use of skills. Of course people with Rett are at least as likely as any healthy person to develop painful and irritating conditions and a careful medical examination is always required to search for such causes of distress. Frustration and anger at unwelcome changes and events are also to be expected in sensitive people who cannot express their feelings and signs of distress always require careful review of the circumstances.

Communication

Communication perhaps presents the greatest challenge to the therapist because the expected means of communication are interfered with to such a great extent by the Rett disorder and yet the person with Rett loves to communicate [18]. This means that the usual ways to assess communicative capacities are invalid. Although speech begins to develop in about half of the Rett population it usually disappears with the onset of the regression period and rarely reappears when that abates. Even in the least severely affected people who can talk and answer questions, the understanding and use of speech is severely restricted. Such speech as is possible gives the impression that in these relatively mildly affected people the intellect is also greatly affected by the disease [18].

In marked contrast is the remarkable ability of people with Rett to relate warmly to other people, to enjoy company, to appreciate simple interpersonal jokes and to enter into the spirit of joint activities. They have clear preferences and can use their own repertoire of actions and expressions very effectively to indicate these [30]. Personality is well preserved throughout life and reactions to situations are often age appropriate. This area of competence provides enormous rewards for both therapist and 'client' but demands great patience, sensitivity and ingenuity to observe and exploit the possibilities. Music has been described as the "genius" for Rett work [30]. Not only has music the potential to provide the relaxed environment that facilitates spontaneous actions but also through active participation it offers the individual at any age rich possibilities for choice and self-expression [31]. It should be understood however that to be of value music must be used just as carefully as speech. Loud or continuous sound of any kind becomes a source of stress and should be avoided. Since vision and hearing are usually normal in Rett there should be periodic routine assessments to ensure that any necessary support provided.

Conclusions

Some problems for the therapist have been discussed that may be improved by physical, pharmacological or surgical treatment but otherwise must be accommodated by the therapist:- reduced use of the hands, stereotyped hand movements and other unwanted involuntary movements, irregular breathing with episodes of altered awareness, feeding difficulties, epilepsy, periods or agitation, altered sense of body position and therefore reduced ability to stand and walk, tendency to develop contractures and scoliosis, the lack of speech and intellectual restriction.

Coexisting with these severe and complex difficulties and often obscured, is the potential for learning and the use of skills, present at all ages provided that the individual is maintained in good health. The challenge to the therapist is to discover these competences and find means by which they can be enjoyed: the capacity for spontaneous movements such as reaching, touching, swimming, swinging, dancing, riding; taking pleasure in mutual activities and sociability and the capacity for specific and maintained relationships; the special sensitivity to musical cadence and rhythm; the introduction of sensual experience through their good vision and hearing with evident enjoyment of visual, tactile and auditory experiences. This will retain the capacity to learn and to acquire new skills throughout life.

Acknowledgments

The author wishes to acknowledge collaboration over many years with the colleagues listed in the references, individuals with Rett Syndrome and their families. The work has been part-funded from several sources including RSAUK, RSA Scotland, IRSA, RSRF and Quarrier's Homes. The University of Glasgow department of Psychological Medicine provided the base for my activities during the last 10 years.

The author has produced an illustrated teaching DVD to show the range of problems in Rett, copies of which may be obtained from the UK Rett Association Langham House West, Mill Street, Luton LU1 2NA. Dr Kerr's 2006 doctoral thesis on Rett Syndrome "A critical account of clinical and physiological studies in Rett syndrome" is available for the University Library of Edinburgh.

References

[1]   Amir RE, Van Den Veyver, IB, Wan M, Tran CQ, Franke U, Zoghbi H. Rett Syndrome is caused by mutations in X-linked MECP2, encoding methyl CpG binding protein 2. Nature Genetics 1999;23:185-8.

[2]   Amir RE, Van den Veyver IB, Schultz R, Malicki DM, Tran CQ, Dahle EI, et al. Influence of mutation type and X chromosome inactivation on Rett syndrome phenotypes. Ann Neurol 2000;47:670-9.

[3]   Ravn K, Bieber-Nielsen J, Skjeldal OH, Kerr AM, Hulten M, Schwartz M. Large genomic rearrangements in MECP2. Hum Mut 2005;25(3):324.

[4]   Rett A. Uber ein eigenartiges hirnatrophisches Syndrome bei hyperammonamie im Kindsalter. Wiener Medizinische Wochenschrift 1966;116:723-6. [German]

[5]   Hagberg B, Aicardi J, Dias K, Ramos O. A progressive syndrome of autism, dementia, ataxia and loss of purposeful hand use in girls: Rett's syndrome - report of 35 cases. Ann Neurol 1983;14:471-9.

[6]   Trevarthen E, Moser HW, Opitz JM. and the Rett Syndrome diagnostic criteria work group. Diagnostic criteria for Rett syndrome. Ann Neurol 1988;23:425-8.

[7]   Kerr AM, Nomura Y, Armstrong D, Anvret M, Belichenko PV, Budden S, et al. Guidelines for reporting clinical features in cases with MECP2 mutations. Brain Dev 2001;23(4):208-11.

[8]   Schanen C, Franke U. A severely affected male born into a Rett syndrome kindred supports X-linked inheritance and allows extension of the exclusion map. Am J Hum Gen 1998;63:267-9.

[9]   Einspieler C, Kerr AM, Prechtl HFR. Is the development of girls with Rett disorder really normal? Pediatr Res 2005;57:696-700.

[10]   Einspieler C, Kerr AM, Prechtl HFR. Abnormal general movements of girls with Rett disorder: the first 4 months of life. Brain Dev 2005;27(1):8-13.

[11]   Kerr AM, Belichenko P, Woodcock T, Woodcock M. Mind and brain in Rett disorder. Brain Dev 2001;23:S44-9.

[12]   Kerr AM. A critical account of clinical and physiological studies in Rett syndrome. MD thesis. Edinburgh: Univ Edinburgh, 2006.

[13]   Kerr AM, Prescott R. Predictive value of the early clinical signs in Rett disorder. Brain Dev 2005;27:S20-24.

[14]   Kerr AM, Burford B. Towards a full life with Rett Syndrome. Paediatr Rehabil 2001;4(4):157-68.

[15]   Armstrong DD. Neuropathology of Rett syndrome. Ment Retard Dev Disabil Res Rev 2002;8(2):72-6.

[16]   Armstrong DD, Deguchi K, Antallfy B. Survey of MeCP2 in the Rett syndrome and the non-Rett syndrome brain. J Child Neurol 2003;18(10):683-7.

[17]   Shahbazian MD, Antalffy B, Armstrong DL, Zoghbi HY. Insight into Rett syndrome: MECP2 levels display tissue and cell-specific differences and correlate with neuronal maturation. Hum Mol Gen 2002;11(2):115-24.

[18]   Kerr AM, Archer HL, Evans J, Gibbon F. People with MECP2 mutation positive Rett disorder who converse J Intellect Disabil Res 2006;50(5):386-94.

[19]   Saunders K, McCulloch D, Kerr AM. Visual function in Rett syndrome. Dev Med Child Neurol 1995;37:496-504.

[20]   Julu POO, Kerr AM, Apartopoulos F, Al-rawas S, Witt Engerstrom I, Engerstrom L, et al. Characterisation of breathing and associated autonomic dysfunction in the Rett Disorder. Arch Dis Child 2001;85:29-37.

[21]   Kerr AM. Individuals with Rett disorder and the role of the physician. Prim Psychiatr 2003;10(2):59-62.

[22]   Kerr AM, Webb P, Prescott R, Milne Y. Results of surgery for scoliosis in Rett syndrome. J Child Neurol 2003;18:703-8.

[23]   Kerr AM, Montague J, Stephenson JBP. The hands, and the mind, pre-and post-regression in Rett syndrome. Brain Dev 1987;9:487-90.

[24]   Wright M, Van der Linden ML, Kerr AM, Burford B, Arrowsmith G, Middleton RL. Motion analysis of stereotyped hand movements in Rett syndrome. J Intellect Disabil Res 2003;47(2):85-9.

[25]   Lindberg B. Understanding Rett syndrome, 2 ed. Toronto, Hogrefe Huber, 2006.

[26]   Kerr AM. Outcome in Rett Syndrome. In: Goodyear I, Howlin P, eds. Outcomes in neuro-developmental and genetic disorders. Cambridge: Cambridge Univ Press, 2002:241-71.

[27]   Julu POO. The central autonomic disturbance in Rett syndrome. In: Kerr AM, Witt Engerstrom I, eds. Rett disorder and the developing brain. Oxford: Oxford Univ Press, 2001:131-81.

[28]   Cooper RA, Kerr AM, Amos PM. Rett syndrome: critical examination of clinical features, serial e.e.g. and video-monitoring in understanding and management. Eur J Child Neurol 1998;2:127-35.

[29]   Blue ME, Naidu S, Johnston MV. Development of amino acid receptors in frontal cortex from girls with Rett syndrome. Ann Neurol 1999;45:541-5.

[30]   Kerr AM, Belichenko P, Woodcock T, Woodcock M. Mind and brain in Rett disorder. Brain Dev 2001;23:S44-S9.

[31]   Elefant C. Speechless yet communicative: revealing the person behind the disability of Rett syndrome through clinical research on songs in music therapy. In: Aldridge G, DiFranco G, Ruud E, Wigram T, eds. Music therapy in Europe. Rome: Ismez, 2004.

In: Rett Syndrome: Therapeutic Interventions
Editors: Meir Lotan and Joav Merrick

ISBN: 978-1-61728-080-1
©2011 Nova Science Publishers, Inc.

Chapter III

Rett syndrome: The Israeli Rett Syndrome Center model. A transdisciplinary play-based assessment

Meir Lotan, MScPT, PhD[*]*, Iris Manor-Binyamini, PhD,*
Cochavit Elefant, MT, MEd, PhD, Judy Wine, SLP, EdD,
Einat Saraf, MEd and Yael Yoshei, BOT, HT

Israel Rett Center, National Evaluation Team, Chaim Sheba Medical Center, Tel
HaShomer, Ramat Gan, Israel

Rett syndrome (RS) is a neuro-developmental syndrome of genetic origin, which mainly affects females. Individuals diagnosed with RS exhibit a variety of functional difficulties, which impair their quality of life. The variety of impairments and the differences between each child makes it necessary to administer skilled treatment, individually tailored to each client. Since the foundation of proper intervention is based on a structured, well administered, insightful assessment, the individual with RS with her complex array of difficulties should benefit from such a procedure. This notion has led to the establishment of the Israel Rett Syndrome Center. The center includes a medical branch located at the Safra Children's Medical Center at Tel Hashomer and an education/rehabilitation team, who performs assessments in special educational facilities and residential settings throughout Israel. The assessment team works by means of arena assessment according to the concept of play-based assessment. This chapter presents the working model used by the education/rehabilitation team at the Israeli Rett Syndrome Center. The principles and working characteristics of the Israel Rett Syndrome Center team are suggested here as a potential model for establishing additional teams, presenting similar evaluation services for other individuals with RS as well as for similar populations.

[*] Correspondence: Meir Lotan, BPT, MScPT, PhD, Department of Physical Therapy, Ariel University Center of Samaria, IL-40700 Ariel, Israel. E-mail: ml_pt_rs@netvision.net.il

Introduction

Rett syndrome is a genetic disorder that primarily affects females [1,2]. Approximately one in every 10,000 females will develop Rett syndrome (RS), a severely disabling neuro-developmental disease [3]. Individuals with RS present an array of phenotypes. Patients with more severe phenotypes might show early symptomatology without the period of normal development and have congenital hypotonia and infantile spasms. Patients with a milder variant may retain some speech and motor functions without seizures [4-6]. This phenotypic variability is mainly the result of different mutation types and locations and distinct patterns of X chromosome inactivation [7]. The phenotypic versatility presented by individuals with RS necessitates a specific knowledgeable evaluation as the cornerstone for a proper management program to be administered for this population. In order to assess the proper model for the evaluation of individuals with RS one must first review existing models of evaluation for individuals with multiple disabilities.

Development of evaluation models

The concept that integrated teamwork can enhance the efficacy of services delivered to individuals with multiple disabilities is not new. This idea was first proposed by Whitehouse in 1951 [8]. Today, more than 50 years later, Health related professionals still find it difficult to be involved in integrated-type treatment, mostly due to the fact that each member of the educational/therapeutic staff was trained to work as an independent, therapeutic provider [8].

The variety of physical, cognitive, therapeutic, educational and mental needs of patients with developmental disabilities presents challenges to the paraprofessionals responsible for their treatment. Accepting this point of view has led support services for pupils with special educational needs to change drastically during the past few decades. Today strong pressure is being exerted by support services to develop cooperative transdisciplinary teamwork. In many countries such as Australia, England, the United States, France and Holland, teamwork has become the guiding component for establishing the policies of education and welfare services. This in turn has led to comprehensive changes such as the development of cooperative assessment by a number of support services. In a broader sense, this process has also led to legislation obligating cooperation between different support services [9]. The rationale behind this policy is based on the fact that solving "complex problems" demands a wider scope of knowledge and more advanced capabilities usually not attainable by a single therapist [10,11]. In actuality, this policy has brought about a process of change and a transition from treatment methods based on the medical model (such as the multidisciplinary and interdisciplinary approaches) to methods such as the transdisciplinary model better suited for the educational environment. The transdisciplinary model was first developed in 1976 by the United Cerebral Palsy Association's service for infants with cerebral palsy. After its assimilation this working model was recognized by health related professions in fields of: occupational therapy [12], physiotherapy [13], special education [14], nursing [15], medicine [16] and rehabilitation advisors [17].

This model was also recommended as a preferred approach for treating populations with multiple disabilities by care providers' organizations in the United States such as: ASHA (American Speech-Language-Hearing Association), AOTA (American Occupational Therapy association), APTA (American Physical Therapy association and TASH (The Association for persons with Severe Handicaps).

Youngson et al [18] described three types of transdisciplinary teams whose objectives encourage cooperation: application teams, discussion teams, and assessment teams. The present chapter deals with an assessment team (for more background on transdisciplinary assessment see Linder [19]) providing services for individuals with Rett syndrome.

Rett syndrome is a neuro-developmental syndrome, characterized by severe dysfunctions such as loss of manual function and speech abilities as well as cognitive, communicative, social, behavioral and functional disabilities. These disabilities first appear at age 6 to 18 months, following an initial period of apparently normal development [3]. Rett syndrome is considered the second most common syndrome causing multiple disability among females - the first being Down syndrome [21]. The individual with RS presents a complex clinical picture requiring an evaluation using a transdisciplinary type approach. At this point in time, there is no known medical prevention or cure for RS, but the reversal of Rett syndrome signs in a mouse model [22] gives hope for future cure for individuals with RS. In the meanwhile effective, supportive treatment can ameliorate the symptoms that characterize the syndrome [23].

The numerous and varied educational and therapeutic needs of individuals with RS, together with their relatively long life span; approximately 50 years [24], demand a professional, transdisciplinary approach. Unfortunately individuals with RS and their families do not always receive the best possible treatment [25]. Therefore, there seems to be a need to develop and improve appropriate management programs for this population. The Israeli model was developed under such circumstances with the aim of addressing the wide range of difficulties presented by this syndrome.

The israeli model

In 2003 the association known as the Israel Rett Syndrome Center (IRSC) was established by families of individuals with RS. It is also managed by the families. The main goal of the Rett Syndrome Center was to improve the quality of life for individuals with RS and their families. This goal was meant to be attained through several routes:

- By promoting awareness of RS among the general public and among the medical and health related professional community, in view of the fact that it is a rare disorder
- By providing support and counseling for parents of individuals with RS
- By assessing of individuals with RS by a team of experts
- By providing guidance for educators and therapists working with individuals with RS
- By promoting and funding research on RS [26].

Two organizations were established for this purpose: the Rett Syndrome Medical Clinic at the Safra Children's Hospital, Sheba Medical Center, Tel-Hashomer and the Rehabilitation/Education Assessment and Counseling group of the Israel Rett Syndrome Center.

The Rett clinic

The aim of the RS clinic is to provide comprehensive medical services for individuals with RS and their families in an effort to meet their medical, therapeutic, and educational needs, while taking the unique characteristics and requirements of each child and her family into consideration. These services are aimed at helping the child to attain optimal function. Diagnosis and assessment at the facility inform guidance in areas such as:

- Counseling for the family and other supportive frameworks
- Recommendations and guidance for a holistic treatment program within the community framework
- Regular follow-up of each client's condition and treatment program

Description of activities

Since the present chapter focuses mainly on the center's health related paraprofessional assessment and guidance team, the activities of the medical arm of the Rett Syndrome Clinic will only be briefly described here.

The Rett Syndrome Medical Clinic treats all girls in Israel who have been diagnosed with Rett syndrome (as of today there are approximately 140 known individuals with RS in Israel). The clinic is located in the Sheba Medical Center, Tel Hashomer and the Director is a senior pediatric neurologist. The team includes an orthopedic surgeon, a gastroenterologist, an endocrinologist, a geneticist and a dietician. During each medical evaluation the child and her parents meet with the head of the team, who examines the individual with RS and provides the parents with information regarding the syndrome and the child's expected prognosis and direction for intervention according to each client's needs. Each child undergoes orthopedic, gastroenterological, and dietetic examination and evaluation. If the child has not yet undergone a genetic diagnosis she is also referred to a geneticist for genetic counseling and evaluation. Due to the erratic nature of RS, the family is encouraged to contact the head of the medical team by phone or by e-mail and to seek immediate counseling in dealing with daily difficulties or emergencies that might arise. The Rett syndrome clinic continues to follow each individual's progress on an annual or semiannual basis, depending on the age of the client and the severity of her phenotypic expression.

The evaluation and guidance team

The Evaluation and Guidance Team was established with the objective of assessing individuals with RS and for counseling the therapeutic, educational and rehabilitation staff, who supports the individual with RS on a daily basis.

The Rett Center assessment team (RS team) is a transdisciplinary team consisting of a special education teacher/advisor, a music therapist, a speech therapist, an occupational therapist and a physiotherapist. The aim of this team is to conduct assessment and advise on services for each child within her special education facility\residence in the presence of the educational staff and the family. In certain cases, such as when the child is too small to be integrated into a kindergarten or is in transition between special education facilities, assessment and guidance are conducted at the Tel Hashomer clinic. All of the assessments are fully funded by the Israel Rett Syndrome Center. The RS team has developed a unique assessment model that provides answers to the comprehensive needs of individuals with RS. The structure of the model is described below.

Assessment structure

A. Pre-evaluation

Weeks before the meeting in the educational facility, a summary of the child's evaluation at the Tel Hashomer medical clinic is sent to all team members. Preliminary working contacts are established between the RS team coordinator, the parents and the educational facility staff. This period of time enables an exchange of information and helps to structure expectations towards the meet.

B. Assessment

The assessment itself is a fluent yet ever changing process (see figure 1). However, for the purpose of simplification the model is presented here in more detail and in a much more structured way than it is actually performed on site.

The first objective is for the family to get acquainted with the team and be presented with the objectives of the meeting. On the day of the evaluation, before the assessment begins, a short meeting is held by the RS team with the educational/therapeutic staff of the child's special education facility and the parents. During this meeting expectations are clarified and missing information regarding the child's level of functioning is provided by parents and the educational/therapeutic staff. In some cases rejection may arise when an alien\outsider team is introduced into a special education or rehabilitation facility. Therefore, this stage must be carried out with sesitivity and proper attention to details [27]. This stage enables members of the RS team and the members of the staff of the special education facility to become acquainted. Sufficient time is allotted for constructing preliminary cooperative working relationships and agreeing on objectives that suit the expectations of the parents and the educational/therapeutic staff.

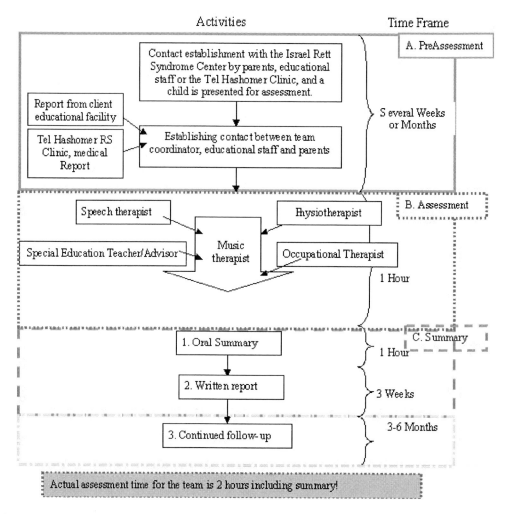

Figure III-1. Chronological flowchart of the assessment of individuals with RS.

After this stage, the RS team initiates contact with the individual with RS. Since individuals with RS have difficulty adapting to unfamiliar people and situations [28-30], the first encounter takes place between the child and the music therapist, who serves as a moderator between the individual and the rest of the RS assessment team.

After this first meeting the assessment will take place using the "play-based assessment" model. During the assessment various members of the team direct the proceedings and engage in activities with the child, by means of mediation through the music therapist, or by joining in on the activity. The special emotional bond that individuals with RS have with music is a well known phenomenon that has been described at length in research literature [28,30-35]. In light of this special affection for music, it is seen as the optimal therapeutic tool for establishing good initial contact, maximizing function and enhancing cooperation. Therefore the music therapist is the key person to establish the initial connection with the child.

Oral summary discussion – At the termination of the assessment a summary discussion is held where the major findings of the RS team are clarified and discussed and the main suggestions for intervention are summarized and agreed upon.

Written summary report - Several weeks after the assessment, a written summary report is issued to the parents as well as to the educational/therapeutic facility, which includes the main suggestions presented at the meeting, but with an elaboration of clinical recommendations regarding intervention options.

Follow-up - an additional follow-up meeting is held between memebers of the RS team and adjacent colleagues from the educational/therapeutic staff of the special education facility, 3-6 months following the presentation of the written summary report. During this meeting the recommendations are reviewed and their implementation within the daily routine of the special education facility is evaluated. If problems have arisen in the process of implementing the recommendations, efforts are made by all those involved to solve those problems. We find such meetings an important component of the model.

Fundamental aspects of the team work

In order for this model to work and for the reader to sense the complexity of this approach, the guidelines according to which the assessment team works are laid out. These guidelines have been assembled by the assessment team of the Israel Center for Rett Syndrome and are constantly being compiled and reviewed:

Accessibility
- Physical accessibility - Since the child spends most of her day in the special education facility, it is considered to be the child's natural surroundings and the assessment is therefore carried out there. An exception to this would occur where the child is still too young to be integrated into a special education facility, or when there is an urgent request from the parents to see the child during a transition phase between educational facilities.
- Online accessibility - The RS team is accessible by telephone or by e-mail to both parents and the educational/therapeutic staff.
- Financial accessibility - Assessment is fully funded by the Israeli Rett Syndrome Center (IRSC). The aim of this aspect of the team is to prevent a situation were a child is denied the assessment due to financial difficulties.

Family directed assessment
Assessment usually takes place following a request from the parents of the individual with RS to the IRSC or following a request by the staff of the special education facility. Meetings are usually held at the child's special education center. In several cases special consideration requires that the venue and manner in which the meeting is conducted will be adapted to each family and child according to their objectives and expectations (see table 1).

Table III-1. Assessment location and objectives as defined by the child's parents

Child's Name	Location	Objectives Defined by Parents
A.B.H.	School	Offering feedback and points of emphasis for the child's Individual Educational Program (I.E.P).
A.E.	Child's Home	Offering activities and promoting motor skills and communication in the framework of the home.
G.O.	Tel Hashomer hospital (Rett clinic)	Initial directions for activities and assisting the parents in locating and organizing the management program for the child (a young child recently diagnosed with Rett syndrome)

Coordination

Each assessment meeting is meticulously coordinated between the coordinator of the RS team, the parents and the staff of the special education facility. For each child previous medical, educational, and developmental assessments are sent to the members of the RS team. These reports inform the agenda and type of meeting which is strutured according to the unique needs of each client, the special education facility, and the parents.

Flexibility

Because of the different character, structure and needs of each client with RS, her parents and the differences between various special education facilities, each meeting begins and progresses in a different manner. The RS team adapts itself to these differences in order to offer an appropriate response to each scenario.

Comprehensiveness

Our ability to supply comprehensive assessments stems from the cooperation between the RS team members and the Transdisciplinary model of the assessment, which enables us to refer to the variability of needs, wishes and abilities of the child, the parents, and the special education facility.

Each assessment/guidance meeting is usually held with all members of the paramedical team in the form of transdisciplinary assessment. Assessment is performed by means of play-based assessment methods. The aim of this comprehensive assessment method is for parents and members of the educational/therapeutic staff to participate. Our professional opinion is that an individual with RS will function at her best, when she feels included and senses that she is supported, fully contained and accepted empathically. The central lead in the assessment team is usually the music therapist, who adjusts her approach to each child's emotional situation and level of communication. Initial contact is usually achieved through the use of live music such as familiar songs or improvised modes of communication. The contact initiated by the music therapist provides the child with a protected and secure framework that enables her to enjoy herself and cooperate to the fullest. Another member of the RS team, usually the physiotherapist, holds the child and provides physical support and mobility when needed (see figure 2). After the establishment of rapport with the child, other activities are added to the musical activities according to the objectives of the assessment team. During the entire assessment other members of the team observe and are actively involved in the interaction.

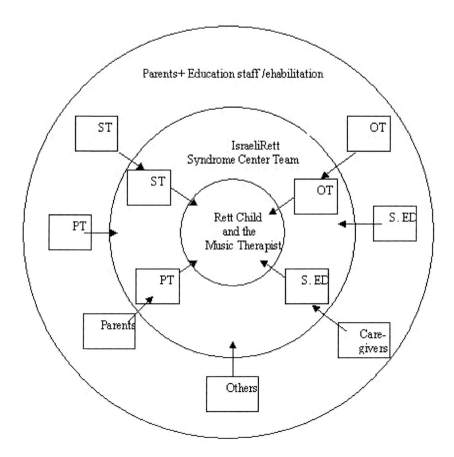

Figure III-2. Evaluation model.

For example, if a problem in handling food was identified or observed during the assessment, the occupational (OT) and speech therapist (ST) will lead the evaluation process at stages, when such intervention is warranted. In addition, there is constant gathering of information regarding the child's capabilities from educational/therapeutic staff and parents and this information is immediately integrated into the evaluation process. At the same time, the team coordinator narrates the meeting in real time -mainly to the parents - regarding the goals and interactions which are being implemented.

In cases where the educational staff members request that intra- professional meetings are held, each member of the RS team consults with his corresponding discipline member among the educational/therapeutic staff.

It is important to reiterate that the formal written description of the model is very structured and presented pragmatically. In actuality, however, there is a constant flexible flow that enables spontaneous assessment in a friendly atmosphere. This is important in promoting cooperation and adapting the assessment process to the needs of the individual with RS, her family and her educational staff. Such an atmosphere has direct impact upon the degree to which we can become acquainted with the child, the level of trust that is established, and the degree of openness that is attained.

Continuity

Continuity is ensured by adhering to the following elements: A detailed report is issued 3-4 weeks following the meeting with the individual with RS. This report is sent to the parents and educational staff and includes the findings of the transdisciplinary team. A copy of the report is also added to the child's medical records at the Sheba Center at Tel-Hashomer. This report emphasizes concrete clinical and educational recommendations. Furthermore the family can receive a video film that was taken during the assessment. The movie can also be viewed by the educational/therapeutic staff. Continuity is also achieved through follow-up meetings, held several months after the initial assessment and after the recommendations suggested by the RS team have been applied by the educational staff. Members of the RS team meet once more with the client's parents and educational/therapeutic staff. This meeting is designed to answer any questions that remain unanswered, to clarify findings that were presented during the previous meeting and to brainstorm regarding difficulties that have arisen during the application of the recommendations.

Follow-up and feedback

Following the evaluation by the RS team, a feedback form is sent to the parents and to members of the educational team. This form evaluates the efficiency and performance of the RS team and enables the center to supervise the work of the team. The members of the RS team are also required to fill out a self-evaluation form regarding every meeting in order to learn and draw conclusions regarding their function. The degree of compatibility between the answers that the RS team provided and the ones filled by the parents/educational facility team enables a cross correlation of the efficacy of the team and constantly improves the quality of the services that are offered. In this manner the team can improve its work towards future meetings.

Interaction methods

The Israel Rett Syndrome team employs several interaction approaches that allow full coverage of the needs of the person with RS:

- Assessment - the most common method of interaction is assessment of the individual with RS at the request of the parents or educational staff. This method was fully described in the previous section. However, there are instances in which different forms of interaction are needed. In these cases the team is prepared to provide solutions in other areas, such as consultation or problem solving.
- Consultation - The members of the RS team have comprehensive knowledge regarding developmental syndromes. Therefore, parents (particularly young ones) can be given guidance in various subjects such as suitable special educational facilities near their place of residence, agencies for renting equipment for the home or school, and therapists or care providers with knowledge about RS (for example, the fact that equipment can be purchased from various suppliers with different price

levels, or on the other hand attained for free through different volunteer organizations, is not always known by the parents).

- Mediation and problem Solving - When specific problems arise between parents and the child's educational facility, members of the RS team might be called upon to negotiate and bridge the gaps. In this way the unbalanced system can return to a situation in which it provides agreed upon supportive, care for the individual with RS in which she can progress. Examples of this type of intervention are:

Case one

A child who was placed in a special education facility by the municipal education board, while the local educational team was opposing the decision. The controversial decision resulted in opposition among the educational/therapeutic staff. This resulted in mistrust and severed relations between the child's parents and the educational/therapeutic facility (rejecting their daughter). Following a meeting between the educational/therapeutic staff, the parents and the coordinator of the RS team, understanding and cooperation was restored between the staff and the family and the child could once regain receive proper care mainly due to restoration of trust relationship between parents and the educational facility.

Case two

Another example of this form of intervention was a case in which a child with RS fell and was slightly injured, while exercising on a treadmill at her educational facility. After the incident her parents instructed the educational facility to refrain from engaging their child in any type! of physical activity at the special education facility. The physiotherapist from the RS team met with the parents and the educational staff and the result of this meeting was a mutual agreement on an exercise program that was shared between the home and the special education facility.

Discussion

The Israel Rett syndrome Center (IRSC) administers a team of experts who work in a unique manner in accordance to the principles described in this chapter: Accessibility, family-directed assessment, coordination, flexibility, comprehensiveness, continuity of connections and communication, follow-up and feedback. These principles are designed to meet the needs of individuals with Rett syndrome and their families and to help paraprofessional teams working in special education facilities to acquire knowledge of the unique characteristics of girls with RS in order to offer them the comprehensive care they require. The unique teamwork described in this chapter originates from a combination of the following factors:

- Cost effectiveness – the actual assessment for each child according to the above described model takes only two hours. An additional few hours is invested in writing and submitting the written report for each child.
- Natural surroundings - The RS team works by visiting the child's natural environment and by offering individual advice and support for the members of the educational staff who care for the child on a permanent basis.
- Manner of assessment – the evaluation of the client's condition is based on transdisciplinary play-based Assessment (TPBA) which is a pleasant form of assessment for the individual with RS and her family as well as transparent and comprehensive.
- Holistic manner of evaluation - the entire RS team assesses the child abilities and needs and presents the educational staff and the parents with a complete therapeutic management program. Since the PT is also acquainted with the Snoezelen approach and adapted seating and due to the fact that the OT is also a hydrotherapist and the team coordinator is an aunt for a person with SR, the team covers a variety of therapeutic fields suitable for this population.
- The human factor - Members of the RS team possess a shared belief in the potential abilities of individuals with RS and therefore a shared view of the treatment/ education goals for this population. In addition, all of the members of the RS have experience of clinically caring for girls with Rett syndrome for more than 15 years. This accumulated professional experience has enabled the team members to form a professional identity. We believe that this is one of the critical elements which make the working model described here, possible.
- Clinical approach – the RS team provides both the parents and the educational facility's staff with "down to earth" clinical suggestions ready for implementation.
- Feedback and follow-up - a child who has undergone initial diagnosis and received recommendations regarding intervention is visited again several months after the recommendations are implemented in order to obtain feedback and make adjustments as necessary. This facilitates the construction of a management plan for each child which is acceptable and accessible to the educational staff. All members of the RS team are easily contactable by the educational staff and the parents via e-mail or by phone.

All the points mentioned above make the working methods of the Israeli Rett Syndrome Center team a unique model both in Israel and as far as we know also abroad.

Conclusions

The working model presented in this chapter is unique both in respect to the work methods used by the assessment team and in respect to the age (1-50) and the level of disability of the target population – children and adults with Rett syndrome. Today the work methods used by the assessment team are being explored more thoroughly in order to identify factors which will enable optimal use of the model and to continue to improve the team's performance. The authors recommend that other national or regional centers adopt a similar working model in order to promote knowledge and improve the quality of services for individuals with RS.

References

[1]   Amir RE, Van den Veyver IB, Wan M, Tran CQ, Francke U, Zoghbi HY. Rett syndrome is caused by mutations in X-linked MECP2, encoding methyl-CpG-binding protein 2. Nat Genet 1999;23(2):185-8.

[2]   Amir RE, Van Den Veyve IB, Schultz R, Malicki DM, Tran CQ, Dahle EJ, et al. Influence of mutation type and X chromosome inactivation on Rett syndrome phenotypes. Ann Neurol 2000;47:670-9.

[3]   Hagberg B. Rett Syndrome clinical and biological aspects. London: Mac K Press, 1993.

[4]   Weaving LS, Ellaway CJ, Gecz J, Christodoulou J. Rett syndrome: clinical review and genetic update. J Med Genet 2005;42(1):1-7.

[5]   Neul JL, Zoghbi HY. Rett syndrome: a prototypical neurodevelopmental disorder. Neuroscientist 2004;10(2):118-28.

[6]   Glaze DG. Rett syndrome: of girls and mice: lessons for regression in autism. Ment Retard Dev Disabil Res Rev 2004;10(2):154-8.

[7]   Gibson JH, Williamson SL, Arbuckle S, Christodoulou J. X chromosome inactivation patterns in brain in Rett syndrome: implications for the disease phenotype. Brain Dev 2005;27(4):266-70.

[8]   Rainforth B, York J, York-Barr C. Collaborative teams for students with severe disabilities: Integrating therapy and educational services. Baltimore: Paul H Brookes, 1997.

[9]   Davis J, Rendell P, Sims D. The joint practitioner- a new concept in professional training. J Interprof care 1999;13(4): 395-404.

[10]   Benierakis CE. The function of multidisciplinary team in child psychiatry- clinic and educational aspect. Can J Psychiatry 1995;40: 348-53.

[11]   Heinemann GD. Teams in health care setting. In: Heinemann GD, Zeiss AM, eds. Team performance in health care: Assessment and development. New York: Kluwer Acad/Plenum, 2002.

[12]   Dunn W. Models of occupational therapy service provision in the school system. Am J Occup Ther 1988;42(11):718-23.

[13]   York J, Rainforth B, Giangreco MF. Transdisciplinary team work and integrated therapy: Clarifying the misconceptions. Pediatric Physical Therapy 1990;2(2):73-9.

[14]   Campbell PH. The integrated programming team: An approach for coordinating professionals of various disciplines in programs for students with severe and multiple handicaps. Journal of the association for persons with severe handicaps 1978;12(2):107-16.

[15]   Hutchinson DJ. The transdisciplinary approach. In: Curry JB, Peppe KK, eds. Interdisciplinary approach to human services. Baltimore: Univ Park Press, 1987:65-74.

[16]   Bennet FC. The pediatrician and the interdisciplinary process. Except Child 1982;48(4):306-14.

[17]   Szymanski EM, Hanley-Maxwell C, Asselin S. Rehabilitation counseling, special education, and vocational special needs education: Three transition disciplines. Career Dev Except Individ 1990;13(1):29-38.

[18]   Youngson-Reilly S, Tobin M, Fielder A. Multidisciplinary teams and childhood visual impairment: a study of two teams. Child Care Health Dev 1995;21(1):3-15.

[19]   Linder TW. Transdisciplinary Play-Based Assessment (TPBA) A functional approach to working with young children, rev ed. Baltimore, MD: PaulH. Brookes, 1990.

[20]   Armstrong DD. The neuropathology of Rett syndrome – overview 1994. Neuoropediatrics 1995;26:100-4.

[21]   Ellaway C, Christodoulou J. Rett syndrome: Clinical characteristics and recent genetic advances. Disabil Rehabil 2001;23:98-106.

[22]   Guy J, Gan J, Selfridge J, Cobb S, Bird A. Reversal of neurological defects in a mouse model of Rett syndrome. Science 2007;315(5815):1143-7.

[23]   Hunter K. The Rett Syndrome handbook, Washington, DC: Int Rett Syndr Assoc, 1999.

[24]   Percy AK. International research review. Paper presented at the IRSA 12th annual conference. Boston, MA: 1996 May 24-27, tape 622-15, 1996.

[25]   McDonnell S. Balancing family needs. Presentation, Ann Rett Syndr Conf, Baltimore, MD: 2004 May 30.

[26]   Israely Rett syndrome center. What is Rett syndrome? An information leaflet, 2004. [Hebrew]

[27]   Middle States Commission on Higher Education. Handbook for evaluation teams, sixth ed. Philadelphia, PA: Middle States Comm Higher Educ, 2000.

[28]   Elefant C, Lotan M. Rett syndrome: Dual intervention – music and physical therapy. Nord J Music Ther 2004;13(2):172-82.

[29]   Lotan M, Hadar-Frumer M. Aquatic Rehabilitation in Rett Syndrome. Rett Gazette 2000 Spring:1-7.

[30]   Lindberg B. Understanding Rett Syndrome: A practice guide for parents, teachers and therapists. Toronto: Hognefe Huber, 1991.

[31]   Merker B, Bergstrom-Isacsson M, Witt Engerstrom I. Music and the Rett disorder: The Swedish Rett center survey. Nord J Music Ther 2001;10(1): 42-53.

[32]   Elefant C. Speechless yet communicative: Revealing the person behind the disability of Rett syndrome through clinical research on songs in music therapy. In: Aldridge D, di Franco G, Ruud E, Wigram T, eds. Music therapy in Europe. Rome: ISMEZ, 2001.

[33]   Wigram T. Assessment and Treatment of a Girl with Rett Syndrome. In: Bruscia K, ed. Case studies in music therapy. Gilsum, NH: Barcelona Publ, 1991.

[34]   Wigram T, Cass H. Music therapy within the assessment process for a therapy clinic for people with Rett syndrome. Presentation, Rett Syndr World Conf, Sweden, 1996.

[35]   Takehisa K, Takehisa-Silvestri G. Intermediate results of music therapy in interdisciplinary work with Rett syndrome in institut Haus der Barmherzigkeit. Vienna, Austria: Institut Haus der Barmherzigkeit, 1997.

In: Rett Syndrome: Therapeutic Interventions
Editors: Meir Lotan and Joav Merrick

ISBN: 978-1-61728-080-1
©2011 Nova Science Publishers, Inc.

Chapter IV

Rett Syndrome: Guidelines for Individual Intervention

Meir Lotan, BPT, MScPT, PhD[*]

Israeli Rett Syndrome Association, National Evaluation Team, National Rett Syndrome Clinic, Chaim Sheba Medical Center, Ramat-Gan; Zvi Quittman Residential Centers, Israel Elwyn, Jerusalem and Department of Physical Therapy, Ariel University Center of Samaria, Ariel, Israel

Rett Syndrome (RS) is a neurological disorder affecting mainly females. RS is considered the second most frequent cause for severe and complex neurological dysfunction in females after Down's Syndrome. Patients with RS are characterized by having an array of neurological and orthopedic difficulties that require an intensive therapeutic intervention program for the duration of the individual's life. Many aspects of the client's well-being and functional status depend on the therapeutic intervention she receives and on her compliance with it. This chapter will briefly review common intervention approaches for individuals with RS and their present day application. Due to the notion that individual intervention is the foundation on which progress and development of the client's functional gains rests, the present chapter will set out basic guidelines for individual intervention with clients with RS. The chapter is mainly based on the clinical experience of the author and others working with individuals with RS.

Introduction

Rett Syndrome (RS) is a neurological disorder found mainly in females [1,2], characterized by normal birth and apparently normal psychomotor development during the first 6-18 months of life [3]. The child then enters a short period of developmental stagnation, followed

---

[*] Correspondence: Meir Lotan, BPT, MScPT, PhD, Department of Physical Therapy, Ariel University Center of Samaria, IL-40700 Ariel, Israel. E-mail: ml_pt_rs@netvision.net.il

by rapid regression in language and motor skills. The trademark of the disease is the repetitive stereotypical hand movements appearing when the child enters stage II of RS. Additional characteristics at the breakthrough of the disorder include Autistic-like behavior, panic-like attacks, bruxism, breathing irregularities, episodes of apnea and/or hyperpnea, gait ataxia and apraxia, tremors and acquired microcephaly [4]. After this period of rapid deterioration, despite the relatively stable manner of the disease. the child with RS is likely to develop dystonia and if not ambulant, might also develop foot and hand deformities [5] as she grows older. Seizures occur in 50%-85% [3,6] of individuals with RS and females with RS typically survive into adulthood and their estimated life expectancy is about 50 years [7].

The difficulties presented by the individual with RS and their longevity, necessitate individual adaptation of intervention in all educational and therapeutic areas. Research shows that brain development continues after the onset of RS [8] and that cognitive and communicative abilities of the individual with RS does not deteriorate over the years. Therefore, the setting of proper and achievable therapeutic educational and communicational goals for the individual with RS is vital [9]. Since overcoming all the above-mentioned impediments requires therapeutic intervention through the course of the person with RS's lifes, it is imperative that such treatments be delivered to the individual with RS and her family with outmost proficiency. Therefore, treatment planning should be related to assessment of the individual's current level of functioning as well as her strengths and weaknesses, yet this basic primary component will be left outside the scope of the present chapter.

General Comments Regarding Therapeutic Intervention

A growing body of research recommends that intensive, sustained treatment is important in improving the long-term outcome in syndromes under the umbrella term of PDD [10]. Intervention planning should, on the one hand, be grounded in the present functional and medical reality but on the other, should focus on the long-term vision\prognosis for the client's potential. Planning entails attention to educational interventions, residential situations and vocational programs [11-13]. A well-functioning intervention program must also include appropriate involvement and collaboration with the individual's family [14]. Intervention should be focused and individualized and must be broadly implemented to relate to the full range of impairments shown by the client. Regardless of the individual's age, treatment planning should include provision for structured opportunities for learning and for generalization of what is learned. Individuals with RS require high-level general medical and para-professional care which includes provision for routine preventive health measures and for the special needs of the multi-handicapped person.

Usually many disciplines are involved in different aspects of the treatment of the clients with RS, therefore it is important that one clinician be primarily involved with the parents to develop a plan of care for the child. This individual must also be responsible for service co-ordination and advocacy [10]. Clinicians should help to co-ordinate services and work with parents to obtain appropriate educational programs, be an advocate for services such as respite care and support for the family and provide consultation regarding prognosis of the disorder, therapeutic medical and pharmacology management [13].

Creating a therapeutic net around the client

Educational services are a central and integral aspect of the treatment of children and adolescents with RS. In most Western countries, the law provides for the provision of an appropriate educational plan for all children, including those with special needs. As part of these educational programs, additional services such as: speech/language therapy, occupational therapy, physical therapy and others are often required. Whilst early intervention undoubtedly is very helpful [15,16], it should be administered while gathering information and addressing issues such as:

- What features of the treatment are most important, and to whom?
- Should those issues be enhanced?
- What characteristics of the child are associated with greatest improvement?
- Should the management program focus on specific issues or address all difficulties?
- What are the present and future targets goals for the client?

It is agreed that, for this population, sustained and continuous, rather than episodic programming is more effective (meaning that the option for Summer programming should be positively considered because children under the umbrella term of pervasive developmental disorder (PDD) might regress in the absence of appropriate services [10].

Supplementary therapeutic services or stretching a therapeutic net around the client with RS means that a group of therapeutic approaches are needed when aiming at fully supporting the individual's and her family's needs. Such therapeutic agents might be conventional or unconventional but it is advised that they collaborate to support jointly the full-scale needs of the individual with RS. A partial list of intervention approaches are:

- Special education (SE) – The concept of "least restrictive environment" implies the integration of students with disabilities in mainstream school programs. The importance of the educational environment, lies in the fact that school represents many academic and social learning opportunities, beyond traditional classroom instruction. Students who are integrated into the mainstream educational environment are exposed to those opportunities. All students require support from teachers, classmates, family and friends, in order to thrive and to gain full benefit from their school experience. Students with RS have special needs that require additional support beyond those ordinarily received in the school setting. Students with RS must have access to an education that will enable them to develop the knowledge and skills they need in order to participate to their fullest ability in their surrounding society. The SE teacher is the heart of the educational system in charge of implementing the theoretical concepts into an actual, achievable daily curriculum. The SE teacher role is to mediate between the child's educational and family surroundings and to deliver the educational plan to her/his class. Furthermore, the SE teacher should integrate all intervention programs for pupils with RS through the construction of the IEP (Individual Educational Plan) and should supervise its execution throughout the academic year by interweaving it into the pupils' daily activities [17].

- Physical therapist (PT) – Individuals with RS struggle to overcome a vast array of orthopedic and neurological difficulties. Coping with such difficulties and overcoming the associated limitations is a wearisome task for the individual with Rett and for her family. The PT can enhance the child's physical fitness and functionality [18], thus reducing the secondary dangers of immobility. The PT can also design and implement a functional intervention plan applied by the therapist him/herself or by others. Within the educational surrounding, the PT is responsible for integrating his/her program in the child daily educational curriculum by means of the IEP. An appropriate and intensely applied physical therapy régime can help the child to cope and even overcome some of the above-mentioned limitations. The PT should advise other team members regarding issues within her\his field of expertise. Joint intervention sessions with other professions are highly recommended [19], as are the use of alternative therapeutic environments, such as the Snoezelen [20, 21].

- Music therapy (MT) - Andreas Rett (1924-1997) recognized the potential of music therapy to penetrate the heavy shield of disability masking the hidden abilities of individuals with RS [22]. Music therapists use their applied musical skills of improvisation and singing to establish rapport with the child, utilizing them as bridges to bond and engage in non-verbal forms of communication. Music therapy can open channels which, through musical sounds; can offer a child new opportunities. With such support, the individual with RS can express emotions and feelings, further enabling some communication and learning to take place. Current knowledge of the use of music therapy as an intervention for the individual with RS, suggests that it can enhance functional hand use and reduce stereotypic hand movements, develop possibilities for choice making, enhance vocalization, improve attention and eye contact and develop emotional-communicative channels that can engage, relax or sooth the child [23-31].

- Speech therapist (ST) – The vast majority of individuals with RS present difficulties in expressive language (talking) and it is believed that their ability to internalize (understand) incoming information is far more greatly achieved than their ability to express themselves verbally. The ST can increase expressive communication of the individual with RS by using different assistive augmentative communication (AAC) devices. Eating is a function on which speech therapists are highly trained and since most individuals with RS present some forms of difficulty in this area [32] the therapist can help the child overcome Apraxia and other basic motor difficulties which interfere with the complex task of eating. It is advised that the ST work jointly with other therapists, staff and family to explore all potentially successful means of communication, and to use effective positioning so that the individual may be fully free to reach her up-most abilities.

- Occupational therapist (OT) – Individuals with RS shows difficulties in areas of manual activities; sensorial perception and processing; in activities of daily living (ADL), such as eating, self care and toileting. Occupational therapists are trained in making the unachievable task attainable. The OT provides ways to help the individual with RS to increase the use of her hands and body by adapting the client's environment. Enhancing the individual's function will improve her satisfaction, confidence and will offer her increased ability to control her own world. The lack of sensory mastery of the nervous system by the individual with RS leaves her with an inability to correctly interpret the world around her. The OT can help the client with RS to better organize the information she receives by using varied therapeutic approaches and techniques such as sensory integration (SI), brushing, swinging, tactile activities and deep tissue compression. As one of the team members embracing the individual with RS, in many daily situations the OT can make recommendations to other team members regarding adjustments to the child surroundings.

- Hydrotherapist (HT) – Hydrotherapy offers pleasant engulfment in warm water whilst at the same time is helpful in reducing spasticity and in softening rigid tissues. The HT can use the water to provide the individual with RS with intense stimulation, thus enabling a better sensory input. The use of warm water might calm the child who is afraid of motion. The person with RS is able to move easily and freely in the water, without fear of falling. Furthermore, spending time in a pool places the individual with RS at a normative place where she can associate with peers and family. Other advantages suggested by hydrotherapy are the pleasure of new and exciting experiences through water activities and the ability to function in ways in which she might not be able to do on land. In some cases, the water enables the child with RS to express her lost and sometimes latent motor skills [33].

- Pharmacological and related interventions - Although not curative, medication may be useful for relieving symptoms which interfere with participation in intervention [34] or alleviate sources of impairment or distress experienced by the individual with RS (constipation, seizures, osteoporosis, etc.).

- Alternative treatments - Given the chronic nature of RS and the lack of knowledge regarding a cure, it is not surprising that putative cures surface quite frequently, many without substantial background. Not uncommonly, initial reports relate to an individual child or a handful of cases. Such reports are difficult to interpret as the many aspects of the intervention approaches described might be vague or highly uncertain. Usually, such reports are not followed by more rigorous, controlled studies in the peer-reviewed scientific literature. Families should be helped in making informed decisions about their use of alternative treatments. Treatments that pose some risk to the individual and her family, should be actively discouraged.

- Follow-up assessments and on-going treatment – Due to the fluctuating nature of RS, therapeutic services must be flexible and possess the ability to change at different points during the client's development (e.g. due to an increase in anti-epileptic medication, the child who could walk independently a week ago might now find it hard to stand). To provide the specific care needed for this population, co-ordination of services and family support is an imperative aspect of on-going care. The nature and intensity of therapeutic contacts depend on the clinical situation and needs of the individual and should be monitored constantly and adjusted. In the light of all the above theoretical background, it would be appropriate, at this point, to evaluate the present state of therapeutic intervention actually presented for the individual with RS.

Therapeutic interventions for rett syndrome

The present state of therapeutic interventions for individuals with RS was investigated by Leonard et al [35]. Their inquiry entailed an investigation of 86 families of children with RS, at various ages, from infancy to adulthood and in different countries around the globe. Their findings suggest that individuals with RS receive an array of therapeutic interventions, according to the following specification:

Table IV-1. Therapeutic interventions for individuals with Rett syndrome

Occupational therapy	Physical therapy	Speech therapy	Hydrotherapy	Hippotherapy	Music therapy
84.9%	77.9%	76.7%	29.1%	17.4%	9.3%

The full scale of these findings was discussed in the original article, but some points should be emphasized. The findings suggest that 36% of parents were dissatisfied about the intervention suggested for their daughters, because of insufficiency of intervention or inappropriateness to RS. Music therapy, which has been described repeatedly as of the utmost value to this population [22,28-30,36,37], is only available for fewer then 10% of individuals with RS.

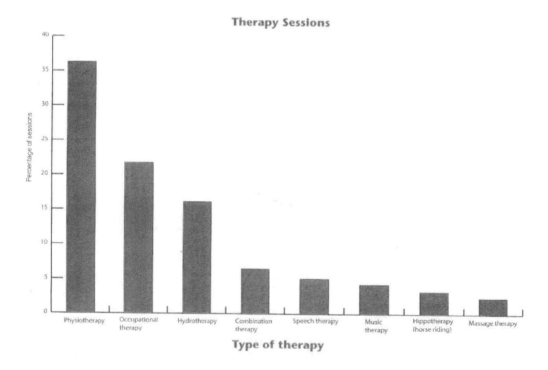

Figure IV-1. Therapeutic intervention for individuals with RS. Published with permission [38].

Possible conclusions that might be drawn from the article of Leonard et al [35] is that, despite the high functional dependency presented by most individuals with RS (as compared to individuals with Down's Syndrome), intervention is not administered to all. In most cases the intervention is not perceived within the medical milieu to be a rehabilitative concept and the intervention delivered is often insufficient and inappropriate. The data presented by Leonard et a [35] revealed that intervention services were insufficient in relation to a complex condition such as RS and should be increased by the active efforts of care-givers and parents.

In the light of the findings by Leonard et al [35], the next section will suggest insights into intervention for individuals with RS.

We encourage therapists to apply multi-disciplinary models of intervention for individuals with RS [39], whether they are delivered as individual intervention [40,41] or in other forms [19], but with attention to the special features of RS.

Insights to intervention with Rett syndrome

It is important to restate that individual intervention is not perceived as the ultimate intervention method but merely one basic step to support integration and independence of the individual. The individual intervention is the foundation upon which progress is based, especially for individuals with RS or as Abraham Harold Maslow (1908-1970) said, the "ordinary (individual) therapy may be conceived as a miniature ideal society of two" [42:263]. By reference to this concept, the present chapter submits guidelines for individual intervention with the client with RS.

Adopting the suggested guidelines will help to advance the individual with RS in her struggle to overcome all the debilitating challenges put forward by RS. The one-on-one intervention may start in the therapy room but must simultaneously develop in the classroom, the residential environment of the child and among her peer group and community. At first encounters, the individual with RS might present difficulties typical of all new students. Such times have been reported as periods of anxiety both for the individual and parents [43].

It is recommended that initial contact between the client with RS and her therapist be conducted in a familiar, quiet place, with a care-giver/family member with whom the child is familiar and trusts. In such a favorable environment, bonding between the individual with RS and her therapist will create the necessary milieu for her later functional advancement. Achieving rapport during the few first encounters is not always easy and even after the establishment of such a connection, the advancement of the intervention with the individual with RS is slow and demanding, requiring much patience by the therapist.

The connection between client and therapist is sometimes influenced by the emotions of the therapist working with the individual with RS [44]. In new and unfamiliar situations or when the therapist is tired, depressed or nervous, results are seldom achieved [44]. If the therapist is attentive to him/herself and to the individual with RS, therapeutic results are much more easily gained. A deeper acquaintance with the person with RS, with her daily program and her physical and human environment will enable improved communication and meaningful attachment and, therefore, is highly recommended. Such bonding will enable the therapist to better decipher the client's signs and his/her reactions to her signals will improve.

As a result, the communicative "output" of the individual with RS might improve, helping in overcoming barriers in education and personal contact [43,45,46].

Despite the fact that, it is probably a well-known feature to any therapist/educator, the author would like to reiterate that "individual intervention" does not mean that every therapist is totally devoted to his private therapeutic agenda and completely oblivious to other team members. Any therapist/educator working with an individual with RS must maintain professional relationships with their client's parents and other health related professionals contributing to her curriculum. It is advised that all team members (working according to a multi/trans-disciplinary approach) join together and decide on combined goals for the client with RS, grouping their efforts and knowledge to advance the treatment of the individual with RS according to the collectively-decided intervention plan. In some cases, parents will seek additional treatments outside the educational setting and it is important that providers of such services co-ordinate their work with that of the educational facility [10].

Intervention goals are built in accordance with each client's abilities and needs and are lead by the combined intention to achieve the highest functional level and the best quality of life attainable. Lewis and Wilson [43] have contributed the obvious, yet important, statement that individuals with RS are complete human beings. Therefore, the intervention for the individual with RS should be holistic, integrating all aspects of treatment, leading to the achievement of maximal functional gains [43]. All therapeutic interventions should address challenges in the performance of the individual in daily activities (eating, drinking, communicating, standing, walking, communicating and socializing).

The recommendations suggested thus far might be agreed upon for many individuals with complex disabilities. The next section will specifically address insights into intervention with RS and it represents the gathered clinical/educational/therapeutic experience by professionals working with this population over the years.

Guidelines for individual intervention

The aim of this last part of the chapter is to establish a body of knowledge, which will help the clinician to approach the client with RS. Despite the fact that every individual with RS is a unique entity, differing from others with RS, while not forgetting that each treatment is a consequence of a thoroughly considered evaluation, there are similarities among individuals with RS, which the following guidelines seek to take in to account.

1. The cognitive ability of individuals with RS is unclear. Conventional intelligence quotation (IQ) tests rely mainly on manual ability or on oral expression, thereby highlighting the weakest abilities of this population. Until appropriate tests are administered, the therapist should believe in the ability of individuals with RS and work with them with respect and on the assumption that they perceive much more than they are able to produce.

2. In order for the intervention process to achieve maximal results, the health related professional is advised to acquire the trust and confidence of the client with RS. Therefore, it would be wise for the therapist/educator to invest in developing strong

rapport before and during intervention implementation. Such connection may later prevent rejection and discomfort [47].

3. It would greatly benefit the individual with RS if all care-givers (siblings, parents, therapists and educational staff) could be involved or at least familiarized with the intervention program. Systematic meetings are recommended to enable information transfer (data regarding the individual's natural forms of communication, her preferences in colors, food, drinking, activities and more) from the educational arena to the client's residence, and vice-versa. Keeping constant open communication paths between meetings is advised.

4. When handling the individual with RS, it is of outmost importance to understand her world. Most individuals with RS can open up to the therapist, using their developed emotional capacities. If the therapist/educator remains sufficiently attentive, he will be able to detect the client's signals.

5. It is preferable to keep the individual with RS calm and to maintain quiet, familiar surroundings. Employing consistency in applying the intervention program is advised.

6. Presenting the individual with RS with proper motivational factors might greatly enhance her co-operation, thereby upgrading her functional abilities (e.g. an individual with RS usually showing typical poor hand function, who was given physical therapy sessions by the author, had the ability to eat a sandwich with chocolate spread or drink a whole glass of Coca-Cola, but only these specific food items, holding both the sandwich and the glass firmly with both hand, for the whole duration of her meal).

7. It is for the best if the individual with RS views her world as safe and comprehensible before attempting to actively participate in it. Therefore, the advice is to:
    - Apply therapy sessions at pre-set times
    - Explain what is likely to happen, in advance
    - Give the individual ample time to accustom herself to the situation (the room, equipment, therapist)
    - Construct each session from familiar components
    - Support the individual when she seems baffled\disoriented
    - Announce the end of therapy in advance.

8. If the individual with RS is extremely attached to a person\object that gives confidence (a care-giver, pacifier, a corner of the room) the therapist should consider using those as a safe starting-point when new demands or exercises are initiated.

9. Individuals with RS love music and songs [48]. They react much better to songs than to a directly spoken instruction. They enjoy whispers in their ears and different voice games and prefer live singing over instrumental music. Using music during therapy could greatly motivate the person with RS to participate actively in individual intervention [49]. If the person with RS does not seem enthusiastic about the music played for her, do bear in mind that each individual with RS has a personal taste in music, not necessarily compatible with that of the therapist.

10. Most individuals with RS do not communicate verbally but this does not mean they have nothing to say. Since body language and eye gaze are silent ways of communicating, it is the responsibility of the therapist to be alert and attentive to the client's signs. If it is known that a specific individual with RS has some distinct gestures with specific meaning, such knowledge should accompany the individual throughout her daily encounters with peers and adults. When the individual with RS is using such a gesture, proper acknowledgement is due, even if her needs cannot be answered at that specific time (e.g. the individual with RS is signaling that she would like to watch a video film during lunch or a family trip – "Yes. I can see that you want to watch a video but we can't do it right now. We can watch a video film when we get home/to class/finish eating"). More information regarding personal communication dictionary can be found in chapter 8.

11. Most individuals with RS can communicate through facial expression. The attentive therapist/care-giver will be able to react to their fear, curiosity, anxiety, enjoyment, anticipation, rejection and much more.

12. Individuals with RS might sometime present vocal abilities after they are acquainted with their surrounding and have accepted the therapist. The therapist should react with their own voice and initiate a mutual "conversation'. When the individual with RS feels that her human environment is responding to her messages, she will increase her output and an on-going dialogue could develop.

13. Routine is important for the individual with RS. It is advised that she be supplied with constant familiar rituals matched with verbal or visual symbols (before food is served, those involved might sit around the table talking about food, laying plates and eating utensils on the table, and looking at pictures of different food items that will be delivered shortly; before going to the swimming pool they can get undressed, wear a bathing suit, look at a picture of the pool and talk about doing hydrotherapy….).

14. Routinely addressing the individual's daily curriculum is more likely to make her fill safe and confident, thus encouraging her fully to express her abilities. If a change in her regular activities is planned, it would be for the best to inform the individual with RS and try to make the change as gradual as possible to allow her time to adjust.

15. The individual with RS finds it difficult to generalize, due to her apraxia. (For instance, an individual who might put her hand on the care-giver's arm at lunch time to signal for more food may not use such a gesture to signal the need to go to the bathroom). It is recommended that an existing gesture be used to generalize a communicative act from one situation to another.

16. When implementing a program for an individual with RS make sure that it:
    - Is clear to the client as well as to the therapist (what is intended to be implemented; what are the primary and final goals);
    - Is structured (the method, the location, other participants, appliances);
    - Entails opening and closing rituals;
    - Keeps the individual interested and involved during all parts of the program;
    - Maintains and supports the client's level of confidence;
    - Changes (if change is due) gradually.

17. When constructing a therapeutic intervention program it is recommended that the program be as comprehensive as possible, involving the individual's home (the home as a support unit for the therapeutic program - whilst it is important for the parents to participate fully in the individual's intervention program, they can only do so in accordance with their emotional state. The therapist should bear in mind that they are, first and foremost, the child's parents, responsible mainly for offering love and care) as well as the educational/rehabilitation facility. It is my experience that without such wide-range support, most programs are likely to bear negligible results or just fade, in time.

18. The recommended duration of therapeutic sessions that is acceptable for most individuals with RS is around 20-30 minutes. Nevertheless, the timetable of therapeutic interactions should not be, a priori, reduced but rather should depend on the capability of the individual with RS. When music and warm, loving care are inter-twined within the therapeutic interaction, the individual with RS can sometimes be kept attentive for hours. When she decides she has had enough, she will show the therapist, in her specific way (closing her eyes, rolling her eyes backwards, falling asleep, losing interest, etc.), that the session has come to its end.

19. Individuals with RS are capable of learning [49]. Therefore, decide on the skill that the person with RS is to acquire and repeat the chosen activity for the amount of time needed for her to internalize this new skill.

20. Due to apraxia, the individual with RS will find it difficult to learn new skills and to perform motor acts [50]. Continuous repetition is advised to reduce the individual's need to organize and plan her performance, thus reducing her reaction time by making the execution of a motor act automatically performed. When results are slow to emerge, on many occasions there is nothing to do but be patient. The Apraxic individual sometimes requires a few months to learn to handle a new task.

21. On the other hand, I have witnessed situations in which the therapist was asking the individual with RS to perform an act repeatedly (e.g. touch named pictures or objects over and over) until the child revolted by suddenly refusing to co-operate. In such cases the therapist\educator should rest assure that she did not suddenly forget everything she previously knew. I believe such situations can be avoided if interactions are planned in a more versatile and challenging way and the therapist shows her/his partner with RS some acceptance and belief in her abilities.

22. Daily activities are best examples for spontaneous learning experience for the individual with RS. (Eating is a chance to talk about farming and food making; bathing is a chance to develop body schema and reduce sensorial sensitivity, by applying massage).

23. Individuals with RS might show some difficulties with regard to sequence acquisition. In such cases it is recommended that the learning program for the learner be adjusted by breaking it into simple steps.

24. It is recommended that general remarks (such as: "go up the stairs") be used, instead of direct, specific instructions demanding exact motor-functional planning (such as: "put your hand on the railing"). Using the former mentioned form of speech might speed up the individual's reaction.

25. When instructing the individual with RS, it is recommended that she is guided by the use of the same instructions. The therapist is advised to refrain from changing the way he/she phrases guidance, since it might confuse the individual, distracting her from achieving her goal.

26. Due to long reaction times of individuals with RS, the therapist is advised to wait patiently for the client to perform following instructions (during that time the person with RS might appear distracted, will accelerate her breathing pattern, look to both sides and perform intense body rocking and hand stereotypical movements). All these behaviors are just her way of preparing her reaction. Repeating the former request during that time will cause her to reset her intention and start planning her reaction from the beginning, causing her to further elongate her reaction time or even neglect her desire to participate.

27. One of the strengths of people with RS is their visual system. The use of pictures should be much encouraged [47] as communication and educational channels, and as means to enable choice in daily situations and (when using pictures of familiar characters) as a motivational factor. The constant use of pictures is most empowering for the individual with RS.

28. Integrating different aspects of one experience is highly recommended and is of great importance. (e.g. how can we expect a child to identify and associat between a picture of a big round apple with those half-moon shaped white slices on her plate if she has not seen an apple sliced into pieces).

29. Some individuals with RS are so handicapped by the combination of ataxia, apraxia, distonic muscles and long reaction-time that performing an accurate manual task might be found to be impossible. For theses individuals, any initiation and attunement towards the requested goal should be praised, even if the action itself was "unsuccessful"(e.g. the individual was asked to get a doll from the table and instead struck it to the ground: "Good!! you tried to take the doll, let me help you a bit"), so she will not be discouraged from trying again.

30. On the other hand, automatically and intensively congratulating an individual with RS for anything she does might cause the praise gradually to become redundant.

31. It is important to note that sleeping patterns of the individual with RS are sometimes immature (waking very early in the morning, disrupted sleep sequence [51]) causing the individual to drowse off during day-time. The use of anti-convulsive medications might also cause the individual to become drowsy and slow to react. It is advised that such circumstances be taken in to account a priori, when planning the individual intervention for the person with RS, introducing such interactions during periods where she is usually known to be at her functional peak.

32. Individuals with RS are famous for their functional fluctuations. During moments in a period of activity (but sometimes even for hours or days) the individual with RS seems lost and disconnected "It is as if her mind is covered by clouds" [47:77]. In some recorded cases, such a behavior was found to reduce staff (care-givers and therapists alike) confidence in the abilities of the individual with RS. One must not give up on the client with RS! This phenomenon is caused by numerous factors

associated with this disorder and the therapist should have confidence in the fact that the individual with RS will reconnect and return to her previous functional abilities.

33. Most individuals with RS will find it very hard to split their attention among several issues. If we are trying to work on one of our therapeutic/educational goals while the individual is trying to convey a different message, she will not pay any attention to story-telling, computer games or whatever task we had in mind. On such occasions it is better to take time out, detect and address her topic of interest and then it might be possible to return to the former planned task.

34. In some cases the individual with RS could be in the "wrong place" (e.g. she is sitting in the kitchen and wants to see a video movie in the living room). Her wishes, in such circumstances, will be difficult to understand. If the wishes of the individual with RS are unclear, try and introduce many options and do a lot of trial and error tests (using questions to and responses from the individual with RS) until her wishes become clear. Such episodes (if successful) are the best communication enhancers.

35. When assisting the individual with RS to perform a task, timing is everything. If we try to hurry her performance she will probably react by clenching her fists and resisting our "push" or she might let go and let us do the action for her. On the other hand assisting too slowly might discourage the child. It is more helpful and productive if the care-giver/therapist/educator is familiar with the client's rhythm and is attentive to the individual's movements, offering assistance with the right timing, direction, force and pace.

36. The siblings of the child with RS are usually her natural therapists. They share remarkable bonding with one-another and the therapist might consider incorporating them into the therapeutic sessions or at least learn from the way they handle themselves with their sister.

37. Age-appropriate intervention should be advocated, as well as enabling the individual with RS to participate in peer activities.

38. Various difficulties impede the individual with RS from achieving independent function. It is advisable that an "independence intervention" be created at regular points in time and place. In these situations, the individual with RS will set the rules of the interaction. This form of intervention will empower the individual, encourage her to initiate and expose her true potential.

Summary

Many individuals with RS are extremely debilitated and handicapped by the vast array of neurological, orthopedic and functional limitations posed by the Rett disorder. Since the aim of the therapist is to improve the client's quality of life by overcoming or reducing these limitations, an individually-tailored intervention program should be implemented.

Such a program should be the result of a well-performed evaluation, holistically employed by a group of care-givers and therapists. The intervention program originating from such an evaluation should create a continuous network of human support around the individual with RS.

It is clear that some of the insights in the above guidelines might contradict one-another. Such contradictions might only be avoided if the therapist is attentive to functional and emotional alterations and applies a flexible therapeutic régime that constantly adapts to the changes presented by the client with RS. It is the belief of this author that individuals with RS can exceed many of their limitations if such a comprehensive, individually tailored and well suited therapy program is to be implemented.

References

[1] Amir RE, Van den Veyver IB, Wan M, Tran CQ, Francke U, Zoghbi HY. Rett Syndrome is caused by mutations in X-linked MECP2, encoding methyl-CpG-binding protein 2. Nat Genet 1999;23(2):185-8.

[2] Amir RE, Van Den Veyver IB, Schultz R, Malicki DM, Tran CQ, Dahle EJ, et al. Influence of mutation type and X chromosome inactivation on Rett Syndrome phenotypes. Ann Neurol 2000;47:670-9.

[3] Hagberg B. Rett Syndrome: Clinical and biological aspects. London, Mac Keith, 1993.

[4] Hagberg B, Aicardi J, Dias K, Ramos O. Progressive syndrome of autism, dementia, ataxia and loss of purposeful hand use in girls: Rett's syndrome: Report of 35 cases. Ann Neurol 1983;14:471–9.

[5] Sponseller P. Orthopedic update in Rett Syndrome. Rett Gazette 2001 Spring:1,4-5.

[6] Glaze D. Epilepsy. Paper presented at the IRSA 12th Annual Conference, Boston, MA: 1996 May 24-27, tape 622-18.

[7] Percy AK. International research review. Paper presented at the IRSA 12th annual conference. Boston, MA: 1996 May 24-27, tape 622-15.

[8] Kaufmann WE, Johnston MV, Blue ME. MeCP2 expression and function during brain development: implications for Rett Syndrome's pathogenesis and clinical evolution. Brain Dev 2005;27(Suppl 1):S77-S87.

[9] Cass H, Reilly S, Owen L, Wisbeach A, Weekes L, Slonims V, Wigram T, Charman T. Findings from a multidisciplinary clinical case series of females with Rett Syndrome. Dev Med Child Neurol 2003;45(5): 325-37.

[10] Volkmar F, Cook EH Jr, Pomeroy J, Realmuto G, Tanguay P. Practice parameters for the assessment and treatment of children, adolescents, and adults with autism and other pervasive developmental disorders. J Am Acad Child Adolesc Psychiatry 1999;38(12 Suppl), 32S-54S.

[11] Gerhardt PF, Holmes DL. Employment: Options and issues for adolescents and adults with autism. In: Cohen DJ, Volkmar FR, eds. Handbook of autism and pervasive developmental disorders, 2nd ed. New York: Wiley, 1997:650-64.

[12] Harris SL, Handleman JS. Helping children with autism enter the mainstream. In: Cohen DJ, Volkmar FR, eds. Handbook of autism and pervasive developmental disorders, 2nd ed. New York: Wiley, 1997:665-75.

[13] Marcus LM, Kunce LJ, Schopler E. Working with families. In: Cohen DJ, Volkmar FR, eds. Handbook of autism and and pervasive developmental disorders, 2nd ed. New York: Wiley, 1997:631-49.

[14] Siegel B. Coping with the diagnosis of autism. In: Cohen DJ, Volkmar FR, eds. Handbook of autism and and pervasive developmental disorders, 2nd ed. New York: Wiley, 1997:745-66.

[15] Ulrich BD, Ulrich DA, Collier DH, Cole EL. Developmental shifts in the ability of infants with Down's Syndrome to produce treadmill steps. Phys Ther 1995;75(1):14-23.

[16] Warfield ME, Krauss MW, Hauser-Cram P, Upshur CC, Shonkoff JP. Adaptation during early childhood among mothers of children with disabilities. J Dev Behav Pediatr 1999;20(1):9-16.

[17]   Lotan M. Management for Rett Syndrome. Grapho-soft; The Israeli Rett Syndrome Center, Tel-Aviv, Israel, 2006. [Hebrew]

[18]   Lotan M, Isakov E, Merrick J. Improving functional skills and physical fitness in children with Rett Syndrome J Intell Disabil Res 2004;48(8):730-5.

[19]   Lotan M, Elefant C. Physiotherapy and music therapy for a girl with Rett Syndrome. A dual treatment approach. Fysioterapeuten 2006;2:15-20. [Danish]

[20]   Lotan M, Merrick J. Rett Syndrome Management with Snoezelen or controlled multi-sensory environment; A review. Int J Adolesc Med Health 2004;16(1):5-12.

[21]   Lotan M, Shapiro M. Management of young children with Rett disorder in the controlled multi-sensory (Snoezelen) environment. Brain Dev 2005;27(Suppl 1):S88-S94.

[22]   Rett A. Grundlagen der Musiktherapie und Music-Psychologie. Stuttgart: Fischer, 1982. [German]

[23]   Allan I. Rett Syndrome: A view on care and management. Washington, DC: Natl Rett Syndr Assoc, 1991.

[24]   Coleman KA. Music therapy in Rett Syndrome. In: Educational and therapeutic intervention in Rett Syndrome. Clinton, MD: IRSA, 1987:93-110.

[25]   Elefant C, Lotan M. Rett syndrome: Dual intervention – music and physical therapy. Nord J Music Ther 2004;13(2):172-82.

[26]   Hadsell NA, Coleman KA. Rett syndrome: A challenge for music therapists. Music Ther Perspect 1988;5:52-6.

[27]   Hill SA. The relevance and value of music therapy for children with Rett syndrome. Br J Special Educ 1997;24(3):124-8.

[28]   Wesecky A. Music therapy for children with Rett syndrome. Am J Med Gen 1986;24(suppl 1):253-7.

[29]   Wigram T. Assessment and treatment of a girl with Rett Syndrome. In: Bruscia K, ed. Case studies in music therapy. Gilsum, NH: Barcelona Publ, 1991.

[30]   Wigram T. A model of assessment and differential diagnosis of handicap in children through the medium of music therapy. In: Wigram T, Saperston B, West R, eds. The art and science of music therapy: A handbook. Chur, Switzerland: Harwood Acad, 1995: 181-93.

[31]   Wigram T, Cass H. Music therapy within the assessment process for a therapy clinic for people with Rett Syndrome. Presentation, Rett Syndr World Conf, Sweden, 1996.

[32]   Budden SS. Management of Rett Syndrome: A ten-year experience. Neuropediatrics 1995;26(2):75-7.

[33]   Lotan M, Hadar-Frumer M. Aquatic rehabilitation in Rett syndrome. Rett Gazette 2002 Spring:1-7.

[34]   McDougle CJ. Psychopharmacology. In: Cohen DJ, Volkmar FR, eds. Handbook of autism and and pervasive developmental disorders, 2nd ed. New York: Wiley, 1997:707-29.

[35]   Leonard H, Fyfe S, Leonard S, Msall M. Functional status, medical impairments, and rehabilitation resources in 84 females with Rett Syndrome: a snapshot across the world from the parental perspective. Disabil Rehabil 2001;23(3-4):107-17.

[36]   Elefant C. Music, choice making and communication in Rett Syndrome. Presentation, Int Course Rett Syndr, Ostersund, Sweden, 2003 Jun 16-18.

[37]   Elefant C. Speechless yet communicative: Revealing the person behind the disability of Rett syndrome through clinical research on songs in music therapy. In: Aldridge D, di Franco G, Ruud E, Wigram T, eds. Music therapy in Europe. Rome: ISMEZ, 2001.

[38]   Leonard S. The Australian Rett Syndrome study inaugural report. Perth, Aust: Telethon Inst Child Health Res, 2002.

[39]   Parry TS. The effectiveness of early intervention: a critical review. J Paediatr Child Health 1992;28(5):343-6.

[40]   Mahoney G, Robinson C, Fewell RR. The effects of early motor intervention on children with Down syndrome or cerebral palsy: A field-based study. J Dev Behav Pediatr 2001;22(3):153-62.

[41]   Siebes RC, Wijnroks L, Vermeer A. Qualitative analysis of therapeutic motor intervention programmes for children with cerebral palsy: an update. Dev Med Child Neurol 2002;44:593–603.

[42]   Maslow A. Motivation and personality, 2nd ed. New-York: Harper Row, 1970.

[43]   Lewis JE, Wilson CD. Pathways to learning in Rett syndrome. Teleford, Shropshire: Wozencroft Printers, 1996.

[44]   Rett A. Rett syndrome. An address at United Kingdom Rett Syndr Assoc Conference, Coleshill, 1985.

[45]   Woodyatt GC, Ozanne A. Communication abilities and a case of Rett Syndrome. J Intellect Disabil Res 1992;36:83-92.

[46]   Woodyatt GC, Ozanne AE. A longitudinal study of cognitive skills and communication behaviours in children with Rett Syndrome. J Intellect Disabil Res 1993;37(Pt 4):419-35.

[47]   Lindberg B. Understanding Rett syndrome: A practice guide for parents, teachers and therapists. Toronto: Hognefe Huber, 1991.

[48]   Merker B, Wallin NL. Musical responsiveness in the Rett disorder. In Kerr A, Witt Engerstrom I, eds. The Rett disorder and the developing brain. Oxford: Oxford Univ Press, 2001:327-38.

[49]   Elefant C, Wigram T. Learning ability in children with Rett Syndrome. Brain Dev 2005;27(Suppl 1):S97-S101.

[50]   Ayres JA. Sensory integration and the child, 5th ed. Los Angeles, CA: Western Psychol Serv, 1982.

[51]   Nomura Y. Early behavior characteristics and sleep disturbance in Rett syndrome. Brain Dev 2005;27(Suppl 1):S35-S42.

In: Rett Syndrome: Therapeutic Interventions
Editors: Meir Lotan and Joav Merrick

ISBN: 978-1-61728-080-1
©2011 Nova Science Publishers, Inc.

Chapter V

Rett Syndrome: Osteoporosis, a Research Investigation and Clinical Suggestions

Lilit Zysman BSc RN[*1] *and Meir Lotan, MSc, PT, PhD*[1,2]

[1]Israel Rett Center, Chaim Sheba Medical Center, Tel HaShomer, Ramat Gan and
[2]Department of Physical Therapy, Ariel University Campus, Ariel, Israel

Osteoporosis is the reduction of calcium density levels in the bones, usually evident in post-menopause females, yet the tendency for osteoporosis can be identified at a young age, especially in patients with chronic diseases and disabilities and those chronically using anticonvalsant medication. Individuals with Rett syndrome (RS) have been found to show signs of osteoporosis at a young age. This condition may cause pathological fractures, inflict pain and seriously damage the child's mobility and quality of life. The present chapter reviews the current knowledge of the phenomenon of RS and osteoporosis. We also presents findings from a screening test of bone strength of 35 individual with RS at different ages, performed by the first author using the sunlite omnisense 7000P ultrasound apparatus, which took place at the medical RS center located at the Safra Children's Medical Center, Sheba Medical Center, Ramat-Gan. The findings specified within the content of the chapter support the need to implement a comprehensive anti-osteoporotic preventive management for this population. Therefore, The third part of the chapter is clinical in nature, presenting the reader with practical suggestions for implementing such a program.

Introduction

Osteoporosis (Osteo= bone, Porosis = Pores) was defined at a 1993 consensus conference as "a systemic skeletal disease characterized by low bone mass and micro-architectural deterioration of bone tissue with a resulting increase in fragility and risk of fractures" [1]. The usual populations at risk of osteoporosis are women at menopause age, yet the tendency for osteoporosis can be identified at a young age, and the tendency for osteoporosis at adulthood can now be associated to lack of achievement of maximal bone mass at a young age [1].

Other findings support the fact that children suffering from chronic disease are also a population at risk for osteoporosis [2]. It was found that 10% of children diagnosed with chronic disease might develop osteoporosis at a young age (ages 3-18 years) due to immobility and minimal exposure to sunlight [3]. Due to the above mentioned conditions, this population is at high risk of bone fractures [4].

Osteoporosis and fractures are major causes of injury, long term disability and even death [5], especially for individuals with disability [4,6]. Children with disabling conditions are prone to fractures of the long bones, which occur with minimal trauma [4,6]. Bone mass density (BMD), a proxy for bone strength, was found to be reduced in children with disabilities compared with their healthy peers [7-9]. Similar findings have been found in the population of children with RS [10].

Osteoporosis and rett syndrome

The general risk factors for developing osteoporosis are: women and men of advanced age, slim body build, smoking, menstrual irregularities, high caffeine consumption, high consumption of alcoholic drinks, a family history of osteoporosis, low calcium nutrition, high salt and protein consumption, a sedentary life style, an early menstrual termination, women who have not delivered, the use of certain drugs such as anti-convulsive medication.

Besides belonging to this group of children with chronic disease, children with RS are exposed to the following risk factors: They do not exercise (especially the non-ambulatory ones), they are usually very slim presenting a mean BMI of 17.5 [11], 30-90% of them are expected to develop epilepsy and will need the use of anti-convulsive medication [11- 15], many of them show menstrual irregularities[16].

When considering the risk of developing fractures due to osteoporosis, it appears that individuals with RS are again disadvantaged. In his article, Heaney [17] mentions falls, lack of soft tissue padding, inappropriate postural reactions, lack of bone strength, and poor nutrition as major contributors to fractures and these factors are common among individuals with RS.

Actually, the fact that individuals with RS are at risk of developing osteoporosis was established by Haas and her associates. This group of researchers has compared mineral bone density, mineral bone content, and mineral density of the spine of 20 young females with RS with those of 11 females with CP and 25 controls with no pathology and found significantly reduced measurements presented by individuals with RS. When differences in age and weight were adjusted, it was found that individuals with RS showed lower bone density at the level of osteopenia (see explanation below), in comparison to the other groups [10]. Their findings

---

* Correspondence: Meir Lotan, BPT, MScPT, PhD, Department of Physical Therapy, Ariel University Campus, IL-40700 Ariel, Israel. E-mail: ml_pt_rs@netvision.net.il

were supported by other groups as well [18,19]. Budden and Gunness found similar results in a study of five children with RS. They suggested that slow bone creation at a young age in individuals with RS eventually causes low bone density in this population. They hypothesized that MECP2's (the gene responsible for RS) influence is not restricted to damaging brain tissues, and that these abnormal findings in bone development are caused by direct effect of MECP2 mutated gene on bone development [20]. Their hypothesis was recently supported by findings presented by Xiao and his associates [21].While the frequency of fractures has not been studied clinically in this population, it appears that there is a higher incidence in relation to individuals without RS [22].

Diagnosis

In the absence of methods of measuring bone quality, the diagnosis of osteoporosis tends to be made on the basis of low bone density [23]. Since 75% of bone strength is determined by bone density, it is considered a good indicator for diagnosing osteoporosis.

Degrees of osteoporosis are defined according to the ratio between the actual bone density found in a client and the expected bone density of his peer population (T-score).

- Normal BMD is defined as a T-score between +2.5 and −1.0 (i.e. the patient's BMD is between 2.5 standard deviations (SDs), above the young adult mean and one SD below the young adult mean).
- Osteopenia (low BMD) is associated with a T-score between −1.0 and −2.5, inclusive. Osteopenia is also a term used by radiologists to indicate that the bones on a plain x-ray film appear to be of decreased mineral content.
- Osteoporosis is defined as a T-score lower than −2.5 [24].

It is estimated that a drop in one SD around the spine increases the chance for a fracture by 190%. A drop in one SD around the neck of the femur increases the chance for a fracture by 240%. It is estimated that a drop of two and a half SD increases the chance for a fracture by 600-800% of that expected in the normal peer group.

The common methods for diagnosing osteoporosis

The techniques for measuring bone may be divided into those that measure the central skeleton (spine, proximal femur, whole skeleton, etc.) and those that measure some part of the peripheral skeleton. Measurements of the skeleton are most widely carried out using:

- Dual-energy x-ray absorptiometry (DEXA/DXA). It is based on low level X-ray radiation. In this method, bone density is measured at two sites (the spine and the hips).There is Level 1 evidence that DXA bone measurement is the most effective way to estimate fracture risk [26].

- Strength measurement in the peripheral skeleton by quantitative ultrasound (QUS) is a widely reported technique. It is achieved by measuring the speed of sound waves along the measured bone. There is evidence that QUS provides measurements of bone density that can be used to estimate risk with accuracy similar to DXA in elderly populations [25], as well as in children with CP [27].
- Other techniques for measuring peripheral bone density such as peripheral quantitative tomography (pQCT), calcaneal and radial DXA, radiographic absorptiometry, have been found to differentiate between those with and those without prevalent fractures in postmenopausal Caucasian women [28].

Table V-1. Personal details of the participants

# of participant Age on examination	Ambulation Yes	No	Phenotype	Mutation
3		+	Classic	R255X
5	+		Classic	T158M
8	+	+	classic	macro_delition
3	+		Classic	Q244fs258x
10		+	Classic	R255X
15	+		Classic	252258x
11	+		Forme Fruste	WT
9		+	Classic	4.2KB_Del
13		+	Classic	R168X
15		+	Classic	R133C
4		+	Classic	62+1delGT
13	+		Angelman-like	A201V polimofism
19	+		PSV	P152Rmis
15		+	Classic	R133C
3		+	Classic	R306C
7		+	Classic	R255X
2		+	Classic	R255X
10	+		Classic	R168X
21	+		Classic	S134C
13	+		Classic	1303t400 deletion insertion P
10	+		Classic	P360fs365X
13	+		Classic	T158M
20		+	Classic	R168X
5	+		Classic	R106W
17	+		PSV	L386-S401 Deletion 15
4	+		classic	WT
34	+		PSV	R133C
12	+		Classic	R270X
20		+	Classic	WT
11		+	Classic	T158M
19		+	Classic	R255X
4	+		Classic	A2059fs266X
39		+	Classic	T158M
10		+	Classic	R168X
3		+	Classic	L386fs431X

Bone strength in rett syndrome

The present part of this chapter describes a research that took place at the Sheba medical center during the Rett syndrome clinic routine evaluation. The research population included 35 individuals with RS (table 1). Age range: between 2-39 years of age with a mean age: 12.8±8.8

The QUS equipment used in this study was an Omnisense 7000P, produced by sunlight company. The Omnisense 7000P device measures the speed of sound of ultrasound waves propagating along the bone [29]. The Z-score calculations are being done by comparing the Speed Of Sound (SOS) with the mean SOS results of a young age, gender matched, control population [29].

Every child with Rett syndrome in Israel visits the Rett clinic at least annually. The research was held over a period of two years (January 2004- December, 2005) during routine annual and semi annual checks at the Sheba hospital Rett clinic. During those follow-up a standard bone strength measurements were taken by the first author.

The QUS test is non painful and non intrusive and requires placement of a US transducer on the distant part of the tibia (when the child is lying down in bed) and the forearm (when the child is seated at a table) according to a pre-determined procedure. Data regarding the general disposition of each patient was collected using a scale by Alison Kerr [30] were 0=good 1=fair 2=worse.

ANOVA procedure was employed through a General linear model using a Statistical Analysis System (SAS) program. Spearman correlation was employed on Statistical Analysis System (SAS) to detect existing connections between different variables.

Our findings

For the whole group of participants the mean bone T-score values over the radius were found at -1.05, placing the research population in the osteopenia range. On the other hand the results from the tibia were found only slightly lower than the norm putting them within the normal range. As expected and according with manufacturer's charts a significant positive connection was found between measurements values and age (P< 0.02; β= 57; N=27) Yet the bone strength of females with RS was found to deteriorate with age in comparison to normal values of females of the same age according to manufacturer data (see figure V-1).

The ANOVA procedure was executed in order to detect possible connections between: bone strength (SOS measurements) and bone Z-values to all other parameters. The ANOVA procedure failed to detect any significant findings. Nevertheless an effect bearing a trend towards statistical significance was noted: Bone strength (at the tibia location) was found connected to MBD mutations (R133; T158) and SOS units. Individuals with MBD mutations have shown on average 206 units higher than other mutations, with a value close to being significant at P=0.083. This finding calls for further investigation with larger populations. No other significant findings could be drawn through the use of the ANOVA procedure.

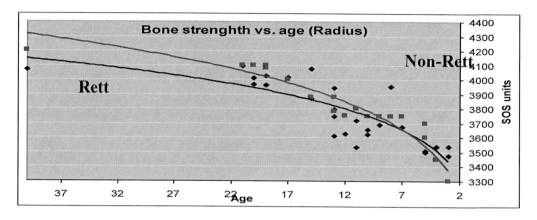

Figure V-1. A comparison of bone strength values for Rett and non-Rett populations.

Table V-2. Significant findings

Spearman Correlation Coefficients Prob > |r| under H0: Rho=0 Number of Observations

Independent variables		Dependent variables			
		Radius	Tibia	Radius Z value	Tibia Z value
Birth year	Correlation	-0.799	-0.631	-0.023	0.282
	Statistical significance	<0.001**	0.004**	0.90	0.242
	N*	N=27	N=19	N=29	N=19
Age	Correlation	0.567	0.647	0.121	-0.270
	Statistical significance	0.002**	0.003**	0.53	0.26
	N*	N=27	N=19	N=29	N=19
Weight	Correlation	0.685	0.443	0.118	-0.158
	Statistical significance	0.000**	0.074	0.573	0.544
	N*	N=23	N=17	N=25	N=17
Height	Correlation	0.775	0.592	0.041	-0.158
	Statistical significance	<0.001**	0.016*	0.852	0.573
	N*	N=21	N=16	N=23	N=15
Calcium	Correlation	0.077	-0.721	0.013	-0.879
	Statistical significance	0.885	0.169	0.980	0.050*
	N*	N=6	N=5	N=6	N=5
Scoliosis	Correlation	0.320	0.448	-0.041	0.139
	Statistical significance	0.116	0.047*	0.836	0.582
	N*	N=26	N=20	N=28	N=18
Epilepsy	Correlation	-0.020	-0.294	0.138	-0.311
	Statistical significance	0.921	0.222	0.484	0.209
	N*	N=26	N=19	N=28	N=18
Speech	Correlation	-0.524	-0.233	-0.220	0.223
	Statistical significance	0.010*	0.351	0.289	0.389
	N*	N=23	N=18	N=25	N=17
Breathing abnormalities	Correlation	-0.269	-0117	-0.489	-0.066
	Statistical significance	0.213	0.644	0.013*	0.800
	N*	N=23	N=18	N=25	N=17
Fractures	Correlation	-0.7977	-0.774	-0.028	0.124
	Statistical significance	0.031*	0.225	0.918	0.659
	N*	N=7	N=4	N=16	N=15

Statistical significance was below 95-99%* above 99%**

N* - Not all participants were integrated in all calculations due to missing data

Correlation in Spearman was executed in SAS software in order to detect primary correlative trends among different elements related to the present investigation. A list of dependent variables (bone strength at tibia and radius, bone Z values at tibia and radius sites) were searched for correlation with potentially influencing variables (height, age, birth year, weight, calcium intake, caloric intake, vitamin D consumption, mobility, fractures in the past, scoliosis, constipation, reflux, epilepsy, speech, level of breathing abnormality, manual functional level head circumference and genetic mutation type). Table V-2 on the previous page presents the significant findings.

Calcium intake was found highly connected (P<0.0001) with bone strength in measurements at both the tibia and radius, when neutralizing age and weight parameters. Calcium was found connected with positive Z values in measurements at the radius (P< 0.05; β= -0.87; N=5) but not the tibia, these results were not significant when neutralizing age and weight parameters (see figure V-2)

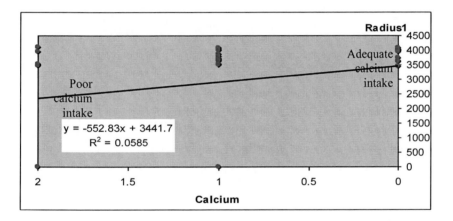

Figure V-2. A correlation between calcium intake and bone strength.

For all participants (N=35) low age (-0.08; P=0.075) (see figure V-3) and weight (-0.46; P= 0.067) variables (young children) were closely connected (yet not statistically significant) with higher tibial Z values.

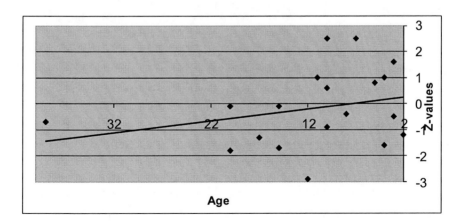

Figure V-3. A connection between ageing and low Z-values.

For all participants (N=35) high caloric intake was found highly connected with bone strength values in measurements of the radius (P<0.0007) (see figure V-4) and the tibia (P<0.005), when neutralizing age height and weight.

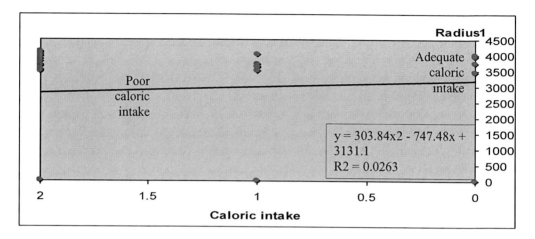

Figure V-4. The connection between caloric intake and bone strength.

Fractures were found connected with reduced SOS units representing bone strength values in measurements of the radius (P<0.0001) and the tibia (P<0.004), when neutralizing age, height and weight. A strong and significant negative correlation was found between fractures and bone density Z values (N=7; Correlation =-0.8; P=0.032) (see figure 5).

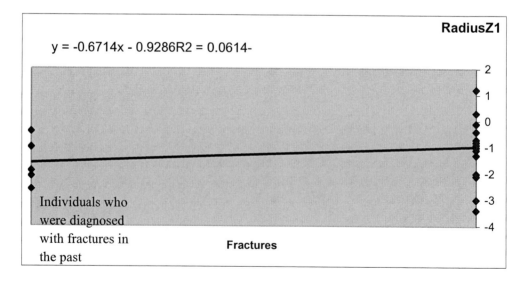

Figure V-5. The connection between previous fractures and bone strength.

Mobility was found positively connected with bone strength values in measurements of the tibia (P<0.007), but not the radius when neutralizing age height and weight (see figure V-6).

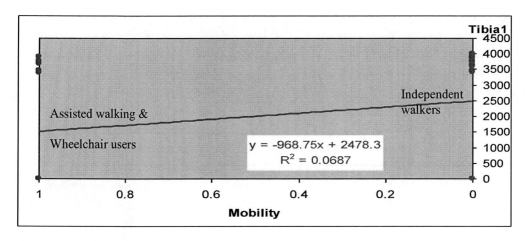

Figure V-6. The connection between mobility and tibia bone strength.

Scoliosis was found negatively connected with bone strength values in measurements of the radius (P<0.001) and tibia (P<0.013), when neutralizing age, height and weight (see figure V-7).

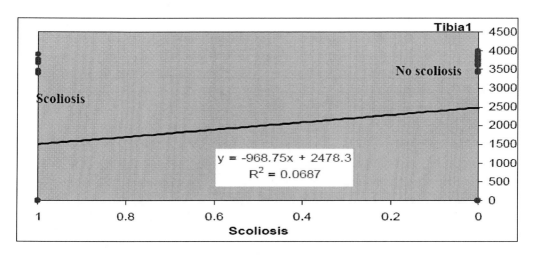

Figure V-7. The connection between scoliosis and tibia bone strength.

Abnormal breathing was found negatively connected with bone strength values in measurements of the radius (P<0.001) and tibia (P<0.003), when neutralizing age height and weight.

Epilepsy was found negatively connected with bone strength values in measurements of the radius (P<0.001) and tibia (P<0.0003) when neutralizing age height and weight.

Discussion

The information presented within the scope of the present chapter suggests some insights as to osteoporosis in individuals with RS. An overwhelming result was that out of 35 participants only four showed positive Z values over the radius. Most of the findings support the results reported by others as to the fact that individuals with RS show reduced levels of bone strength and bone density at the level of osteopnia in comparison to normative values. Yet our findings showed that bone strength levels showed normative value at a young age and a deteriorating tendency, escalating with age. These findings might collide with the hypothesis made by Budden and Gunness, who suggested that the osteopenia of individuals with RS is connected to the activity of MeCP2 [20]. Unless we assume that the inactivity of MeCP2 in the skeletal system becomes apparent only at age higher than 7 years (the age when Rett bone strength is becoming inferior compared to normative findings).

The most important finding is the fact that fractures in individuals with RS were found to negatively correlate with bone strength values as well as bone density Z values. This is an expected yet alarming result that necessitates proper intervention by therapists and caregivers.

The fact that calcium intake was found highly connected with bone strength, as well as with positive Z values emphasizes the importance of calcium intake as preventive intervention for the development of osteoporosis in individuals with RS.

The fact that worse Z values were correlated with advanced age is not surprising and reiterates the importance of an anti-osteoporotic intervention for this population from a young age. The finding in the present research also supports the importance of proper high caloric nutrition as part of such an intervention. The correlation found between mobility and Tibia strength vs. reduced tibial strength and reduced mobility reiterates the importance of maintaining walking abilities in this population. These findings correspond with the findings of Cepollaro and associates [31]. It should be mentioned however that ambulatory status was not found connected with level of (bone mineral content) BMC by a second group of researchers [19].

Abnormal breathing as well as epilepsy and scoliosis (all related to a more severe phenotype of RS) were found to correlate with reduced bone strength. These findings suggest that applying an anti-osteoporotic intervention plan is highly warranted when the individual with RS is showing worse phenotypic expression.

The results of the present research urge the implementation of a comprehensive anti-osteoporotic intervention from a young age for individuals with RS. Therefore the basic components of such an intervention are here by presented.

No difference was found in SOS measures between individuals with and without epilepsy at all ages. These findings are inconsistent with the findings of Cepollaro and associates [31], but correspond with the findings of Motil and her associates [19].

The present findings support previous researchers in their call to use QUS (as the equipment transmits less radiation) to discriminate between healthy and osteopenic subjects [32-34].

Osteoporosis intervention in rett syndrome

Osteoporosis is a multi-disciplinary problem requiring proper diagnosis and organized intervention. In order to achieve good management, the appropriate experts should be consulted with (a physician, a dietitian, and a physical therapist). The basic steps of such an anti-osteoporotic regime should include: A thorough evaluation of the individual with RS to sustain or eliminate a diagnosis of osteoporosis/ Osteopenia (and in case the situation necessitates) the introduction a comprehensive program. Such a program should include:

- Appropriate dietetic changes,
- Increased mobility, movement, and strengthening according to the individual's limitations (if the client is non mobile, an intensive daily standing exercise program should be applied) and,
- Exposure of the child to sunshine.

The authors join the call of previous researchers to implement a multi-component anti osteoporosis program for individual with RS starting from a young age.

Management of osteoporosis

About 80% of bone mass is determined by hereditary elements, while the other 20% are dictated by environmental causes and life style. Despite the fact that only one of many factors contributing to bone health is within our control, these factors can have a significant effect on the bone construction at young age [30].

In the normal population, two main elements determine bone calcium level and later the level of osteoporosis. Maximal bone mass achieved during adolescence and the rate of calcium loss at adulthood [35].

Fractures caused by osteoporotic fragility may be prevented with multidisciplinary intervention programs [36]. Bone substance is made out of protein and mineral. Not surprisingly therefore, the foundation of any preventive or therapeutic medical regimen is an adequate dietary intake of the following bulk materials: high quality protein, calcium, phosphor [17], accompanied by physical exercise.

The clinical characteristics of Rett syndrome require aggressive intervention to maximize the quality of life of the affected individuals [19]. There are 3 important factors that may affect bone strength and therefore should be included in an intervention program:

- Medication
- Nutrition (especially that including calcium and vitamin D)
- Exercise

Medication

This chapter will not go into detailed description of appropriate medication in the case of osteoporosis, but will mention common possibilities.

Estrogen hormonal treatment

Estrogen consumption was found to prevent further bone deterioration and even prevent fractures, but this treatment must exceed three years in order to become effective. Due to recent knowledge that this form of intervention may be involved in increasing the risk for other diseases, it is no longer considered the treatment of choice for osteoporosis reduction and prevention.

Kalcytonine hormone management (Miacalcic)

This hormone, originating from the pituitary gland, stops the osteoclasts (cells that are in charge of destroying the bone tissue), thus preventing bone absorption. This treatment is effective as the estrogen treatment, as well as reduces back aches caused by fractured or cracked vertebrae. It is also highly recommended for non-mobile populations, making it even more attractive for the population with RS.

Raloxifen (evista)

This family of drugs enhances bone density by 2% over a period of two years in 60-70% of the patients. It also reduces the chance (between 10-50% according to different sources) of bone fractures [30].

Bifasfonates

This group of Anti-reabsorptive medications is usually recommended only when a severe drop in bone mass is observed, or when hormonal treatments show no improvement. These drugs have been found to reduce vertebrae and femur neck fractures by 45-50%. These medications (especially Foslan) are not easily absorbed through the digestive system and their consumption should be carefully evaluated prior to prescription, especially for individuals showing swallowing and digestive difficulties (as is the case for many with RS) [15,37,38]. In this family of medication, one can find Pamidronate, Alendronate and Opadronate, which has been found useful in decreasing the risk of fractures [39]. Despite the fact that Bisphosphonates have been in use with children and adolescents for the last 25 years, its use was not consistent and was mainly reported as case studies. Nevertheless, the use of these drugs has been reported with patients with RS [40]. According to new findings researchers warrant the use of bone reabsorption medication for individuals with RS [19].

Anabolic agents

Anabolic agents are considered an important development in anti-osteoporosis therapy within recent years [17]. This agent is given subcutaneously on a daily basis. When supported with adequate calcium and vitamin D supplements, teriparatide production increases bone mass by 10% to 15% annually [41,42]. More importantly, it reduces the risk of all vertebral fractures by two-thirds, and of severe and multiple vertebral fractures by approximately 85% [41]. It also reduces non-vertebral fracture rates by approximately 50%. When given combined with estrogen, teriparatide increased spine bone density by 30% and hip bone density by 12% during a period of two years [42]. Because the agent is so new, there is virtually no practice experience to describe; it is likely that the use of teriparatide will be concentrated initially in patients with severe osteoporosis, with treatment duration of probably 18 to 24 months and a transition to an anti-reabsorptive agent at the end of that time [17].

Nutrition

Even with adequate medication, bone restoration will not occur if a negative nitrogen and mineral balance is sustained due to inadequate intake of these nutrients [17]. A well-balanced nutrition includes a wide range of provisions that may assist in keeping the strength and health of the bones in a constant, optimal state.

Calcium

Calcium contains 67% of the bone weight and therefore plays an important part in maintaining bone strength. Calcium is an important part of the rebuilding process of long bones and its presence in the bones also serves as storage for other body organs/systems requiring this element (e.g. heart, muscles, blood and nervous system). Therefore it is important to maintain high levels of calcium intake in order to help establish bone mass during childhood and maintain it during adolescence and adulthood to ensure proper functioning of vital organs. Despite the fact that calcium on its own cannot prevent bone mass reduction, it is a crucial part of every management program aimed at preventing and treating osteoporosis. The recommended dosages of calcium at different ages are specified in the following table in accordance with international guidelines (http://www.nap.edu) (see table. V-3).

Table V-3.Normative calcium levels at different genders and ages

Category	Age	Calcium (mg)
Children	1-3 yrs	500
	4-7 yrs	800
Girls	8-18 yrs	1300
Women	19-54 yrs	1000
	51+ yrs	1200
Boys	8-11 yrs	1300
	12-15 yrs	1300

In order to help the individual with RS attain proper calcium intake the following chart presents the different food items rich with calcium (table. V-4).

Table V-4. Different food items with high calcium content

Food	Quantity	Calcium (mg)
Milk		
Regular	1 Cup (250ml)	285
Skim		375-440
Goat's Milk		290
Cheese	Per 35g	
Parmesan		385
Swiss		300
Brie		165
Feta		125
Ricotta		80
Cottage		25
Soy Cheese		140
Yogurt	Per200g (1 tub)	
- regular		340
- low fat		420
Ice Cream	Per 50g (1 Scoop)	
Vanilla/Flavoured		70-80
Soy Products		
Tofu	100g	336
Soy Beans (dry, cookied)	100g	76
Spreads and Dips		
Sesame Paste		148
Tahini		65
Tzadtziki	1 Tblsp (20g)	30
Hummus		5
Nuts		
Almond		240
Brazil		150
Walnut	per 100g	90
Hazelnut		90
Pistachio		90
Peanut butter		50
Seeds	Per 10g (1Tblsp)	
Sesame		7
Sunflower		10
Fruits	average serving	
Orange	1 Medium	50
Dried Fig	1	25
Prunes	6 Large	30
Vegetables	Per100g	
Sliverbeet		70
Cabbage		60`
Spinach		93
Kale		179
Broccoli	30g	30
Miscellaneous		
Chocolate(Milk)	5 Squares (20g)	75
Breads and Cereals		
Muesli (swiss)	60g	60
Fish	per100g	
Sardines, Canned		300
Salmon, Canned		200-300
Prawns		100-135

Edited from [42]

Vitamin D

Vitamin D is produced in the kidneys. It is an important element of calcium absorption through the intestines. Vitamin D is supplied to the body by supplementing food items such as fish preserved in oil, eggs, milk, and margarine. The best way to enhance production of vitamin D is to expose the skin to sunlight; Yet it is advisable to restrict exposure to early morning and late afternoon hours in order to prevent skin damage, typical of overexposure.

Vitamin D is an important supplement for inactive individuals. The recommended intake of vitamin D is 200 IU (5 mg), suited for individuals up to age fifty [44]. Substantial reductions in extremity fractures were found within 18-36 months of initial intakes of calcium and vitamin D [44].

Food supplements

Food supplements other than calcium and vitamin D which are recommended as preventive intervention and even as means to improve osteoporotic state are: Magnesium, vitamin B6, folic acid, vitamin B12, silica, fluoride, fito estrogens.

Food elements which should be avoided – Several food items and supplements have been found to prevent calcium absorption and their reduced intake should be considered. Here are some examples:

- Phytates- can be found in different fibers (e.g. unprocessed whit)
- Tannins – exist in tea
- Oxalate – can be found in spinach
- Caffeine – can be found in coffee and cola-based soft drinks
- Alcohol – in large amounts
- Phosphate – can be found in soft drinks
- Some food elements cause enhanced calcium urination. These are: salt, protein-rich foods, and caffeine.

It is reiterated that changes in food consumption should only be made after consolation with a dietitian.

Exercise

Musculoskeletal rehabilitation should be considered in conjunction with pharmaceutical medication and proper nutritional intake in order to optimize musculoskeletal health, improve quality of life, and reduce the risk of fracture and fracture recurrence [36]. It has long been established that the boney structures in the body need nourishment and appropriate mechanical stress from physical activity in order to remain strong and healthy [46]. Daily exercise helps to keep bones and muscles strong, maintain flexibility, and reduce the chances of injury.

It was found that women who are more active, have greater bone density and less of a chance for fractures, than women at the same age that were inactive [47]. In cases of individuals with disability such as RS, ample activity from a young age will be hard to achieve, exposing this population to a poor initial boney start. Therefore it is the responsibility of the caregivers to supply enough chances to partake an active life style in order for the child to reach her maximal level of activity. Nevertheless, it should be mentioned here that low magnitude mechanical loading [48] has been found to enhance bone density and that such a program actually improved bone mass density in a group of disabled children [49]. Despite accepted conception that bone density improvement occur only when a minimal intensity of 2 hour daily standing program is executed, an average standing time of less than 4.5 hours a week per participant has also been found to improve BMD in the spine of children with cerebral palsy [50].

For individuals without disability, two types of exercise are particularly beneficial for the development of young bones – weight bearing and strength-training. Examples for such exercises are: walking, jogging, netball, dancing, tennis, golf, strength-training or resistance-training. Unfortunately, individuals with RS will not be able to perform most or all of the above mentioned exercises.

If an exercise program is to be applied for individuals with RS it should:

- be accompanied by proper nutrition – consult a dietitian.
- be started slowly and progress gradually.
- be performed or supervised by a physical therapist.
- include exercises that puts stress on the bones, causing the boney structures to build and strengthen themselves (swimming has all the positive elements of exercise but does not promote boney strengthening or growth).
- include back muscle exercise in order to enhance back strength due to the connection found between persons with osteoporosis and weak back musculature [51,52].
- include a proprioceptive dynamic posture training (PDPT) program to improved posture and balance [53].
- become a routine (physical activity should be executed for at least three hours a week)
- taking in to account the medical limitations of the individual with RS).
- be strenuous (at least on a minimal level – try and get the child to put in some effort herself).
- be varied (every once in a while change the exercises to make the program more interesting as well as to change the pressure they apply on the bones).
- include fall prevention strategies in case the child is ambulant (due to conjunction of inactivity and impaired neuromuscular function found in causing fall related fractures) [54]
- be fun (e.g. sing to the child, add a dog to the program, etc.).
- be done in a group (e.g. add peers or family members).
- not cause pain (pay attention to the child's face) [35].

For individuals who have already suffered from pathological fractures in the past: it was established (for senior adults) that rehabilitation after fractures caused by osteoporosis should consist of exercises intended to: improve muscle strength, decrease the risk of falls, include back strengthening exercises to improve posture and apply sedative physical therapy to decrease postural related pain [36]. Such exercises should be considered as a base line for individuals with RS in the case they were diagnosed with an osteporotic fracture.

In addition, it is most likely that the child will show fear of movement, in which case she will fixate her body by applying muscular resistance over the fragile bones. This is a complex situation requiring delicate intervention.

- A balanced program should be agreed upon between the parents and the care giving team.
- This program should establish maximal movement while maintaining maximal caution.
- Proper balance should be kept between nutritional and medicational administration.
- The program should include a preparatory stage for calming the child and relaxing her tight muscles.
- The child should be verbally cautioned before every movement is performed.
- Performing the program in a relaxed atmosphere such as in the Snoezelen environment [55,56] is recommended.
- Daily routines (such as bathing, dressing and undressing) should be included as part of this program and include limb and trunk movements.
- Slow, careful and various positioning of the child should be performed throughout the day (e.g. using standing frames, benches, pillows, etc.) [57].

Conclusions

Osteoporosis is a multi-disciplinary problem requiring proper diagnosis and organized intervention. The present chapter as well as previous reports suggest that individuals with RS should be considered as a population at risk for osteopenia/osteoporosis and should be suggested a proper intervention program from a young age.

In order to achieve good management, the appropriate experts should be consulted with (a physician, a dietitian, and a physical therapist). The basic steps for an anti-osteoporotic regime should include: A thorough evaluation of the individual with RS to sustain or eliminate a diagnosis of osteoporosis and, in case the situation necessitates, the introduction of a comprehensive program.

Such a program should include appropriate dietetic changes, application of increased mobility, movement, and strengthening according to the individual's limitations (if the client is non mobile, an intensive daily standing exercise program should be applied) and exposure of the child to sunshine.

References

[1]   Consensus development conference. Diagnosis, prophylaxis, and treatment of osteoporosis. Am J Med 1993;94:646-50.

[2]   Zacharin M. Current advances in bone health of disabled children. Curr Opin Pediatr 2004;16(5):545-51.

[3]   Hartman C, Brik R, Tamir A, Merrick J, Shamir R. Bone quantitative ultrasound and nutritional status in severely handicapped institutionalized children and adolescents. Clin Nutr 2004;23(1):89-98.

[4]   Gray B. Fractures caused by falling from a wheelchair in patients with neuromuscular disease. Dev Med Child Neurol 1992;34:589-92.

[5]   Sahaf M. (2005) Osteoporosis - The disease, diagnosis and management. Shenbon, The religious college for education 2005;8:152-3. [Hebrew].

[6]   Lingam S, Joester, J. Spontaneous fractures in children and adolescents with cerebral palsy. BMJ 1994;309:265.

[7]   Kovanlikaya A, Loro M, Hantgartner T, Reynolds R, Roe T, Gilsanz V. Osteopenia in children: CT assessment. Radiology 1996;198:781-4.

[8]   Henderson R. Bone density and other possible predictors of fracture risk in children and adolescents with spastic quadriplegia. Dev Med Child Neurol 1997;39:224-7.

[9]   Loro M, Sayre J, Roe T, Goran M, Kaufman F, Gilsanz V. Early identification of children predisposed to low peak bone mass and osteoporosis later in life. J Clin Endocrinol Metab 2000;85:3908-18.

[10]   Haas RH, Dixon SD, Sartoris DJ, Hennessy M.J. Osteopenia in Rett syndrome. J Pediatr 1997;131(5):771-4.

[11]   Leonard S. The Australian Rett syndrome study inaugural report. Aust: Telethon Inst Child Health Res, 2002.

[12]   Nieto MA, Candau RS, Prieto P. Contribution to studies of seizures in Rett Syndrome analysis of critical forms of four cases. Review Neurology 1995;23:1185-9.

[13]   Glaze D. Epilepsy. Presentation, IRSA 12th Ann Conf, Boston, MA: 1996 May 24-27, tape 622-18.

[14]   Hagberg B. Rett Syndrome clinical and biological aspects. London, MacKeith Press, 1993.

[15]   Ellaway C, Christodoulou J. Rett syndrome: Clinical characteristics and recent genetic advances. Disabil Rehabil 2001;23:98-106.

[16]   Hunter K. The Rett syndrome handbook. Washington, DC: Int Rett Syndr Assoc, 1999.

[17]   Heaney RP. Advances in therapy for osteoporosis. Clin Med Res 2003;1(2):93-9.

[18]   Leonard H, Thomson M, Glasson E, Fyfe S, Leonard S, Ellaway C, Christodoulou J, Bower C. Metacarpophalangeal pattern profile and bone age in Rett Syndrome: Further radiological clues to the diagnosis. Am J Med Genet 1999;12(83):88-95.

[19]   Motil KJ, Schultz RJ, Abrams S, Ellis KJ, Glaze DG. Fractional calcium absorption is increased in girls with Rett syndrome. J Pediatr Gastroenterol Nutr 2006;42(4):419-26.

[20]   Budden SS, Gunness ME. Bone histomorphometry in three females with Rett syndrome. Brain Dev 2001;23(Suppl 1):S133-7.

[21]   Xiao P, Chen Y, Jiang H, Liu YZ, Pan F, Yang TL, et al In vivo genome-wide expression study on human circulating B cells suggests a novel ESR1 and MAPK3 network for postmenopausal osteoporosis. J Bone Miner Res 2008;23(5):644-54.

[22]   Hanks SB. Why Physical Therapy? Rett Gazette 2001;1-2:4-6.

[23]   WHO. Guidelines for preclinical evaluation and clinical trials in osteoporosis. Geneva: WHO, 1998.

[24]   WHO Study Group. Assessment of fracture risk and its application to screening for postmenopausal osteoporosis: report. Geneva, WHO, Tech Rep Series, 1994.

[25]   Marshall D, Johnell O, Wedel H. Meta-analysis of how well measures of bone mineral density predict occurrence of osteoporotic fractures. BMJ 1996;312:1254-9.

[26]   Hui SL, Gao S, Zhou XH, Johnston CC Jr, Lu Y, Gluer CC, Grampp S, Genant H. Universal standardization of bone density measurements: a method with optimal properties for calibration among several instruments. J Bone Miner Res 1997;12:1463-70.

[27]   Wilmshurst S, Ward K, Adams J, Langton C, Mughal M. Mobility status and bone density in cerebral palsy. Arch Dis Child 1996;75:164-5.

[28]   Brown JP, Josse RG. 2002 clinical practice guidelines for the diagnosis and management of osteoporosis in Canada. CMAJ 2002;167(10 Suppl):S1-34.

[29]   Sunlight Medical Technical Support. Omnisense 7000p bone Sonometer, Technical Overview, 2002.

[30]   Sela B. On prevention and management of osteoporosis 2004. Extracted on December, 2004 from web site: http://tevalife.com/article.asp?id=1556. [Hebrew]

[31]   Cepollaro C, Gonnelli S, Bruni D, Pacini S, Martini S, Franci MB, et al. Dual X-ray absorptiometry and bone ultrasonography in patients with Rett syndrome. Calcif Tissue Int 2001;69:259–62.

[32]   Gluer CC. Quantitative ultrasound techniques for the assessment of osteoporosis: expert agreement on current status for the International Quantitative Ultrasound Consensus Group. J Bone Miner Res 1997;12:1280–8.

[33]   Jaworski M, Lebiedowski M, Lorenc RS, Trempe J. Ultrasound bone measurement in pediatric subjects. Calcif Tissue Int 1995;56:368–71.

[34]   Daly RM, Rich PA, Klein R. Influence of high impact loading on ultrasound bone measurements in children: a crosssectional report. Calcif Tissue Int 1997;60:401–4.

[35]   Qroitaro S, Volodarsky A. Osteoporosis - The disease, and management 2006. Extracted on September, 2006 From internet site [Hebrew]: http://www.physiotherapist.co.il/reviews/ osteoporosis.htm

[36]   Pfeifer M, Sinaki M, Geusens P, Boonen S, Preisinger E, Minne HW. ASBMR Working Group on Musculoskeletal Rehabilitation Musculoskeletal rehabilitation in osteoporosis: a review. J Bone Miner Res 2004;19(8):1208-14.

[37]   Reilly S, Cass H. Growth and nutrition in Rett syndrome. Disabil Rehabil 2001;23:118-28.

[38]   Budden SS. Management of Rett Syndrome: A ten-year experience. Neuropediatrics 1995;26(2):75-7.

[39]   Cummings SR, Black DM, Thompson DE, Applegate WB, Barrett-Connor E, Musliner TA, et al. Effect of alendronate on risk of fracture in women with low bone density but without vertebral fractures: Results from the Fracture Intervention Trial. JAMA 1998;280:2077-82.

[40]   Zacharin M, Cuindy T. Osteoporosis pseudoglioma syndrome: Treatment of spinal osteoporosis with intravenous bisphosphonates. J Pediatr 2000;137:410-5.

[41]   Neer RM, Arnaud CD, Zanchetta JR, Prince R, Gaich GA, Reginster JY, et al. Effect of parathyroid hormone (1–34) on fractures and bone mineral density in post-menopausal women with osteoporosis. N Engl J Med 2001;344:1434–41.

[42]   Arnaud CD, Roe EB, Sanchez MS, Bacchetti P, Black DM, Cann CE. Two years of parathyroid hormone 1–34 and estrogen produce dramatic bone density increases in post-menopausal osteoporotic women that dissipate only slightly during a third year of treatment with estrogen alone: Results from a placebo-controlled randomized trial. Bone 2001;28:S277.

[43]   Diamond T, Bennell K, Babic Z, eds. Everybody's bones. A handbook for the prevention and management of osteoporosis, 3rd ed. Victoria: Osteoporosis Victoria, 2001.

[44]   The Food and Nutrition Board, Institute of Medicine. Dietary Reference Intakes for Calcium, Magnesium, Phosphorus, Vitamin D, and Fluoride. Food and Nutrition Board, Institute of Medicine. Washington, DC: Natl Acad Press, 1997.

[45]   Chapuy MC, Arlot ME, Duboeuf F, Brun J, Crouzet B, Arnaud S, et al. Vitamin D3 and calcium to prevent hip fractures in elderly women. N Engl J Med 1992;327:1637–42.

[46]   Jones H, Priest J, Hayes W, Tichenor C, Nagel D. Humeral hypertrophy in response to exercise. J Bone J Surg Am 1977;59:204-8.

[47]   Gregg EW, Cauley JA, Seeley DG, Ensrud KE, Bauer DC, for the Study of Osteoporotic Fractures Research Group. Physical activity and osteoporotic fracture risk in older women. Ann Intern Med 1998;129:81-8.

[48]   Rubin C, Xu G, Judex S. The anabolic activity of bone tissue, suppressed by disuse, is normalized by brief exposure to extremely low magnitude mechanical stimuli. FASEB J 2001;15:2225-9.

[49]   Ward K, Alsop C, Caulton J, Rubin C, Adams J, Mughal Z. Low magnitude mechanical loading is osteogenic in children with disabling conditions. J Bone Miner Res 2004;19(3): 360-9.

[50]   Caulton JM, Ward KA, Alsop CW, Dunn G, Adams JE, Mughal MZ. A randomised controlled trial of standing programme on bone mineral density in non-ambulant children with cerebral palsy. Arch Dis Child 2004;89(2):131-5.

[51]   Sinaki M, Itoi E, Wahner HW, Wollan P, Gelzcer R, Mullan BP, Collins DA, Hodgson SF. Stronger back muscles reduce the incidence of vertebral fractures: A prospective 10 year follow-up of postmenopausal women. Bone 2002;30(6):836-41.

[52]   Sinaki M, Khosla S, Limburg PJ, Rogers JW, Murtaugh PA. Muscle strength in osteoporotic versus normal women. Osteoporos Int 1993;3:8-12.

[53]   Sinaki M, Lynn SG. Reducing the risk of falls through proprioceptive dynamic posture training in osteoporotic women with kyphotic posturing: A randomized pilot study. Am J Phys Med Rehabil 2002;81:241-6.

[54]   Dargent-Molina P, Favier F, Grandjean H, Baudoin C, Schott AM, Hausherr, E, Meunier PJ, Breart G. Fall-related factors and risk of hip fracture: The EPIDOS prospective study. Lancet 1996;348:145-9.

[55]   Lotan M, Merrick J. Rett syndrome: Management with Snoezelen or controlled multi-sensory environment. A review. Int J Adolesc Med Health 2004;16(1):5-12.

[56]   Lotan M, Shapiro M. Management of young children with Rett disorder in the controlled multi-sensory (Snoezelen) environment. Brain Dev 2005;27(Suppl 1):S88-94.

[57]   Lotan M. Management for Rett syndrome. Israeli Rett syndrome center, Israel, Tel- Aviv, 2006. [Hebrew].

In: Rett Syndrome: Therapeutic Interventions
Editors: Meir Lotan and Joav Merrick

ISBN: 978-1-61728-080-1
©2011 Nova Science Publishers, Inc.

Chapter VI

Rett Syndrome: Clinical Insights at Meal-Time

*Judy Wine, DSPA, EdD[1,2], Yael Yoshei, OT, HT[1,3,4] and Meir Lotan, BPT, MScPT, PhD[*1,5,6]*

[1]The Israel Rett Center, National Evaluation Team, Chaim Sheba Medical Center,
Tel Hashomer, Ramat Gan
[2]The Mish'aul Center for Augmentative Communication and
Assistive Technology, Jerusalem
[3]Beit Issie Shapiro Educational Facility, Raanana
[4]Kalisher School for Special Education, Tel-Aviv
[5]Zvi Quittman Residential Centers, Israel Elwyn, Jerusalem
[6]Department of Physical Therapy, Ariel University Campus, Ariel, Israel

Rett syndrome (RS) is a genetic disorder affecting mainly females. The individual with RS may present a variety of eating disorders, regularly leading to a very small and slim physique. Given that increased food consumption can yield positive results on both the functional abilities and the emotional state of individuals with RS, it is important that focused attention be given to the feeding ability of these individuals. The present chapter will address the principles of eating with individuals with RS. The chapter is an amalgamation of up-to date knowledge on feeding for individuals with disabilities and the authors' clinical experience with individuals with RS. The chapter suggests different ways to evaluate and to positively influence the activity of eating with persons with RS by discussing the person herself, the setting, and the handling by caregivers.

* Correspondence: Meir Lotan, BPT, MScPT, PhD, Department of Physical Therapy, Ariel University Campus, IL-40700 Ariel, Israel. E-mail: ml_pt_rs@netvision.net.il

Introduction

Rett syndrome (RS) is a genetic disorder that primarily affects females [1,2]. The disorder causes a neurological and developmental arrest that manifests itself in a variety of disabilities such as loss of functional hand use, loss of acquired speech, apraxia, ataxia, autonomic system dysfunction, epilepsy, breathing abnormalities, failure to thrive, orthopedic problems and muscle tone irregularities [3-5]. One of the issues that affect the functional ability of the individual with RS, in addition to affecting her appearance and stature, is that related to the individual's eating abilities. The present chapter addresses the difficulties with feeding typically exhibited by individuals with RS and suggests possible intervention techniques; the information is derived both from the limited existing literature on clinical issues relating to RS and from the authors' experience.

There is a multitude of factors involved in the eating habits of individuals with RS that influence its correctness and speed. In order to decide on appropriate intervention, all of these factors must be taken into consideration (Fig. 1). In order to emphasize the severity of this issue among individuals with RS, it may be noted that 74% of the individuals with RS present gastroenterological problems [6].

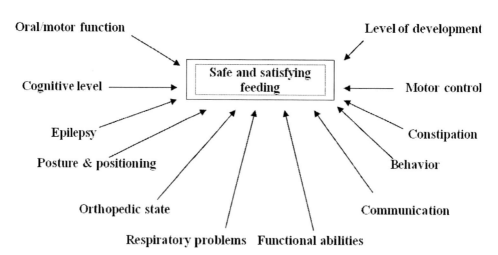

Figure VI-1. Factors affecting the feeding ability of the individual with RS

When considering the issue of feeding as it relates to people with developmental disabilities in general and to individuals with RS in particular, it is recommended that the subject be approached according to the following four headings (based on Evans and Klein [7] adapted for RS):

- The execution of a comprehensive assessment.
- The use of a problem-solving approach.
- The individual's functioning within the overall framework of her disabilities and challenges.

- Mutual discussion and consent among therapists and caregivers (including parents) regarding the intervention regime.

The assessment of the individual with RS can be divided according to the three main purposes of eating intervention:

- Safe eating
- Sufficient food intake
- Social acceptability/esthetics.

Safe eating relates to a state where the individual is not in danger of aspiration or penetration of food items into her air passages while eating or drinking. A decision regarding the danger in eating is considered after gathering data from different sources, such as:

- Medical history (past lung infections and their frequency)
- Medical examination (examination of the respiratory system before and after eating).
- A questionnaire which has been completed by the staff members familiar with the individual's eating habits and functional abilities.
- Observations regarding the ability to intake different food and liquid items.
- Evaluation of the swallowing mechanism (in instances where the initial non-intrusive evaluation indicates that the individual is experiencing some difficulties in handling food intake, the execution of a video-fluoroscopy examination should be considered)
- Evaluation of the state of the respiratory system (when suspicion arises regarding the proper functioning of the swallowing mechanism due to recurrent lung problems, lung x-rays at random or on a regular basis should be taken).

Sufficient food intake is measured by the amount and type of food that the individual with RS consumes, together with its compatibility with her daily caloric expenditure and her growth curve. Deviation from the norm should provide the impetus for the initiation of a process intended to identify the difficulties exhibited by the person with RS and the application of appropriate measures aimed at improving the individual's condition.

Therapeutic intervention during mealtime

Swallowing, or the ability to swallow food and fluids, is a complex action which depends on an array of mechanisms. The tongue's motion and the closing of the lips begin the swallowing process, as they move the food to the rear area of the mouth and pharynx. Sensory receptors in the pharyngeal area transfer information to different nerve centers, which start the reflexive swallowing process, while the food continues from there to the esophagus. A large number of persons with swallowing problems, including many individuals with RS, are not capable of halting the respiratory process during the swallowing process (as most people with a normally functioning system do). If there is food inside the individual's mouth that she is not able to swallow between breaths, she must be able to block the entry of food to the esophageal area before attempting to swallow again. This action demands skilled and separate tongue movements, which generally cannot be executed by people with swallowing problems as part of their complex neurological profile. In such cases the joint air and food inhalation is expressed by coughing and could lead to suffocation. If the individual cannot achieve good lip closure, the formation of negative pressure which is necessary for the efficient flow of food to the esophagus while swallowing is affected. If the head and neck are not in the correct position (for example, hyperextension of the neck) then swallowing efficiency is affected and a high risk for aspiration exists. It may be stated that the most important physiological assistance for normal swallowing is a slight forward flexion of the neck. Many individuals with RS present postural problems such as a kyphotic thorax, and therefore may have a hyper extended neck when sitting. This position causes the cervical vertebrae to protrude forward and press on the end of the esophagus, thus blocking the food pathway to a certain extent. However, exaggerated flexion (forward bending) of the neck also interferes with the closing of the epiglottis and causes food to be shoved into the bronchioles.

Aspiration can be either active (coughing, interruption in breathing, cyanosis, noisy breathing) or without external indication (silent aspiration). Slow swallowing can derive from sensory abnormalities, oral-motor problems, reaction to medication, or a decreased state of awareness. Aspiration might occur when the eating process is slow and it becomes necessary to inhale before the food has completely left the mouth/pharynx area (in such cases spooning small amounts might be the solution).

Additional eating problems which might interfere with swallowing are manifestations such as vomiting, spitting, gagging, and coughing. These problems, when reoccurring, may cause issues of malnutrition and/or dehydration. It is important to diagnose the cause and not to loosely hang the blame on personal or behavioral issues ("Joanne doesn't like the rice", "Tami is really stubborn today").

Vomiting (gag reflex)

Abnormal gag reflex was found among 20% of individuals with RS [8]. The gag reflex is usually located in the last third of the mouth, i.e. in the soft palate area, in people without neurological problems; the purpose of the gag reflex is to prevent unwanted and/or undesirable substances from being swallowed.   The reflex can be produced by either internal stimulation (e.g. sickness) or external stimulation, for example, pressure or weight of different foods and substances in the mouth. Some individuals with RS have an inappropriately strong gag reflex and may feel ill as a result of stimulation in the area, in some cases, without the ability to cough. The therapist or caregiver should be sensitive to such a problem and if vomiting movements are noticed, a wash with water (if the food is the apparent cause) can be helpful. An opposite problem is the lack of the gag reflex, which implies that the bronchioles of the person with RS are defenseless. A postural change of the eater that will create a change in head position (forward or backward) will cause movement of the food in the mouth, and may positively affect the pattern of movement of the head and shoulders, thus reducing the recurrence and severity of the gag reaction.

Spitting

In general, this is defined as a strong emission of food in a voluntary manner from the mouth [9]. In fact in some cases an individual may be defined as a "spitter" even if she did not voluntarily emit the food. It is a well known fact that individuals with RS show respiratory irregularities expressed in some cases as explosive exhalation. A second reason for apparent deliberate spitting is a situation where the person's mouth is full with food and there is a need to inhale. Such a situation might be resolved through the exhalation of air with food particles thereby forcefully spraying food out of the mouth. Additional reasons for the spitting of food can be either sensitivity in the mouth area or excessive drooling. Our clinical experience has shown that in some cases deliberate spitting is behavioral as the individual with RS enjoys the attention she gets as a result of this behavior.

Intestinal problems

Intestinal problems have an effect on swallowing and on eating speed; for example, reflux and the slow emptying of the stomach will extend meal times. Chronic reflux may cause ulcers or bleeding, and pain during mealtime, thereby affecting esophagus/respiratory timing, which will in turn have a jeopardizing effect on the individual's health. The slow emptying of stomach content if later accompanied by lying down will probably lead to reflux, and to the individual's refusal to eat. The slow emptying of the stomach caused by the hypoactive para-sympathetic system [4] is commonly accompanied by constipation problems and/or fecal intestinal blockage (two well known manifestations in the digestive system of individuals with Rett syndrome).

Environment during mealtime

When trying to create the most appropriate environment during mealtime, one should consider the following factors:

- Physical environment – The individual's head, back, and legs should be well supported, and if necessary, the sides of her trunk as well. The head should be erect, in midline, and slightly tilted forward. The caregiver (feeder) should sit in front (if eye contact is desired) or to the side of the individual (if support to the jaw is required). If the individual is actively seeking eye contact with the caregiver yet is in need of support when eating, a mirror can be placed in front of her to enable both eye contact and proper support.
- Sensory environment – If the individual with RS is sensitive to noises (most RS individuals have a sensitive auditory system) a loud environment can cause sensory overflow, thereby leading to muscle tone increase. If the individual's reaction is misunderstood by her caregivers the situation may be incorrectly interpreted as a behavioral problem. If the individual with RS is restless during mealtimes, all types of sensory stimulation which may be considered as possible disturbing elements

(such as different scents, sounds, sights, and tactile stimulations) should be taken into consideration and modified until the individual is calm and is able to function in accordance with her maximal ability.

- Communicative environment – Food is usually an extremely positive motivator for the individual with RS. Thus mealtime is frequently the ideal time to develop and put into practice both manual and communicative skills. For example, the caregiver could wait for the individual to signal her wish to eat or drink, and then respond accordingly by giving the desired item, thereby enhancing her control over the situation and supporting communicative interaction. It is recommended to await the individual's choice in regards to different food possibilities and then to serve her according to her choice. The use of mealtimes is a good opportunity to improve the eater's eye contact, vocal abilities, and hand usage in a communicative manner. A possible recommendation is the preparation of tablemats that present the different utensils and food possibilities and might serve at the same time as mealtime communication boards (appendix 1).

- Facilitating caregiver support– It has been recommended that each person in need of an augmentative communication system have a Personal Communication Passport [10,11] (see chapter on communication), in addition to all his/her other communication tools. The purpose of the Personal Communication Passport is to present important and relevant information about the person in a clearly written and interesting way so that it is accessible to all those who are in contact with the person. Within this Passport there can be a page on "eating" which describes the seating and eating methods, the required utensils, and the handling to be provided by the feeder. On this page the person's personal preferences as well as dislikes in regards to food and drink should be specified. Personal reactions during emergency situations can also be described. The page should be prepared as a joint venture of the parents and habilitation\educational staff in consultation with the RS individual. It will serve to ensure that the same forms of assistance will be given to the individual with RS during mealtimes, even with changing caregivers and across settings.

Of the above mentioned aspects of feeding two are of immense importance as they are potentially the source of many eating problems; dealing with them may in many cases prevent or alleviate these problems themselves. These elements are the positioning and the caregiver's handling of the individual (special attention must be paid to them as they are potential sources of influence on oral- motor function).

Most individuals with RS present a thin and short stature[6]. Despite the fact that they are generally good eaters who enjoy their food, even though they spend an especially long time at their meals, they generally do not put on weight relative to peers. Some even suffer from failure to thrive (FTT), a condition which requires enhancing caloric intake and in extreme cases even using tube feeding through a gastro-intestinal tube (G-tube) [12]. The severity of eating problems of individuals with RS usually escalates until mid-childhood age and thereafter stabilizes [13].

BMI (Body Mass Index) points to the relationship between the body height and weight of the individual (appropriate figures for the general population are 21-26 BMI). Individuals with RS have been found with average BMI values 17.5 (table VI-1)[6]. This figure points to the fact in most cases (especially during childhood) the individual with RS is extremely thin relative to her height.

Table VI-1. BMI values of individuals with RS

Age groups	BMI
All ages	**17.5**
0-7 Year(s)	15.4
7-12 Years	15.5
12-17 Years	16.6
17+ Years	21

[6]

A few studies show that many individuals with Rett syndrome are in fact in a mild to moderate state of malnutrition [14] and that their calorie intake is 70% of normal caloric intake [15]. Studies show that the stereotypical hand movements account for a high burning of calories causing the need for a high caloric intake [16]. Since this imbalance is extended over a period of years, the individual with RS may reach malnutrition with its harmful effects. Often, the duration of mealtime (due to swallowing problems) may bring on the decision for surgery for inserting a G-tube (gastrostomy). The Australian RS research group reported that 12.5% of the individuals use nutritional aids such as G.I. Tubes [6].

Studies have shown that an eating program via a G-Tube helps to put on weight and sustain a proper growth rate in individuals with Rett syndrome. In addition, it has been found that an increase in caloric intake results in a calmer, more sociable disposition, as well as in the ability to become more physically active [12].

On one hand, the goal is having the individual with RS take in as many calories as possible through a balanced diet in order for her to grow properly, be calm, be physically active, and build up her immunity to disease. On the other hand, we are interested in sustaining the self feeding abilities of individuals with RS in order to enhance functional skill and prevent them from loosing those skills which they already possess. Therefore a balanced feeding program should be created for each individual with RS. Such a program must maintain daily exercises aimed at preserving functional eating abilities at the same time as it ensures sufficient caloric intake. It should be emphasized that a normative eating program can be implemented even with the insertion of a feeding tube, by using the G-tube to supplement oral caloric intake and not replace it.

Practical instructions for mealtime

The caregiver involvement begins after proper planning and decisions are made based on the results of the initial evaluation. Factors to be considered include:

- The physical condition of the individual (oral-motor abilities, oral deformities, body movement patterns, level of assistance required at mealtime).
- Behavioral and social abilities.
- Environmental considerations (such as the availability of equipment, training and/or professional knowledge of the caregiving team, etc.).

According to these indicators we determine correct therapeutic posture. One may photograph the individual in the correct position during mealtime and provide proper instructions to caregivers. A good tactic is to write these instructions out on a large placard, preferably with accompanying diagrams; this placard can then be hung on the wall both as a reminder to staff and family, and as a teaching tool in the event that a new caregiver joins the team.

Correct eating posture should:

- Enable correct arrangement of the eating area (of the seating system, position of the individual relative to the table, and the position of the caregiver in relation to the individual).
- Sustain and improve midline orientation.
- Provide support for the back/trunk and for the lower extremities.
- Allow the individual to function at her highest possible level of ability.

Individuals with RS usually love eating, and food can be used as a powerful motivational factor for them, with the intent of reaching additional therapeutic goals through the use of food.

As mentioned above, despite their great appetite, individuals with RS consume about 50 calories less than the average per day, which results in some instances in malnutrition [12]. It is important to remember that the limited communicative abilities of individuals with RS generally prevent them from expressing their hunger. Therefore if the individual with RS is thin, larger amounts of food and high caloric food supplements should be suggested, despite the prolonged mealtime. However mealtime should not exceed 30 to 40 minutes, and therefore it is sometimes necessary to add another meal per day. It is reiterated that individuals with RS who were given sufficient caloric intake were found to be calmer, more aware of their surroundings, and more active; they also displayed proper growth curves [12].

When an individual with RS has been noted to have reached an extremely low weight, despite constant feeding attempts, it is recommended that high-caloric food and liquid supplements be introduced, for example enriched liquid drinks such as Ensure or Pedishure® jello, ice cream, milkshake, whipped cream, olive oil, and more. At times, a high-caloric diet may prevent the use of a G-tube.

It is common for the majority of individuals with RS (also those who have not been evaluated as having swallowing problems) to aspirate occasionally (the intake of food into the respiratory system). This constitutes a dangerous situation, especially if concealed aspiration is performed (when unaccompanied by coughing) as the caregiver is thus unaware of its existence and complications can occur, including pneumonia, a life-threatening illness.

In cases of recurring lung pathology:

- It is important to take the individual with RS for an evaluation by a specialist, in order to determine the occurrence and frequency of aspiration, (The foremost factor to be suspected and examined in individuals with RS presenting lung problems would be aspiration).
- A liquid thickener should be used (such as Thick & Easy, Thick-It® ThickenUp®, or No More Lumps) to reduce the risk of aspiration.

- An individual with RS who aspirates must be fed thickened pureed foods devoid of lumps.
- The positioning of the head should be re-evaluated and backward tilting of the head should be prevented during mealtime (this is the state wherein the bronchioles are at their most open/vulnerable position).
- It is necessary to keep the body erect, with the head stable. If the seating system does not support the required postural modifications, the hand of the caregiver not occupied with feeding can be wrapped around the shoulders in order to support the back of the neck from behind, as a tactic for achieving proper stability and positioning.
- If there is a lack of control of the jaw movements, the jaw may be stabilized to enhance proper chewing and swallowing with the help of the caregiver's free hand. It is important to keep steady pressure via the support and to keep the head and neck at the right position. Examples for the proper support can be found at [17].
- It is important to try to place the food either on the tongue or between the upper and lower molars, as placing the food in these areas will cause complex mouth action involving the teeth, tongue and jaws, for the purpose of encouraging chewing behavior.

It is recommended to keep a food diary tracking the amount of calories the individual with RS consumes. A food diary will also allow for the tracking of unusual events such as the making of strange sounds, epileptic attacks, manifestations of anxiety, or any other strange behavior which has occurred during or after the eating of a specific food, thus preventing needless future suffering.

Previous studies have shown that individuals with RS do not have allergies on a level and frequency beyond the normative level [18]. In spite of this knowledge, there are random reports from parents which point to sensitivity of some individuals with RS to strawberries, wheat products, tomatoes, eggs, chocolate, corn, milk, nuts, and soy [19-21]. It must be remembered that individuals with RS present a variety of phenotypic expressions; this, in combination with their limitations in the area of communication, requires us (the caregiver/parents/therapists) to be attentive and make numerous attempts to improve their care, including on the gastronomical front.

It might be found that an individual with RS is sensitive to a specific food item but not enough to elicit an allergic reaction. In other words, no allergic sensitivity would be found through allergy evaluation, and yet, she will react negatively to a certain food item. We must identify these food items (by conducting the food diary suggested earlier) and if in fact the manifestation escalates, neutralize them from her diet.

It is possible and even common for individuals with RS to present oral sensory issues. Therefore one should pay attention during mealtime; refusal to eat/drink can stem from:

- The food texture is not pleasant (one should try and change the texture in order to verify this assumption).
- The food/drink temperature is not adequate (one should try the same food at different temperatures until reaching the individual's preferred temperature).

Individuals with RS may present low oral muscle tone accompanied by sensory problems. It is therefore advisable to provide oral stimulation prior to mealtime when needed, in order to improve the oral functioning, thereby improving the quality of eating and shortening mealtime duration. Instruction for oral treatment is given by an occupational therapist/speech language pathologist/physical therapist who is familiar with this type of intervention and should be personalized for the needs of every individual with RS [22, 23]. The intervention includes a gentle, yet firm massage of the cheeks, chin, lips, and if possible, the inside of the mouth, using a gentle brush of the kind used to massage a baby's teeth. It is important to remember that some individuals with RS may resist having the therapist's finger or a brush inserted into their mouth; it is paramount that we respect the person's wishes and avoid forcing this intervention if the person feels uncomfortable.

Exercise before and during mealtime can include slow and rhythmic moving of the joints, together with the application of pressure in the direction of the center of support. Such procedures frequently reduce spasticity and give the individual the opportunity to achieve proper eating, as well as reduce her stereotypic hand movements. As opposed to the above mentioned intervention, a hypotonic individual (usually a younger individual) with RS, will actually gain from vigorous movement before/during mealtime. This procedure may include jumping on a physiotherapy ball, dancing (either standing on the floor or in the therapist's arms), jumping while sitting on the therapist's knees (if age-appropriate), or rolling – the person with RS can be positioned in a prone position with the underarms supported with a small cylinder or folded up blanket; the therapist may use gentle backwards and forwards rolling movements which put pressure on the person's hands, arms and shoulder girdle.

Immature tongue movement patterns prevent the individual with RS from performing coordinated tongue movements which are required for the transfer of food from side to side inside the mouth, thus also preventing proper chewing [14]. In order for the individual with RS to initiate proper tongue action, it is important to place the food at one side of the mouth between the molars, thereby enhancing execution of complex mouth, tongue, and lip movement.

RS individuals fixate their trunks in order to prevent the unpleasant sensation which accompanies ataxic shuddering and to improve the slight control they have over their muscles. The negative side effect to this gain of control is prevention of proper active stabilization of the back and head. If this is the case, trunk and neck muscle strengthening exercises are warranted together with manual techniques for the upper torso and neck, aimed at releasing tight tissue and enhancing joint range of movement during treatments in between meals.

Since self-feeding and manual functioning are dependent on trunk control, the basic way to achieve improved trunk stability as well as manual functioning is by activating the trunk muscles. If better functioning can be attained while eating by the use of a specific exercise, it is advisable to plan a practice session of this kind before mealtime and start the meal immediately at the end of the exercise. This way, the individual will be physically prepared; moreover the practice session will serve as a framework for the meal, as she will come to recognize that food is served right after the exercise.

Seating system

Individuals with RS have poor postural control. Therefore it is essential that the individual is properly seated during mealtime. Prior to the meal the therapist and caregivers should check to see that the individual with RS is seated in a proper chair, that her body is well supported, and that the distance and height of the table are individually adjusted to her needs. Without these initial conditions, the chances of enabling the individual with RS to manually function or eat properly are poor.

In order to achieve maximal engagement during meal time, the individual's attention should be focused towards eating. If her body is not supported well enough and she is preoccupied with lack of stability, her oral functions will be inadequate for achieving the control and coordination necessary for the complex action of eating. Therefore the individual with RS should be provided with some form of seating which will enable her to support herself in the position desirable from the therapist's standpoint. Generally this is also the position that is most comfortable for the individual. On the other hand it is important to remember that stabilization prevents movement; therefore we will always aim at achieving functional self-feeding with minimum external support from facilitators as well as equipment.

One must remember that most individuals with RS present low muscle tone, and as such, they become more passive with increased external support. Therefore minimum required support should be provided. For example, using a chest support during mealtime will usually encourage forward leaning with hyperextension of the head and neck; as this is an undesired posture, the use of a chest support should therefore be avoided.

It is recommended that a slight leaning backwards of the seat's back support, which will allow for a slight leaning forward of the head, is (as mentioned before) an ideal posture for eating. This suggestion is general in nature and does not prevent individual problem-solving proceedings when issues such as orthopedic neck problems, skewed sensations in regard to midline, and respiratory problems may in fact lead to the appropriateness of a completely opposing posture.

Some individuals with RS show extremely high muscle tone. In order for such individuals to reduce their spasticity, thereby improving their functional abilities (and this is suggested only for extreme cases showing very high spasticity), it is advised to use slow, rhythmic and soothing movement before and during mealtimes. In such cases a suspended chair might be considered as a proper seating system and might help in reducing the individual's spasticity.

Many individuals with RS show agitation in new unfamiliar situations. Therefore an acclimation period should be allowed when changing the seating arrangement of an individual with RS.

Due to the known communication difficulties of most individuals with RS, it is likely that they will be unable to verbally communicate unease or distress in regard to discomfort caused by the seating system. Therefore when new postures are pursued the therapist should be attentive to the individual's non-verbal messages. Extensive hand mannerisms accompanied by high muscle tone might imply that the individual with RS needs some more time to get accustomed to the seating system or that some alterations are required for the individual to be comfortable and thus enjoy her meals.

When constructing a seating system for individuals with RS, consideration should be given to the correct position of the thighs, hips, trunk and shoulders in order to determine the preferred mealtime posture. Due to sensory dysfunction and faulty body scheme, individuals with RS frequently produce continuous movements of the lower and upper extremities. Such movements tend to distract the individual, thereby reducing her functional level. Due to the need for a careful balance between stabilization and mobilization, the individual with RS should receive a scrupulous evaluation when provided with a seating system. The functional outcome should serve as the guiding principle of the decision making process. It is important to decide what kind of support should be given and at what times; during feeding, for example, some individuals with RS might be in need of maximal support in order to prevent preoccupation with postural issues. At other times, less support enables the achievement of balance reactions and muscle strengthening. For the hypotonic person less support will enhance muscle tone thereby enhancing functional abilities

If the individual presents different needs during mealtime and free time (i.e. a need for massive support during mealtimes but ability to achieve independent seating when individual intervention is not required) the use of two different seating systems might be considered.

The human environment

Therapeutic intervention goals for the individual with RS should always emphasis her independence and maximal achievable function. Due to the fluctuating nature of RS the caregiver should always be informed and updated regarding intervention goals and the appropriate handling required for achieving such pre-set goals.

Individuals with RS are apraxic meaning that they have difficulties in performing a motor act on demand or in learning a new function [24]. Touch is a very meaningful modality for the apraxic individual, and therefore the caregiver's touch is of extreme importance. A sensitive attentive touch by the caregiver can reduce the individual's agitation and enhance function; however if unprofessionally applied this touch may do just the opposite and thus negatively influence the mealtime experience. A touch lacking attentiveness and sensitivity can cause the individual to disengage from the eating situation and thus diminish her cooperation.

Due to the fact that individuals with RS are extremely sociable, the location of the feeder during mealtime is an important consideration. Having the feeder sit in front of the individual is a potent motivational factor since it encourages eye contact and communication. On the other hand sitting at the side of the individual enables the caregiver to achieve better control over her posture. Generally the location of the caregiver is determined by the amount of support required by the individual with RS as well as her interest in her close human environment. In the event that the individual with RS requires massive physical support (therefore suggesting that the caregiver should be situated at her side), but her need for personal interaction calls for direct eye contact, one might consider the option of placing a mirror in front of the individual with RS and her caregiver. Another option could be supporting the person with RS by sitting beside her during meal times, thereby enabling social interaction with other class/family members

Another factor influencing the seating arrangement of the person with RS and her feeder is the need to control stereotypical hand movements which may interfere with feeding. It is preferable for the feeder to sit on the side of the more active hand, thereby being in a position to assist in self feeding. This control is usually given by holding the non-dominant hand.

The orthopedic condition of the person with RS can also determine the position of the feeder. If the individual with RS is diagnosed with scoliosis then the feeder is best to seat on the side of the scoliosis (i.e. at the right hand side of an individual diagnosed with a right scoliosis). In such a case a slight shifting of the plate away from the midline towards the right (of the individual with RS) is warranted. This will facilitate asymmetrical muscle action against the natural curve of the spine (More details regarding the approach to scoliosis might be found within the physical therapy chapter in this book).

The height of the feeder is an important issue as well, especially as the mealtime duration for individuals with RS is generally lengthy. The height of the feeder should allow him to assist for the entire duration of the meal without becoming fatigued in his arms or back

Communication is an important human factor. As it is necessary for a caregiver to be present during mealtimes to assist the individual with RS, the time for communication and interaction is both available and appropriate:

- Communication should be directed at and with the individual with RS; mealtime should not be a time for discussion between caregivers within a classroom setting or family members in the home, without the inclusion of the person who is eating.
- Conversation should be carried on with the person with RS; this conversation can include what food is available, information about the tastes, temperatures and textures of the food, the person's likes and dislikes, what is going to happen throughout the day, what happened yesterday, etc.
- Mealtime is an excellent opportunity for active communication through choice-making. Choices can be made through the use of the food items themselves or through the use of pictures or written words representing those items; even when there is a set menu the person can be asked what she wants to eat first i.e. the vegetable or the chicken, or whether she wants to eat or drink first. The options of "I want more" and "I have had enough, thanks" can also be given. Even when giving a choice between two different foods (the vegetable or the chicken) it is often good to add a third choice, such as "neither of these" or "I have had enough". Frequently, messages such as "more" and "enough" can be uttered through the use of single message voice output communication device such as the BigMack. It must be remembered that persons with RS frequently indicate their choices through the use of eye gaze rather than through hand-pointing.

The food

The fact that each individual should receive only food items and food textures that are appropriate for her chewing and manual abilities is probably very clear to all readers, nevertheless we chose to bring it up as basic as it is. For example, an individual with eating or chewing problems should receive a biscuit or varied pureed food choices rather than a carrot or apple, so she can safely enjoy her food. An individual with good gripping ability should be served long and graspable food items (chocolate bars, grissini sticks) which are easy to hold, instead of small items which might frustrate her (i.e. cheerios).

The same cautious approach should be taken towards liquids. Thickened liquids should be suggested if the individual with RS's oral abilities put her in danger of aspiration when attempting to handle drinks of regular consistency. Thickened liquid can also be used both as a means for enhancing caloric intake and for increasing the sensation it creates when introduced to the mouth (allowing the individual with RS to easily handle the liquid). Thickened liquids also slow down the pace of swallowing, thereby enhancing the individual with RS's efficiency for handling the liquid in her mouth.

Most individuals with RS show clear preferences regarding food items. There are types of food which the individual with RS resists simply due to the fact that she does not like their taste. There are also types of food that are so delicious, that the individual who usually! does not eat independently (not even with her hands i.e. finger feeding) will agree to hold a spoon and eat independently! For example, an individual with RS known to the authors was willing to hold and independently eat a sandwich only if it contained chocolate spread, to independently hold and drink from a cup only if it contained Coca-Cola, and independently eat with a teaspoon only if she was served with a chocolate flavored dairy product. It is important to identify such food items in order to offer the individual with RS an enjoyable treat, as well as to facilitate improvement of her manual functioning based on the motivational element which such products hold. The improvement of manual functioning is a cornerstone in the therapeutic intervention for individuals with RS and should always be pursued. Furthermore a success in one situation may overflow to other situations and therefore the identification and usage of motivational factors is of immense importance.

Due to such clear preferences regarding the taste of food items (and due to staff turnover in educational and residential facilities), it is recommended to list each individual's preferred foods. Different tastes such as salty, spicy, sour, or sweet can be very arousing for the individual with RS and can be served when the individual is "under a cloud" [25:72]. A detailed list of specific food likes and dislikes can be included in the individual's personal communication passport (as described earlier in this chapter); this will empower the individual with RS and will enhance her quality of life. Other items which should be included in such a list are known allergies, food items towards which the individual with RS demonstrates a slight sensitivity, or items that somehow create a negative reaction. A list of this kind will allow the planning of a diet which the individual will truly enjoy, thus turning mealtime into a positive experience.

One should always aspire to enhance the oral abilities of each individual with RS by serving different types of food and introducing interesting textures, always taking into account individual preferences and abilities. On the other hand, many individuals with RS show difficulties in sensory processing in the oral area which may be manifested as either hyper- or hyposensitivity [14]. Therefore foods of mixed textures (like soup), may deter such persons. If the individual with RS is orally hypersensitive, she may be more at ease with mashed foods (puree). On the other hand an individual with oral hyposensitivity may enjoy crunchy textured foods which stimulate the mouth. The food texture and size should be determined according to the oral sensitivity of the individual with RS as well as to her ability to chew and swallow and to her personal preferences. Appropriate food items for the individual with RS with oral hyposensitivity should include long cookies, biscuits, grissini (bread sticks), bananas etc.

For the individual with RS who does not use her teeth for chewing, it is recommended to vary the diet as outlined in the "Non-chew cookbook" [26]. Some diets have been tried with individuals with RS, and the reports by their parents were positive. These diets include:

- The glutton-free diet: was reported to encourage weight gain and reduced constipation [27].
- A combination of the glutton-free and dairy-free diets: was reported to reduce screaming attacks and seizures [28].
- The egg-free diet: was reported to reduce screaming episodes [29].
- The macrobiotic diet which excludes red meat, dairy products, sugar, salt, tropical fruit, and white flour from one's diet: was reported to reduce constipation and to improve the function of the immune system [30].
- The catogenic diet which is a diet based on the exclusive eating of fats (which is very difficult to hold). Its purpose is to improve epileptic conditions for individuals who do not respond well to anti-convulsive medication. For an individual with RS it was reported to improve epileptic conditions, vocalization, and intestinal conditions, while supporting an improved general health state [31]. Another child showed improved awareness and function with this diet (ML).

Food utensils

Assistive equipment mediates between the food and the individual with RS. Specific assistive equipment is prescribed by taking into consideration the position of the individual with RS, as well as her manual, oral, and postural abilities. The goals in using assistive equipment are to improve the independent functional abilities of the individual with RS, to aid the caregiver\feeder in assisting the eater with RS, and to facilitate relaxation so that the individual with RS can increase her food intake and shorten the duration of the meal.

A cup/mug

- In order to prevent the individual with RS from bending her neck back too far thus causing extension of the neck, a slanted cup (such as a flexi cup) should be used (see figure VI-2).

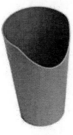

Figure VI-2. A cut-out cup, which prevents extension of the neck during drinking. This picture is taken from http://www.activeforever.com; similar cups may be purchased at different stores and websites carrying items for people with special needs.

- Due the lack of precision typical of ataxic individuals, it is important that the cup be made of unbreakable material and pleasant to bite on (such as thick plastic).
- The size of the cup should be such as to enable eye contact with the individual as she drinks.
- In instances where the person with RS is able to independently hold the cup, it is suggested that the cup be equipped with a mechanism controlling the amount of liquid drawn from a single sip (a holed cover or one with a mouthpiece).
- The individual with RS should be introduced to the possibility of using her hands while drinking (by using a cup with handles).

A straw

If the individual with RS achieves good lip closure it is recommended to teach her to use a straw, which allows better consumption of liquids. Learning how to drink from a straw is an important stage. This ability can usually be acquired with relative ease:

- Use the individual's favorite drink (milkshake, cola, chocolate milk).
- Use a flexible container, with a closed upper tube (the liquid is poured when the bottle is squeezed).
- The liquid is then pressed up the tube to the drinker's mouth provoking her to sip it in.
- Kissing sounds may be made as audible hints for the individual to begin sucking.
- If a straw is used it should be of a type that will not crush under the uncontrolled bite of the ataxic individual.
- A cup with a straw is recommended since it helps in stabilization of the shoulder girdle, the neck, and the head.
- A straw made out of thick and flexible plastic material can make it easier for the individual with RS to grip it with her lips (Fig. VI-3).

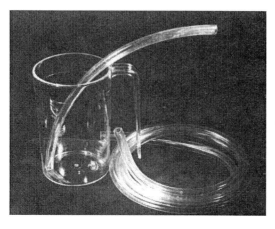
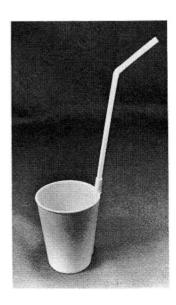

Figure VI-3. Different straws [32].

- Due to the complex integrative abilities needed for drinking out of a cup (co-control of the shoulder girdle, arms, trunk, head and mouth), the use a cup with a long straw, in a way that allows drinking without the need for using the hands is recommended, when manual abilities are lacking. Drinking from a cup placed on the table (with a straw) is functional and it is believed that some individuals with RS will prefer this sort of device rather than investing the effort in learning how to drink. Such a device will enhance the independent abilities of the individual with RS, as well as improve her liquid intake.

Spoons

A flat spoon will allow easy removal of food through the use of the upper lip. The spoon should be unbreakable (thick plastic) and pleasant to chew on (not metal). The size of the spoon should fit the size of the individual's mouth, and the length of the handle should fit the size of the feeder's hand. In some cases when the individual with RS feeds independently or with slight assistance, but lacks the ability to constantly hold the spoon, it is possible to add an upper semi circular strap to the handle of the eating utensil, in order to support the grip, and to enable the completion of a full feeding cycle without the spoon being dropped. The authors would like to caution against the frequent use of this technique which might prevent the individual with RS from taking responsibility for eating independently to the best of her ability.

A heavy, solid thick-handled spoon will provide the individual with clear sensory input, thereby helping the apraxic\ataxic individual in handling the spoon and in progressing towards independent function. Since most individuals with RS have difficulty with complex motor abilities, such as the rotation of the forearm to both supination and pronation, an angled spoon will enhance the possibility of independent eating or at least aid the caregiver feeding the individual with RS.

In some cases the motivation of the individual with RS to hold onto the spoon, thereby improving her hand grip, can be enhanced by either painting the handle of the utensil or attaching a colorful shiny object to it.

Plates

Due to the generally poor manual abilities of individuals with RS, a plate with a high rim can prevent food spilling from it and will facilitate the scooping of food if the eater is independent or in need of slight assistance.

Placement of the plate on a rubber surface (such as Dycem®, a non-slip mat which prevents the plate from being pushed or moved during feeding), or a plate with an adhesive surface is recommended. This will prevent the tipping over of the plate that may occur either by the stereotypical hand movements of individuals with RS or an inaccurate hand reach in the case of an independent eater with RS.

Due to the long duration of mealtime of individuals with RS the food may become cold by the end of the meal. Therefore the use of a double rimmed plate into which warm water can be poured is suggested. The use of this type of assistive utensil will enhance the individual with RS's enjoyment for the duration of the meal. Since it is known that individuals with RS may be orally sensitive [14], keeping the food at a warm temperature may assist in cases where the individuals are sensitive to extreme temperatures (hot\cold). Such plates are found in most department stores selling baby equipment.

Placing the utensils in the mouth of the individual with RS

The following techniques are fundamental and are not unique for individuals with RS. These might be changed according to individual needs and specifications (i.e. if the individual with RS is fed through the use of a bottle or is placed in a tilted way due to the existence of contractures or decubitus (pressure sores).

When feeding individuals with special needs the common practice is to insert the spoon towards the center of the mouth, above the tongue, to press down on the tongue with the spoon, to wait for lip closure over the spoon, and to then remove the spoon from the mouth in a straight horizontal plane. Removal of the spoon in this fashion will facilitate the scraping of the food off the spoon and into the mouth by the upper lip. This procedure is usually similarly executed with individuals with RS.

In drinking, the cup should be placed on the lower lip and lifted in a way that will allow drops of liquid to enter the mouth when it opens.

The recommended amount of food per serving

Due to the oral sensitivity of individuals with RS [14] and their poor oral coordination [6,8,33,34], the amount of food placed in the mouth should be adapted according to the individual's ability to cope with food in her mouth, taking into consideration the type of food, the support of the seating system, and the skill and efficiency of the feeder.

The timing of servings could be important to enable proper coping with food by the individual with RS. It is important to evaluate the time the eater takes to clear her mouth after every serving and to act accordingly. The serving of food too quickly may induce vomiting and/or aspiration, while too slowly may be annoying or produce boredom, thus causing the individual to stop eating with a result of limited food consumption.

The right amount of food should be more than what is needed to initiate the swallowing process but less than the amount the individual with RS can cope with, in between two intakes of air. Giving too little will make the feeding process too long both for the eater and the caregiver; giving too much will prevent the eater from chewing and swallowing properly, thereby causing the food to accumulate in the upper palate, or possibly leading to aspirations. The skilled caregiver will quickly learn what "the right personal amount" is. In order to deal with issues of staff turnover, in cases where "the right personal amount" is a critical issue it is advised that this sort of information be entered into a food journal or personal communication passport including a photo entitled: "Spoon with correct amount of food".

Caregiver intervention during mealtime

As a rule the intervention of the caregiver should aim at maximal independence on the part of the individual with RS and minimal assistance on the part of the caregiver.

The assistance should be given according to the amount required by the individual with RS. An individual in need of substantial support can be helped by the "hand over hand" technique. On the other hand when there is need for minimal assistance only, this assistance can be provided through slight physical hints given at the wrist, elbow, or shoulder level.

It is sometimes possible for the individual with RS to achieve independent eating through continuous training. It is generally a gradual and slow process, progressing from total passivity to finger feeding and in some cases to independent eating with a spoon. Factors which may contribute to the development of independent eating skills include the development of a good rapport between the individual with RS and the feeder, together with the recognition of her abilities, of her sleep and wakeful hours throughout the day, and of her motivational factors. It is the belief of the authors that when the above mentioned factors are included within an intense intervention program, involving all the caregivers supporting the individual with RS, functional progress by the individual with RS can be achieved.

On the other hand we must never forget that individuals with RS consume a diminished caloric intake [12] and therefore it is essential that they eat properly. Since appropriate food consumption is a matter of survival, a balance should be found between the amount of food consumed and independent eating. Therefore the caregiver might consider dividing mealtimes into periods of feeding (for the sake of caloric intake) and periods of practice\self feeding.

As indicated above, communication is an essential aspect of eating; therapists and caregivers must remember to talk with the persons with whom they are interacting during mealtime. Responses through the use of communication strategies can be expected.

Environmental considerations

Due to the strong attraction held by individuals with RS for music [35-40], music can be used to create a relaxed atmosphere during mealtimes. It is advisable to play soft music in accordance with the preferences of the person with RS.

Due to the significance of food for the individual with RS, mealtime can serve as an ideal active learning experience. In order to achieve the maximum gain, close attention should be paid to the individual with RS during mealtimes. Personal conversations among caregivers should be avoided at such times.

A noisy eating environment might prevent successful communication between the caregiver and the individual with RS. Therefore steps should be taken by the caregiver to create a peaceful environment.

The fluctuating nature of RS might affect the feelings, mood, and behavior of the individual with RS, thus causing a distraction during or around mealtime. It is important for the caregiver to be attentive and sensitive to possible distracting factors. The importance of the eating experience to this population (in terms of caloric intake, social and educational experiences, and food as a motivating factor) necessitates that care must be taken to ensure its positive value. Therefore in "bad times" efforts must be made both to detect the cause of this behavior and to find strategies for its resolution.

An example of how the positive experience of mealtimes of the individual with RS can be maximized relates to the issue of smell. Because individuals with RS are often adversely affected by many different smells, different measures should be taken to ensure that the only aromas present during mealtimes are those of the actual food being eaten.

An additional example with regard to environmental influence is the issue of color. Color is a highly potent environmental factor which can have an effect on both general feeling and mood. When considering environmental color and its effect on individuals with RS during mealtime, one must take into consideration whether or not we want the individual to look at her caregivers and the other individuals during mealtime, or at the flashy furniture and classroom walls.

Individuals with RS have good peripheral vision [25]. Movement at the edge of her visual field will draw the individual with RS's attention; therefore in order to ensure a quiet eating milieu, it is suggested that there be as few disturbances around the eating place as possible during mealtime.

If the individual with RS is distracted and cannot fully participate in the eating experience, it is possible to consider moving her to a quiet spot. Such a transfer will allow her the time and conditions she needs for a positive mealtime experience. Such a solution might enable the resolution of different "mealtime associated problems". Despite the above, the therapeutic goal of the eating experience is full integration into community settings. Therefore the therapeutic staff's final goal for individuals with RS is to facilitate their enjoyment of mealtime in a crowded, loud, and provoking environment such as a restaurant.

Conclusions

Despite the fact that individuals with RS present a variety of difficulties, which may arise during and around mealtime, most of these problems can be resolved through the combination of a proper evaluation and a comprehensive prior knowledge of the different typical aspects related to this disorder. Due to the fluctuating nature of RS, evaluations of the individual and her eating environment should be on-going, in order to examine the therapeutic efficiency of previously taken measures. The complexity of RS, of the mealtime situation, and of the actual action of eating can easily hamper the smoothness of this experience. The application of knowledge and sensitivity on the part of therapists and caregivers can turn this from being a repetitive nightmare to being a positive experience for the individual with RS.

The complexity of RS might challenge the caregivers and therapists with unanswered issues which remain outside the scope of the current chapter. In such situations the individual with RS and her family should be referred for consultation with experts in the field of feeding. Full resolution of these challenges might come from collaboration among colleagues in the disciplines of occupational therapy, speech language pathology, nutrition, and gastroenterology.

References

[1]   Amir RE, Van den Veyver IB, Wan M, Tran CQ, Francke U, Zoghbi HY. Rett syndrome is caused by mutations in X-linked MECP2, encoding methyl-CpG-binding protein 2. Nat Genet 1999;23(2):185-8.

[2]   Amir RE, Van Den Veyve IB, Schultz R, Malicki DM, Tran CQ, et al. Influence of mutation type and X chromosome inactivation on Rett syndrome phenotypes. Ann Neurol 2000;47:670-9.

[3]   Hagberg B. Rett Syndrome: Clinical and biological aspects. London: Mac Keith Press, 1993.

[4]   Engerstrom IW, Kerr A. Workshop on autonomic function in Rett Syndrome, Swedish Rett center, Frösön, Sweden. Brain Dev 1998;20:323-6.

[5]   Lotan, M. Management for Rett syndrome. The Israeli Rett Syndrome Center, Rotem publications. Tel- Aviv, Israel, 2006. [Hebrew]

[6]   Leonard S. The Australian Rett syndrome study inaugural report. Aust: Telethon Inst Child Health Res, 2002.

[7]   Evans MS, Klein DM. Pre feeding skills. A comprehensive resource for feeding development. Tucson, AZ: Therapy Skill Builders, 1987.

[8]   Budden SS. Management of Rett syndrome: a ten year experience. Neuropediatr 1995;26:75–7.

[9]   Lotan M. Zysman L. The digestive system and nutritional considerations for individuals with Rett syndrome. ScientificWorldJournal 2006;6:1737–49.

[10]   Millar S. Personal communication passports: Guidelines for good practice. Edinburgh: CALL Centre, 2003.

[11]   Millar S. Personal Communication Passports. The CALL Centre, 2006. Information retrieved on June 2007, from site: http://www.communicationpassports.org.uk/

[12]   Motil K. Nutrition and weight management. Presentation, IRSA 12th Ann Conf, Boston, MA, 1996 May 24-27, tape 622-11.

[13]   Cass H, Reilly S, Owen L, Wisbeach A, Weekes L, Slonims V, Wigram T, Charman T. Findings from a multidisciplinary clinical case series of females with Rett syndrome. Dev Med Individ Neurol 2003;45(5):325-37.

[14]   Hunter K. The Rett syndrome handbook. Washington, DC: Int Rett Syndr Assoc, 1999.

[15]   Thommessen M, Kase BF, Heiberg A. Growth and nutrition in ten girls with Rett syndrome. Acta Pediatrica 1992;81:686-9.

[16]   Motil KJ, Schultz R, Brown B, Glaze DG, Percy AK. Altered energy balance may account for growth failure in Rett Syndrome. J Child Neurol 1994;9:315-9.

[17]   Werner D. Disabled Village Children. A guide for community health workers, rehabilitation workers, and families. Chapter 36, Feeding The Hesperian Foundation, Berkeley, CA. 1999. extracted at November 2006 from site: http://www.dinf.ne.jp/doc/english/global/david/dwe002/dwe00238.htm.

[18]   Hunter K. Food allergies. Personal communication, 1997.

[19]   Personal communication I.: Thyroid, brassering, mucus and questions received through the Rettnett 1997 Mar 13, low@iadfw.net.

[20]   Personal communication II. What's wrong with Haley? Rettnett 1997 Mar 04, LEE@ LSI.MHSCompuServe.COM.

[21]   Personal communication III. What's wrong with Haley? Rettnett 1997 Mar 05, cloudy@ mail.nwlink.com.

[22]   Krigger KW. Cerebral Palsy: An Overview. Am Fam Physician 2006;73:91-100.

[23]   Workinger MS. Cerebral palsy resource guide for speech-language pathologists. Clifton Park, NY: Thomson Delmar Learning, 2005.

[24]   Ayres JA. Sensory integration and the child, 5th ed. Los Angeles, CA: Western Psychol Serv, 1982.

[25]   Lindberg B. Understanding Rett syndrome. New York: Hogrefe Huber, 1991.

[26]   Wilson JR. The non-chew cookbook. Glenwood Springs, CO: Wilson, 1985.

[27]   Holly G. Nutritional Link. RettNett, 1996 Dec 23, retnett@paltech.com.

[28]   Kehler K. What's wrong with Haley? RettNett, 1997 Apr 03, retnett@paltech.com.

[29]   Weisz C. What's wrong with Haley? RettNett, 1997 Mar 05, retnett@paltech.com.

[30]   Curtin M. Springtime illness. RettNett, 1997 Oct 11, retnett@paltech.com.

[31]   Lane I. Ketogenic diet. RettNett, 1996 Oct 11, retnett@paltech.com.

[32]   Pugh M, Stansfield S. Assessment of drinking equipment (cups and straws). DH Disability, undated.

[33]   Budden SS. Rett syndrome: habilitation and management reviewed. Eur Individ Adolesc Psychiatry 1997;6(Suppl 1):103-7.

[34]   Motil KJ, Schultz RJ, Browning K, Trautwein L, Glaze DG. Oropharyngeal dysfunction and gastroesophageal dysmotility are present in individuals and women with Rett syndrome. J Pediatr Gastroenterol Nutr 1999;29(1):31-7.

[35]   Merker B, Bergstrom-Isacsson M, Witt Engerstrom I. Music and the Rett disorder: The Swedish Rett Center survey. Nord J Music Ther 2001;10(1):42-53.

[36]   Rett A. Grundlagen der Musiktherapie und Music-Psychologie. Stuttgart: Fischer, 1982. [German]

[37]   Wigram T. Assessment and treatment of an individual with Rett syndrome. In: Bruscia K, ed. Case studies in music therapy Gilsum, NH: Barcelona Publ, 1991.

[38]   Wigram T. A model of assessment and differential diagnosis of handicap in individuals through the medium of music therapy. In: Wigram T, Saperston B, West R, eds. The art and science of music therapy: A handbook. Chur, Switzerland: Harwood Acad Publ, 1995:181-93.

[39]   Wigram T. The effect of vibroacoustic therapy on clinical and non-clinical populations. Dissertation. London: St Georges Med School, Univ London, 1996.

[40]   WigramT, Cass H. Music therapy within the assessment process for a therapy clinic for people with Rett syndrome. Presentation, Rett Syndr World Conf, Sweden, 1996.

Appendix 1. Mealtime placemat/ communication board

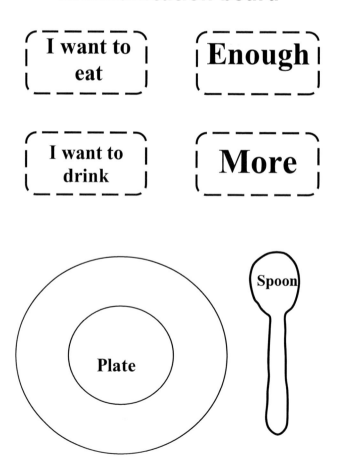

In: Rett Syndrome: Therapeutic Interventions
Editors: Meir Lotan and Joav Merrick

ISBN: 978-1-61728-080-1
©2011 Nova Science Publishers, Inc.

Chapter VII

Rett Syndrome: Digestive System and Nutritional Considerations

Meir Lotan, BPT, MScPT, PhD[*,1,2] *and Lilit Zysman, BSc, RN*[1]

[1]Israel Rett Syndrome Center, National Evaluation Team, Chaim Sheba Medical Center,
Tel HaShomer, Ramat Gan
[2]Department of Physical Therapy, Ariel University Campus, Ariel, Israel

Rett Syndrome (RS) is a neuro-developmental disorder of genetic origin, which mainly affects females. Individuals diagnosed with RS exhibit a variety of functional difficulties that impair their quality of life. One of the affected systems is the digestive system, where 74% of persons with Rett Syndrome have abnormal functioning. The affected digestive system causes this population to present an array of problems such as gastro esophageal reflux (GER), constipation and malnutrition, leading to failure to thrive (FTT), which results in reduced functional ability. By reference to the severe effects of the dysfunctional digestive system on individuals with RS, this chapter will describe the problems common to this population and will suggest some clinical options for intervention.

Introduction

Rett Syndrome (RS) is a genetic disorder that primarily affects females [1,2]. The disorder causes a neurological and developmental arrest that manifests itself in a variety of disabilities such as loss of functional hand use, loss of acquired speech, apraxia, ataxia, autonomic system dysfunction, epilepsy, breathing abnormalities, failure to thrive and muscle tone irregularities [3-5]. Swallowing is a complex process involving a sequence of intricately-timed maneuvers, executed by a large number of muscles (including muscles of the mouth,

* Correspondence: Meir Lotan, BPT, MScPT, PhD, Department of Physical Therapy, Ariel University Campus, IL-40700 Ariel, Israel. E-mail: ml_pt_rs@netvision.net.il

pharynx, larynx, oesophagus, and diaphragm). Therefore, it is not surprising that this choreography is profoundly disturbed by muscle weakness, dystonia, as well as poor co-ordination in neuromuscular conditions, such as occurs in RS [6].

Digestive system dysfunctions are a significant component of the different phenotypic expression of individuals with RS and at least one gastrointestinal problem can be found among 74% of individuals with this diagnosis[7]. It is a known fact that inadequate food intake and bowel management hold severe consequences for this population [7-11] and due to their poor nutritional state, nutritional intervention is an important element in the daily management of individual with RS. Good nutritional management can improve not only the weight of the individual with RS but also her activity level and her functional abilities [10,11], thereby positively effecting her overall quality of life.

It is clear that other characteristics of this population, such as abnormality of the respiratory system, (e.g. apnea and hyperventilation episodes) [12] and orthopedic difficulties (e.g. muscle-tone abnormalities, scoliosis and postural misalignment) [13-15] aggravate the digestive system dysfunction. The handling of all the above-mentioned elements should be addressed by a multi-professional team approach [16] and such a team should preferably include a pediatric dietitian specializing in developmental disabilities. Due to the fact that the overall functional and health situation of the individual with RS is dependent upon her nutritional status, the significance of a pediatric dietician being in position is substantial. The dietitian should check the initial state of each client, set appropriate intervention programs and follow the implementation of these programs in order to ensure that the individual achieves her predetermined weight [17].

Since findings imply that the eating abilities of each individual correspond to her general physical condition [18], the achievement of proper and stable dietary management for the individual with RS sets the base [8] for a healthier living. A well established régime enables her to participate fully in learning experiences and to flourish without setbacks that result from a poor nutritional state. Many individuals with RS develop eating problems at an early age, although, 82% have been found to develop such problems at relatively older ages (8-12½ years) [18]. These findings suggest that early multi-disciplinary evaluation of eating abilities and nutritional state should be performed. A continuous follow-up should commence at an early age and continue as the individual is growing up and aging.

The next section of the chapter will outline some of the common problems attributed to the digestive system of the individual with RS, such as difficulties in eating and swallowing, inappropriate gag reflex, hyper-sensitivity around the mouth, voluntarily food emitting, breathing irregularities, Gastro Esophageal Reflux (GER) and constipation. Intervention methods that have been found appropriate for this population are suggested.

Difficulties in eating and swallowing

Despite their excellent appetite, individuals with RS commonly present an array of eating problems [18]. Only few of them actually develop mature chewing patterns and up to 64% of individuals with RS show moderate to severe oral-motor dysfunction [18]. Of those showing oral-motor dysfunction, 41% of the cases originate from factors influencing chewing, such as:

- Abnormal tongue movements (such movements, especially towards the left side, were noted in all individuals at III-IV stage of RS), usually caused by lack of movement in the central and frontal area of the tongue [19]
- Hypo- or hyper muscular tone of the tongue
- Poor posture of the spine at the cervical and upper torso areas
- Muscular rigidity of the shoulder girdle (usually exhibited by elevated and protracted shoulders)
- Hyper-extension of the neck, usually accompanied by tongue-thrust [20]

One of the expressions of an oral-esophageal problem is the spitting or vomiting of food. One of the main causes for the spitting/vomiting of food is an inappropriate gag reflex.

Inappropriate gag reflex - spitting/vomiting

The gag reflex is usually located at the end section of the mouth, i.e. the soft palate area, in people without neurological problems. It has been found present in 20% of individuals with RS [20]. The reflex is produced by internal stimulation (i.e. sickness) as well as by external stimulation, such as pressure or weight (from different foods inside the mouth). Some individuals with RS are unable to elicit an appropriate gag reflex and may feel uncomfortable as a result of stimulation of the area, forcing them to vomit. An opposite, even more serious, problem is in the case when the individual is unable to cough, despite gag reflex stimulation, leaving the bronchioles defenseless. A change of position forward or backward may cause movement of the food in the mouth and positively affect the pattern of movement of the head and shoulders (i.e. the pattern of movement and the regulation of a high tone), thus reducing the gag reaction.

Hyper-sensitivity around the mouth

The sensory system of individuals with RS has never been thoroughly investigated. Nevertheless, accumulating reports suggest that this system does not function in a normative fashion [21]. The individual with RS may spit hot or cold food items because of hyper-sensitivity in the mouth area or because of food lumps that are too large within a serving. Such problems may be addressed through appropriate sensory stimulation outside and inside of the mouth. Nonetheless, there are differing reasons for spitting besides hyper-sensitivity.

Voluntarily food emitting - spitting

In general, this is defined as a strong emission of food from the mouth in a voluntary manner. In fact, in some cases, an individual may be inclined to spit even if she does not voluntarily emit. It is a well-known fact that individuals with RS show respiratory irregularities [12] expressed in some cases as explosive exhalation. A second reason for apparent deliberate spitting is a situation in which the person's mouth is full of food and there is a need to inhale.

Such a situation may be resolved through the exhalation of air (with food particles), thereby forcefully spraying food out of the mouth. Our clinical experience has shown that, in some cases, deliberate spitting is behavioral as the individual with RS enjoys the attention she gets as a result of such behavior.

Recurrent aspiration

The incidence of recurrent aspiration in selected groups of individuals with intellectual or developmental disability was reported at 26% and 27% cases respectively [22,23]. Individuals with RS present many factors which may interrupt smooth eating and swallowing, such as apraxia, ataxia and breathing abnormalities [3]. Abnormal breathing patterns such as apnea, hyperventilation, breath holding and bloating are presented by 84% of individuals with RS, usually from stage III of the disorder [24]. These incidents are apparent during waking hours alone [25] and, as they interfere with the complex mechanism of eating, they may cause recurrent aspirations.

Thin liquids are particularly prone to be aspirated [26]. Therefore one of the ways of preventing aspirations is liquid-thickening and the serving of puréed food items. In some severe cases of recurrent aspirations, oral feeding should be stopped, yet for individuals with RS who take so much pleasure in eating, the termination of all oral intake seems very harsh as a solution to the prevention of aspirations. The first thing to do in such cases would be to try conventional intervention, such as small- volume meals with puréed food and liquid thickening (elaboration on the subject of puréed food can be found in books such as "Non-chew cookbook") [27].

If surgical intervention (such as a gastro-intestinal tubing (GIT)/Percutanos Endoscopic Gastrostomy (PEG, which is discussed later in this chapter) is required, one should still consider applying small, low-volume "tasters" [28], being careful not to jeopardize the eater, for the sake of the quality of life of the individual with RS.

Gastro-eosophageal reflux (ger)

Gastro-esophageal reflux (GER) is the return of the stomach content to the upper-digestive system. It has been diagnosed in about 15%-25% of individuals with RS [7,20]. This phenomenon is caused when the chain of muscular tissue of the upper digestive system (esophageal, larynx, pharynx and the pyloric sphincter) is dysfunctional. Since the stomach content is acidic, the result of a slight reflux is a bad taste in the mouth and heartburn. However, in severe cases, GER can cause:

- Aspirations – the entry of stomach content into the airways may cause coughing and in more severe, chronic situations, recurrent lung infections.
- Prolonged exposure of the esophageal tissue to stomach acidity, causing discomfort from the penetration of stomach content through the esophageal outer coating and, as a result, the inflammation of the area.

- Esophageal narrowing – a recurrent, daily damage to the esophagus will cause adhesions in the inflamed esophageal tissue, leading to difficulty in swallowing and the sensation of food stuck in the throat.

Such a situation can be identified if the person with RS is fed by a naso-gastro tube and the insertion of the tube to the stomach gradually becomes more difficult. This phenomenon usually occurs together with increased difficulty in handling solid foods. Other recurrent health problems may accompany esophageal narrowing, such as vomiting with dried up brown particles ("coffee ground"), signs of distress before or after meal times, constant and gradual decrease in weight and refusal to eat or loss of appetite.

The incidence of gastro-esophageal reflux is quite high among individuals with developmental disability, as a group and specifically among individuals with RS. Even apart from its high manifestation rate, many individuals with RS will find it difficult to express the fact that they are uncomfortable when in distress. The combination of such dangers necessitates the sensitivity and alertness of the care-giving staff, ensuring that they notify the health-related personnel and the parents and direct the individual with RS for further evaluation [18]. If conventional intervention has produced no alleviation of the eater's discomfort, the intervention for gastro-esophageal reflux is handled by a pediatrician or a gastroenterologist. Intervention is applied according to the following steps:

- Phase A: Postural changes during and following meal-times, dietetic changes and the use of liquid thickeners. This stage is accompanied by the use of acidity neutralizers, such as Losec (Omeprazole), Pepsid (famotidine), Reglan (metoclopramide) and others.
- Phase B: At this stage, the use of pro-kinetic drugs is introduced. These medications are intended to increase esophageal clearance and enhance the muscular tone of the pyloric sphincter.
- Phase C: If the elevation in dosage of the formerly used drugs is ineffective, surgical intervention, such as fundoplication, is suggested.

The fundoplication is a relatively simple invasive procedure requiring general anesthesia and involves the rotation of the stomach around its vertical axis. This procedure is justified in a person with confirmable reflux, unresponsive to maximal medical management and showing troublesome symptoms [28]. This leads to spiraling of the esophagus, causing a mechanical obstruction for up-coming stomach content. In some cases, the side-effects of such an operation are the shrinkage of the stomach size and reduction of food capacity, leading to longer meal-time durations. Since individuals with RS are usually slow eaters, this will probably go unnoticed.

Gastro-intestinal problems

Gastro-intestinal problems have an effect on swallowing and on eating speed. For example, reflux and the slow emptying of the stomach will extend meal-times. Chronic reflux might cause ulcers, bleeding and pain during meal-times, thereby affecting esophagus/respiratory timing, which will, in turn, have a jeopardizing effect on the individual's health. The slow emptying of stomach content, if later accompanied by lying down, will probably lead to reflux and later might be observed as the individual's refusal to be fed. The slow emptying of the stomach, caused by the hypoactive para-sympathetic system [29], is commonly accompanied by constipation problems and/or fecal intestinal blockage (two well-known manifestations of the digestive systems of individuals with Rett syndrome).

It is obvious that due to the complexity of the oral-esophageal challenges presented by individuals with RS, a thorough evaluation and intervention should be applied by a multi-disciplinary team. Such a multi-professional approach can take into account all the possible difficulties and will address them with an holistic approach. In some cases, surgical intervention is required, although in many cases better posture or more appropriate handling during meal times may positively influence the eating abilities of the individual with RS. That said, appropriate intervention in respect to feeding will be discussed within the chapter dealing with feeding and is beyond the scope of the present chapter, which will focus on nutrition.

BMI (Body Mass Index) is a value calculated from an individual's height and weight (kg/m2). It is used as a rough guide to nutritional status [30]. It has been found that individuals with RS show average BMI measurements of 17.5 [7], when the normative healthy findings in the population should be around a BMI of 21-26 [31]. As individuals with RS are so slim and of small stature, any digestive problem can easily cause a rapid deterioration in weight, leading to failure to thrive (FTT).

Failure to thrive (FTT)

FTT is diagnosed in about 85%-90% of individuals with RS and the situation has been found to worsen with increased age [18,32]. This may be due to the fact that individuals with RS receive a daily caloric intake of 66.9% of the normative daily caloric intake [33]. FTT is a symptom, not a sickness per se, with distinct criteria. It seems that individuals with RS are in such poor nutritional condition, that 85% of them fall within the category of "moderate to severe malnutrition" [34]. Malnutrition subjects the respiratory muscles to catabolism, leading to atrophy, weakness, reduced lung-function [35], increasing bacterial colonization of the airways and reduced resistance to infection [36].

This condition may be present despite lengthy meals. Due to the severity of the situation and the functional implications of malnutrition, it is important that a close-eye should be kept on the growth rates of the individual with RS and any noted decline from the norm should be presented to the gastroenterologist/dietitian/child neurologist. Joint input from dietician and speech therapist is essential, implementing appropriate feeding modification and supplements for some individuals, while others require naso-gastric feeding; if this condition persists for long periods, the implementation of a gastrostomy (GIT) is usually advocated [28]. It has been found that in regard to the norm, individuals with RS present a slightly reduced absorption rate of nutrients. Even so, this slight cutback in absorption, combined with a steady reduction in caloric intake, together with the individual's difficulty in reporting her hunger [11], eventually might lead to a constant untreated state of malnutrition [11,18].

The conventional management of FTT is the introduction of supplementary high-caloric intake. Increase in caloric intake is essential for individuals with RS who may suffer from malnutrition and is strongly recommended since it has been found to enhance their resilience to external infections, extend attention-span during educational experiences, reduce agitation and enhance the individual's physical activity (the participants were more active, trying to crawl and walk) [9,10]. One should seek out the advice of a dietitian in order to build a proper diet for the individual with RS and monitor its effects. In order to enhance caloric intake, one may try a high caloric, high fat, low volume diet which follows the guidelines below:

- Increased caloric intake by introducing mostly high-fat yet low-cholesterol food items. Neutral high-caloric ingredients include: Raw Tahina, Avocado
- Avoid food items that contain high- sugar ingredients which may lead to dental decay.
- Include vitamins and minerals to enhance general health
- Include additional meals each day (3 main meals + 3 interim meals)
- Serve as many and as much of the food items of which the individual with RS is extremely fond
- If a food item which the individual with RS likes is a foodstuff which may harm the dental system (such as chocolate or cola), an oral hygiene program should be implemented simultaneously with the new diet
- Decrease fluid intake during meal times
- Restrict the intake of juices, especially fruit juices
- Suggest mainly high-caloric liquids (e.g. Osmolite, Ensure)
- Add high-fat sauces with each meal
- During cooked meals fried food items (such as French fries, Schnitzels/chicken patties, fried eggplants) might be suggested [8].

Recommended food items are: avocado, sausages, butter, meat, whipped cream, margarine, steaks, cream, sour cream, peanut butter, mayonnaise, cream cheese, fish oil, whole yogurt and French fries. If the diet is ineffective and the individual with RS continues to show poor nutritional condition, there may be a need for a percutaneus endoscopic gastrostomy (PEG), (i.e. the surgical procedure to insert a Gastro-Intestinal tube (GI tube).

Percutaneus endoscopic gastrostomy (PEG)/gastro intestinal tube (GI tube)

Feeding through a PEG is an invasive method, which uses a special tube inserted directly through the abdominal wall into the stomach. The tube is inserted following a surgical or an endoscopical procedure. This method is regarded as extremely safe, presenting low risk to the patient, and enables the implementation of a long term proper dietetic management. The PEG is held in place by a balloon inflated after the insertion of the tube inside the stomach. All the PEG systems used today are equipped with a series of uni-directional valves, enabling excess pressure to be released in order to prevent it from building up in the client's stomach, causing reflux. This mechanism is extremely valuable if the person with RS is bloating. The efficiency of the PEG can be initially tested via the use of naso-gastric feeding. Such an experiment will enable evaluation of tube feeding without the need for a surgical procedure. Reasons for using a PEG may be:

- Prevention of aspiration and recurrent lung inflammations
- Prevention of, or improvement in a state of malnutrition (in case this change cannot be achieved through oral feeding) and its consequences (chronic weight loss and recurrent hospitalizations)
- Prevention of dehydration due to multiple vomiting
- Prevention of reflux, thereby preventing its consequences (heartburn, pain and a threat to the integrity of the esophagus)
- Enabling the easy and precise insertion of different medications, thereby simplifying the monitoring of the medical condition of the individual with RS (including such symptoms as constipation, epilepsy)
- Preventing the inconvenience of vomiting
- Changing meal-times to purely pleasurable quality time
- Reducing the time spent on feeding, and using the extra time to achieve other therapeutic goals (e.g. educational or motor activities)
- Simplifying the work of the care-givers
- Enabling the exact monitoring of caloric intake of the individual with RS
- Enabling extra time for the family of the individual with RS, when time-consuming elements are added to the familial frame (e.g a new job or baby)
- Replacement of food additives and food supplements that were found ineffective in achieving their dietetic purpose
- Preventing challenging behavior that may have developed during long periods of rejection of food and liquids.

The insertion of a PEG is a joint decision by the medical staff and the guardians of the individual with RS. Reilly & Cass [18] have constructed a simplified decision-making flowchart, which will help the family in deciding on the proper course of action.

The surgical procedure for the insertion of the GIT is short and easily performed. Following this procedure, there is a constant need to clean the area around the GIT to prevent infections and inflammations. Within the weeks following the operation, excessive gas production is a common side-effect that spontaneously disappears. The daily management of the tube is relatively easy, necessitating the cleaning of the inner and outer walls of the tube with water. There is unanimous agreement as to the success of this procedure, by all parents of individuals with RS who have completed it. Within the Australian RS population, 12.5% of individuals with RS use such a device [7]. There is a variety of GIT "off the shelf" supplements, answering to the nutritional needs of all clients; most of them are available in liquid form. These supplements are recommended, since they are sterile and their nutritional composition and caloric value are known. It is possible on the other hand, to use ground food, which has more emotional and social advantages, although its drawback lies in the fact that it may be infected or present a non-unified texture [37]

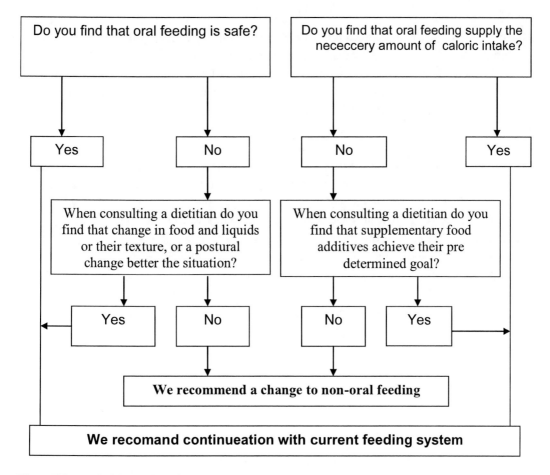

Figure VII-1. A decision-making flowchart to help the family decide on implementation of gastro-intestinal feeding [18].

Constipation

Constipation has been defined as a delay or a difficulty in defecation, present for two or more days, sufficient enough to cause significant distress to the patient [38]. This condition is responsible for an estimated 3 to 5 percent of physician-visits by children[39]. Leonard [7] reports that the most common digestive problem presented by individuals with RS is constipation, affecting almost two-thirds of the Australian RS population. Saavedra, on the other hand, reports that constipation affects 85% of individuals with RS, occurring at least once in their life-span [40].

Reilly and Cass [18] suspected that constipation in individuals with RS was caused by several problems, such as: lack of physical activity, low muscle-tone, diet, medication, small quantities of liquid intake and scoliosis. Constipation may be identified even as early as the child's first-second year of life. Hard, large and rare defecations are usually common in this population and they tend to worsen with time, if left untreated. Besides the findings relating to the under-active para-sympathetic system [12,41], no primary pathological or physiological factors were detected within the neural and muscular structures of the intestines of individuals with RS, and defecation reflexes were normally elicited [40].

Since individuals with RS do not present serious organic anatomical or physiological causes for constipation, their constipation can be referred to as functional constipation (see explanation below). This means that the appearance of constipation may be aggravated by the behavioral reaction of the individual suffering from it. It has been found that approximately 50% of constipated children contract, rather than relax the external sphincter complex during a defecation attempt [42]. If the individual with RS is to react in the same way and does not wish to defecate, she may tighten the external anal sphincter and squeeze the glutei muscles. These actions can push feces higher up inside the rectal vault and reduce the urge to defecate. If the individual with RS frequently avoids defecating, the rectum eventually stretches to accommodate the retained fecal mass and the propulsive power of the rectum is diminished. The longer feces remain in the rectum, the harder they become. Passage of a hard or large stool may cause a painful anal fissure. The cycle of avoiding bowel movements because of a fear of painful defecation may progress to stool retention and infrequent bowel movements, a condition that is termed "functional constipation" [39].

Luckily, early intervention may improve the chances for complete resolution of functional constipation [43]. Treatment goals include dis-impacting the rectum and then maintaining a regular bowel-movement routine. Months of treatment may be necessary before maintenance medications can be diminished[39]. An individual anti-constipation solution should be adapted by a dietitian to every individual with RS suffering from constipation, taking into account her age, type of constipation, medical history and food preferences. Immediate solutions to prevent constipation may be:

- Applying a high-fiber diet, using food sources such as whole-wheat, cereal, breads, pasta, fruits and vegetables (preferably fresh and with its skin). Preferred fruits are plums, pears, peaches, apricots and dried fruits. In regard to dry food items, the use of beans, peas, bran and oats (e.g. popcorn, nuts and different kind of seeds) as a source for a high-fiber diet is sometimes recommended for the general population, yet the authors believe that the use of these food items might be hazardous due to the known eating and swallowing problems characteristic of this population [18, 20] and therefore they should be avoided by individuals with RS.
- Consuming large volumes of liquids: about 8-10 glasses per day (including soup and water-based drinks). In order to achieve the recommended volumes of liquids, it is advisable to insert a regular curriculum of drinking during but mostly in-between meals.

A rough calculation can be done in the following manner: If the individual's weight is below 23kg (50 lbs), then the multiplication of her weight by 125 = minimal daily liquid demand. If the individual's weight is above 23kg (50 lbs), then the multiplication of her weight by 85 = minimal daily liquid demand. Every liquid under room-temperature is accountable as drinking (ice-cream, yoghurt and sour milk). Important factors which should be considered as well are:

Table VII-1. Recommended water requirements per age and weight

Age	Optimal quantity		Weight of the person		# of cups per day
	In OZ	In CC	Libras	Kg.	
1-3	54	1625	29	13	6.75
4-6	71	2125	44	20	8.75
7-10	80	2400	62	28	10
11+	84	2520	101	46	10.5

- Physical activity promotes regular bowel movement and should therefore be a part of an anti-constipation régime.
- A gentle abdominal massage is a simple way to enhance bowel movement and ease abdominal aches and should be considered as one of the primary solutions [18].
- A warm bath sometimes helps, by relaxing the tight anal muscles and reducing pain around this area, thereby encouraging defecation [44].
- Paraffin oil might be used in conjunction with the previous suggestions (when taking in to account the fact that paraffin oil reduces the effectiveness of the intestines absorption capability).
- Food items that are known for their ability to promote constipation (apple sauce, white rice, cooked carrots, etc.) should be avoided.
- The regular use of laxatives should only be applied under the guidance of a physician and is usually not recommended as it could lead to slowing down of intestine activity, thereby attributing to a need for a gradual increase in dosage leading to total dependency [8].

In order to keep track of the bowel movements of the person with RS, to enable continuous and healthy bowel movements and to prevent painful constipation, a defecation chart, completed by the residential and educational facility of the individual, is recommended [45]. The chart, should show the following steps being taken, as shown in table VII-2.

Table VII-2. Management of daily bowel movement in RS

Number of days	Day count	Action
A day with defecation	Day 0	-------------
Next day - no defecation	Day 1	-------------
Next day - no defecation	Day 2	Mineral oil
Next day - no defecation	Day 3	laxatives, preferably natural laxatives such as Metamucil, Fiberall/konsy/Senokot
Next day - no defecation	Day 4	Enema

A day with defecation resets the counts back to day 0. Some dietitians recommend that the use of laxatives and enema should be delayed. Therefore, they might suggest a sequence as per: Days 2+3 - the use of mineral oil, day 4 – laxatives and day 5 - enema. When in doubt as to which anti constipation régime to follow, we suggest that you refer to the child's discomfort as your guide.

Home-made recipes

As part of the research for this chapter, we screened some old correspondence that went over the RettNet a few years ago and we gathered some home-made recipes which were suggested by parents of individuals with RS and have been found to work. One should bear in mind that even when applying these home-made solutions, the advice of a dietitian should be sought. Also important is always to start with only few changes, introducing one new item at the time and to advance slowly while closely supervising the reaction of the child:

- At least one defecation a day was achieved through the use of the following daily recipe: oats with butter and brown sugar (added liquids are mandatory), baby prunes, canned pears, green beans and prune juice [46]
- A daily dose of the following recipe was recommended (along with physical activity) to help regular bowel movements: A teaspoon of Mylanta (an anti-gas ingredient), Simethicone (prevents stomach acidity), A large teaspoon of Metamucil or similar fiber in orange- squash served in a large glass of water. Constant stirring is necessary while the person with RS drinks, to prevent the fibers from settling in the bottom of the glass [47]
- A particular person with RS has been constipation-free for two years, ever since she started the following diet and after trying many other solutions, as a result of drinking a cup of the suggested recipe daily: One cup of fiber, one cup of cereal, 12 oz. apple juice, 8 oz. pitted prunes, two cups of apple-sauce and one cup of yogurt. Soak the cereal and prunes in the apple-juice until they become soft. Process in a food-processor until the mixture becomes a purée; add the apple-sauce and mix (the reader should pay attention to the fact that apple-sauce, a known constipation enhancer, is a major component of the above-mentioned recipe) [48].
- A particular person with RS presenting severe constipation at a young age has been on a macrobiotic diet, which, basically, means no dairy products, no red meat, no sugar or salt, no citrus or tropical fruit and no white (processed) flour. The implementation of the diet has been going on for 15 years, with only seldom episodes of constipation and without the use of any medications [49].
- A milder solution was adopted by a family that reported that they could not get their child with RS to drink enough water, making it problematic to add fibers into her diet. This family is using something called "liquid calcium-magnesium". Each morning, the child in question received a teaspoon of this medication with breakfast [50]. The medication was cleared by the child's physician, yet, due to the impact of magnesium on the heart and the known cardiac irregularities of individuals with RS [51], a consultation with a physician familiar with RS is justified, before commencing the use of the above-mentioned medication.
- Ortisan fruit cubes were also suggested as a great natural way to promote bowel movement. Half a cube is added to the child diet after one day without defecation.

Warnings

Fibers can assist regular daily defecation when presented with water, but if they are given without enough water, they become the worst bowel-blockers. Therefore, their use and dosage should be the subject of consultation with a dietitian and supervision of water quantities consumed by the individual with RS should also be undertaken.

Prunes are natural laxatives and help in the achievement of regular bowel movements, but their active ingredients may cause dependency as much as any medication. Therefore, constant use of prunes should not be pursued as a first option

In patients unresponsive or intolerant to fibers, both osmotic and stimulant laxatives are effective, but the latter must be avoided for long-term use, as they have the potential for adverse effects [52]

An enema can help the individual with RS, as well as her family, to avoid hours and days of suffering from the effects of constipation and bowel impaction, but it does cause dependency by the intestines and, therefore, should not be used too often, if possible

If the individual with RS is on different medication for long periods, especially antibiotic medication, the natural intestine bacteria are destroyed, in which case, the artificial insertion of these bacteria (Acidophilus and Bifidus) is recommended to enhance proper bowel work and nutritional absorption

Some pain-killers (such as morphine or codeine and other medication) cause reduction in bowel movements so therefore the use of such drugs should be avoided. Consultation with a physician familiar with RS is advised, when initiating new medication.

If constipation is not regularly and successfully treated, it may deteriorate into a bowel impaction. Therefore, if recurrent episodes of constipation are present, consultation with a gastroenterologist is highly recommended.

Bowel impaction

When constipation becomes severe, fecal impaction can result with a mass of compressed feces in the rectum and/or sigmoid colon. Standard treatments include various combinations of oral laxatives and enemas and, when or if these fail, manual evacuation is warranted. The symptoms of bowel impaction are:

- Sudden and severe abdominal tension
- Vomiting of gallbladder juices (green or yellow in color)
- Appearance of constant non-relenting pain and discomfort
- Reduction in defecation (if constipation was not present beforehand)
- Diarrhea of bloody excrement

All the above-mentioned symptoms require immediate medical intervention [40]. Your physician may suggest differing intervention approaches for these conditions, but some conventional techniques include:

- Daily treatment of PEG electrolyte solution, given orally at a dose of one liter daily for up to three days. This method is considered to be a highly effective and acceptable treatment for fecal impaction. This treatment was found to be effective for patients presenting a wide age-range and with differing functional and ambulatory states. The stools which passed through patients after treatment were generally of large volume and soft, and most patients (Not with RS) graded the act of defecation as being easy [53]. Absence of the need to strain at stool can be an important positive safety aspect, particularly in patients who will not voluntarily assist the clearance of stools, such as individuals with RS
- Severe constipation or fecal impaction can be resolved through an iso-osmotic laxative, such as Movicol [54], taken orally
- Pulsed irrigation-enhanced evacuation has been found to be a simple, quick, and effective treatment for severe fecal impaction [55].

Additional factors

An additional factor which should be taken into consideration is that 87% of individuals with RS have been found to have decreased bone calcium and mineral density [18,56]. Osteoporosis has been reported in very young girls and patients with RS due to decreased bone mineral density, compared to controls [57]. This finding puts the individual with RS at risk of suffering pathological fractures, due to osteoporosis [57]. It is assumed that this phenomenon results from poor bone formation. It supports the need for routine checks of bone density of individuals with RS since childhood, and the commencement of physical activity (such as intensive standing and walking programs [58]) and nutritional and medical intervention, when the situation necessitates such courses of action.

In few individuals with RS, there seems to be a tendency to over-weight [34]. These individuals should be referred to a dietitian and treated appropriately to achieve weight-loss, to prevent functional deterioration due to over-weight.

Conclusions

The sound state of the digestive system of individuals with RS has a significant effect upon the wellbeing and quality of life of the client herself, as well as on that of her care-givers. Moreover, it has been found that 43% of individuals suffering from feeding and digestive problems similar to those presented by individuals with RS, are prone to suffer from irritable bowel syndrome (IBS), which aggravates the digestive system [59].

Most individuals with RS have very healthy appetites and according to our experience, when compared to their peers, do not normally have unusual nutritional demands. Nevertheless, the array of challenges presented by the gastro-intestinal system of individuals with RS necessitates constant supervision by a multi-professional team, including a gastroenterologist and a dietitian, while regularly:

- receiving nutritional evaluations
- performing feeding assessments
- repeating instructions for care-givers, regarding proper nutritional care.

Sometimes, the nutritional regime necessity to enhance the weight of the individual with RS may consume many hours of the day and contradict with her need to maintain an active anti-osteoporotic régime or with the need to prevent constipation and bowel impaction. Such contradictions should be acknowledged and resolved by the dietitian. Due to the fact that individuals with RS usually lack the ability to specifically pinpoint their level and location of suffering, it is imperative that constant regular care be given to the digestive system of this population.

References

[1]   Amir RE, Van den Bellver IB, Wan M, Tran CQ, Francke U. Zoghbi HY. Rett syndrome is caused by mutations in X-linked MECP2, encoding methyl-CpG-binding protein 2. Nat Genet 1999;23(2):185-8.

[2]   Amir RE, Van Den Veyve IB, Schultz R, Malicki DM, Tran CQ, et al. Influence of mutation type and X chromosome inactivation on Rett syndrome phenotypes. Ann Neurol 2000;47:670-9.

[3]   Hagberg B. Rett syndrome: Clinical and biological aspects. London: Mac Keith Press, 1993.

[4]   Lotan M. Management for Rett syndrome. Graphi-soft; The Israeli Rett syndrome Center, Tel-Aviv, Israel, 2006. [Hebrew]

[5]   Kerr AM, Julu PO. Recent insights into hyperventilation from the study of Rett syndrome. Arch Dis Child 1999;80:384-7.

[6]   Casas MJ, Kenny DJ, McPherson KA. Swallowing/ventilation interactions during oral swallow in normal children and children with cerebral palsy. Dysphagia 1994;9:40–6.

[7]   Leonard S. The Australian Rett syndrome study inaugural report. Aust: Telethon Inst Child Health Res, 2002.

[8]   Rice M. Nutrition care guidelines for Rett syndrome. La Jolla, CA: Neurometab Clinic, Dept Pediatrics, Univ California, 1989.

[9]   Motil K. Gastrointestinal concerns. Presentation, IRSA 12th Ann Conf, Boston, MA, 1996 May 24-27, tape 622-19.

[10]   Motil K. Nutrition and weight management. Presentation, IRSA 12th Ann Conf, Boston, MA, 1996 May 24-27, tape 622-11.

[11]   Motil KJ, Schultz R, Brown B, Glaze DG, Percy AK. Altered energy balance may account for growth failure in Rett syndrome. J Child Neurol 1994;9:315-9.

[12]   Julu PO. Autonomic dysfunction and aspects of pharmacological treatment. Presentation, Int Course Rett Syndr, Ostersund, Sweden, 2003 Jun 16-18.

[13]   Kerr AM. The future for Rett syndrome girls. Int Rett Syndr Assoc Newsletter 1992:13-4.

[14]   Sponseller P. Orthopedic update in Rett syndrome. Rett Gazette 2004; 1:4-5.

[15]   Lotan M, Merrick J, Carmeli E. Scoliosis management in Rett syndrome –A case study. Scientific World Journal 2005;5:264-73.

[16]   Cass H, Reilly S, Owen L, Wisbeach A, Weekes L, Slonims V, Wigram T, Charman T. Findings from a multidisciplinary clinical case series of females with Rett syndrome. Dev Med Child Neurol 2003;45(5): 325-37.

[17]   Krick J, Murphy PE, Markham JF, Shapiro. A proposed formula for calculating energy needs of children with cerebral palsy. Dev Med Child Neurol 1992;34:481-7.

[18]   Reilly S, Cass H. Growth and nutrition in Rett syndrome. Disabil Rehabil 2001;23:118-28.

[19]   Morton RE, Pinnington L, Ellis RE. Air swallowing in Rett syndrome. Dev Med Child Neurol 2000;42:271-5.

[20]   Budden SS. Management of Rett syndrome: A ten-year experience. Neuropediatrics 1995;26(2):75-7.

[21]   Lindberg B. Understanding Rett syndrome: A practice guide for parents, teachers and therapists. Toronto: Hognefe Huber, 1991.

[22]   Arvedson J, Rogers B, Buck G, Smart P, Msall M. Silent aspiration prominent in children with dysphagia. Int J Pediatr Otorhino laryngol 1994;28:173–81.

[23]   Rogers B, Stratton P, Msall M, Andres M, Champlain MK, Koerner P, Piazza J. Long-term morbidity and management strategies of tracheal aspiration in adults with severe developmental disabilities. Am J Ment Retard 1994;98:490–8.

[24]   Mount RH, Hastings RP, Reilly S, Cass H, Charman T. Behavioral and emotional features in Rett syndrome. Disabil Rehabil 2001;23;129-38.

[25]   Elian M, Rudolf ND. EEG and respiration in Rett syndrome. Acta Neurol Scand 1991;83:123-8.

[26]   Mirrett PL, Riski JE, Glascott J. Videofluoroscopic assessment of dysphagia in children with severe spastic cerebral palsy. Dysphagia 1994;9:174–9.

[27]   Wilson JR. The non-chew cookbook. Glenwood Springs, CO: Wilson, 1985.

[28]   Seddon PC, Khan Y. Respiratory problems in children with neurological impairment. Arch Dis Child 2003;88:75-8.

[29]   Engerstrom IW, Kerr A. Workshop on autonomic function in Rett syndrome. Swedish Rett Center, Fröson, Sweden. Brain Dev 1998;20:323-36.

[30]   Dietz WH, Bellizzi MC. Introduction: the use of body mass index to assess obesity in children. Am J Clin Nut 1999;70(1):123S-5S.

[31]   Baumgartner RN, Heymsfield SB, Roche AF. Human body composition and the epidemiology of chronic disease. Obes Res 1995;3(1): 73-95.

[32]   Ellaway C, Christodoulou J. Rett syndrome: Clinical characteristics and recent genetic advances. Disabil Rehabil 2001;23:98-106.

[33]   Thommessen M, Kase BF, Heiberg A. Growth and nutrition in ten girls with Rett syndrome. Acta Pediatrica 1992;81:686-9.

[34]   Hunter K. The Rett syndrome handbook. Washington, DC: Int Rett Syndr Assoc, 1999.

[35]   Sullivan PB, Rosenbloom L. Feeding the disabled child. London: Clin Dev Med, 1999.

[36]   Martin TR. The relationship between malnutrition and lung infections. Clin Chest Med 1987;8:359

[37]   Shetel Z, Arbel N, Nitzan-Kaloski D. Instructions for gastrointestinal feeding: methods, emulsions, and possible complications. Ministry of Health, Public Health Services, Food & Nutrition Services, Central Office, state of Israel, 2003. [Hebrew]. Extracted 29 October, 2006 from site: http://www.health.gov.il/download/pages/pium_kiva.doc

[38]   Baker SS, Liptak GS, Colletti RB, Croffie JM, Di Lorenzo C, Ector W. Constipation in infants and children: evaluation and treatment. A medical position statement of the North American Society for Pediatric Gastroenterology and Nutrition. J Pediatr Gastroenterol Nutr 1999;29:612-26

[39]   Biggs W, Dery WH. Evaluation and treatment of constipation in infants and children. Am Fam Physician 2006;73(3):469-77

[40]   Saavedra JM. Gastrointestinal crisis in Rett syndrome. Int Rett Syndr Assoc Newsletter 1997; Winter:3-5.

[41]   Witt-Engerstrom IW. Autonomic monitoring in Rett syndrome at the Swedish Rett Center, Froson. Fort Washington, MD: Handout, 2001.

[42]   van Ginkel R, Büller HA, Boeckxstaens GE, van der Plas RN, Taminiau AAJM, Benninga MA. The effect of anorectal manometry on the outcome of treatment in severe childhood constipation: A randomized, controlled trial. Pediatrics 2001;108(1):9.

[43]   McGrath ML, Mellon MW, Murphy L. Empirically supported treatments in pediatric psychology: constipation and encopresis. J Pediatr Psychol 2000;25:225-54.

[44]   International Rett Syndrome Association. Parent idea book. Fort Washington, MD: Int Rett Syndr Assoc, undated.

[45]   Personal communication I. Bowel impaction. RettNett, 1996 Dec 20, saw17@whidbey.net.

[46]   Personal communication II. Response to constipation. RettNett, 1997 Jan 18, CAlbrit155@aol.com

[47]   Personal communication III. Constipation. RettNett, 1997 Feb 04, cloudy@mailnwlink.com

[48]   Personal communication IV. Constipation. RettNett, 1996 Oct 21, reece@northweb.com

[49]   Personal communication V. Medication. RettNett, 1997 Jan 17, CURTIN1@ aol.com

[50]   Personal communication VI. Constipation. RettNett, 1997 Feb 09, InHisGrip6@ aol.com

[51]   Sekul EA, Moak JP, Schultz RJ, Glaze DG, Dunn KJ, Percy AK. Electrocardiographic findings in Rett syndrome: An explanation for sudden death. J Pediatr 1994;125:80-2.

[52]   Thompson WG. Laxatives: Clinical pharmacology and practical use. Drugs 19880;19:49-58

[53]   Culbert P, Gillett H, Ferguson A. Highly effective new oral therapy for faecal impaction. Br J Gen Pract 1998;48(434):1599–1600.

[54]   Ungar A. Movicol in treatment of constipation and faecal impaction Hosp Med 2000;61(1):37-40.

[55]   Kokoszka J, Nelson R, Falconio M, Abcarian H. Treatment of fecal impaction with pulsed irrigation enhanced evacuation. Dis Colon Rectum 1994;37(2):161-4.

[56]   Haas RH, Dixon SD, Sartoris DJ, Hennessy MJ. Osteopenia in Rett syndrome. J Pediatr 1997;131(5):771-4.

[57]   Budden SS, Gunness ME. Bone histomorphometry in three females with Rett syndrome. Brain Dev 2001;23:S133-S7.

[58]   Weeks L. Rett syndrome. Presentation, Sydney, Aust, February, 1997.

[59]   Locke RG, Ashok AK. Some indigestion or irritable bowel sufferers likely to have both ailments. Presenattion, 68th Ann Sci Meet Am Coll Gastroenterol, Baltimore, MD, 2003 Oct 12-15.

In: Rett Syndrome: Therapeutic Interventions
Editors: Meir Lotan and Joav Merrick

ISBN: 978-1-61728-080-1
©2011 Nova Science Publishers, Inc.

Chapter VIII

Rett Syndrome: The Use of Augmentative Communication Strategies to Enhance Communication

Judy Wine, DSPA, EdD[*]

Israel Rett Center, National Evaluation Team, Chaim Sheba Medical Center,
Tel HaShomer, Ramat Gan, Israel

This chapter will discuss the communication abilities and intervention possibilities of girls with RS, based on the author's experience (over the past 17 years) in both clinically intervening with this population and serving as the speech language pathologist on the transdisciplinary clinical assessment team of the Israel Rett Syndrome national center (having evaluated over 130 individuals with RS to date). Special emphasis will be given to intervention using Augmentative and Alternative Communication (AAC) strategies. The final part of the chapter will describe C, a client with RS who has developed remarkable communication skills, despite an initial diagnosis of severe cognitive disability.

Introduction

Rett syndrome (RS) is a neuro-developmental disorder, in which the age of onset is typically between 6 and 18 months [1]. In the past it was believed that RS occurs in females only; it is now known that it occurs to a much lesser extent in males as well. The explanation appears to be that the severity of the disorder is much greater in males, thus causing most of them to perish in utero. For the purpose of this discussion we will refer to "girls" with RS, with the acknowledged awareness that it is not an exclusively female disorder.

---

* Correspondence: Judy Wine, DSPA, EdD, POBox 40012, IL-90805 Mevasseret Zion, Israel. E-mail: judywine@ gmail.com

One of the main characteristics of RS is a lack of speech, caused by severe developmental dyspraxia [2,3] together with a strong hypotonic element, particularly evident during the first few years of life [4]. Many girls for whom the onset of the syndrome occurred after they had reached 12 to 14 months of age are reported to have started to speak in single words or, in some cases, even in full short sentences prior to onset (personal communication with parents). For these girls the onset of the disorder represents a loss of a skill which was in the process of being acquired. As pointed out by Lindberg [5], since dyspraxia is a difficulty in motor planning which affects the ability to carry out purposeful movements, the lack of speech typical of girls with RS is not actually due to the loss of the skill but rather the lack of ability of knowing how to do it. A fascinating but as yet unexplored area for investigation would be the amount of memory which girls with RS have with regard to their acquired speech skills and early speech experiences.

Between one to four percent of girls with RS [6,7] display an atypical form of RS insofar as they have retained some speech skills. The nature of the speech appears to differ between girls; some talk using single word utterances while others use full sentences to express themselves. One woman over 40 years of age known to the author talks in full sentences but these are frequently not relevant to the situation; another young girl of four years of age appears to use the word "no" at the beginning of each sentence, not to indicate negation but rather as a starter to enable her to begin the utterance. Still another woman over 50 years of age does not speak at all, but is able to sing a large repertoire of songs, including all the words and the correct melody for each song. Needless to say, traditional speech therapy intervention must be undertaken with all girls with RS, with the aim of enabling them to make as much progress as possible in the area of speech production and expression. However the focus of this discussion is that population of girls with RS who are non-speaking for whom we want to find effective strategies to enable communication, while at the same time working on the development of their speech skills, specific to the abilities of each girl.

Hetzroni, Rubin and Konkol [8] demonstrated that girls with RS can learn to choose between three different symbol pictures from the Picture Communication Symbol (PCS) library (Mayer Johnson) through the use of technology. Elefant [9] in her doctoral study, examined the use of music as an enhancer of communication for girls with RS with positive results. Hetzroni and Rubin [10] stressed the importance of eye gaze as a communication access strategy for girls with RS, while Lariviere [11] discussed tools of access as being the key to communication and learning in girls with RS.

Skotko, Koppenhaver and Erickson [12] examined the consequent communication outcomes resulting from the reading behaviors of mothers of girls with RS and concluded that girls with RS can learn to communicate when they are provided with the tools to do so (assistive technology), together with the appropriate support from their mothers. In their discussion these authors stressed the need for mothers to assume competence and attribute meaning to potentially communicative acts on the part of their daughters. Evidence of the validity of this approach lies in the fact that by the end of their study the girls with RS were demonstrating ability to learn and intentionality to communicate.

In working with girls with RS in the area of communication, two guiding principles must be remembered. Firstly, the lack of speech is not indicative of a lack of ability to understand language. One of the most difficult tasks appears to be that of determining the level of language comprehension of girls with RS. A recent research project has demonstrated just how difficult this task can be. In their study, Elati and Gershenowich [13] attempted to assess the language comprehension of girls with RS between the ages of six and eight years. Seven girls with RS, all non-speaking, from unilingual (Hebrew-speaking) homes, were included in their study. The researchers selected sections of the PLS-3 language assessment tool which focus on language comprehension and adapted these sections to be accessible by either gross hand pointing or eye gaze. All seven girls had an opportunity to interact with the assessors for a short period ranging from five to twenty minutes prior to the assessment session(s). The results of this study indicated a huge discrepancy between the abilities of the girls to perform under assessment conditions; one girl was unable to complete the screening test while another succeeded on all ten sections. The other five girls were able to complete from two to four sections of the protocol. Important to note is the number of sessions which it took the girls to complete the testing; these ranged from two to four sessions, due to factors such as slow response time, short attention span, and fatigue. The researchers concluded that due to the small number of subjects, the wide range of scores, and the non-standardized situation under which the assessments were conducted, this work should be regarded as a pilot study, to be expanded and continued in the future.

However, daily contact with girls with RS indicates that they do understand language – different girls have different levels of language comprehension depending on their level of ability. They continuously give signs of their comprehension through their body, facial, vocal, and emotional reactions – through their sense of humor, their attention to what is going on around them, their eye contact, laughter, anger, crying, etc. For those girls who are already using augmentative and alternative communication (AAC) systems, their responses to questions and situations using their various AAC strategies indicate that they have understood what is being said and being asked of them. For example, M a 20 year old young woman, composed a letter to one of her communication assistants congratulating her on her up-coming marriage and telling her how much she will miss her when she takes time off for her wedding. Another example is of C, a 7 year old, who is able to answer questions relating to the content of a story that has been read to her, indicating that the boy is sad because his balloon has burst. Or N, a 4 year old, who used her ability to indicate her choice from between three different picture possibilities to tell her mother that she wants her to bring her a doll when she goes on a holiday. Lastly there is the example of H, who comes from a Hebrew speaking background, but who has begun to learn English in school. She has recently displayed the ability to correctly answer questions in English when a choice of flashcards with possible answers are placed in front of her; similarly she is able to correctly select the answer to complex arithmetic questions (i.e. multiplication of three digit numbers x three digit numbers) from a choice of three or four possible answers presented on flashcards.

The second principle relates to the fact that just because a person (a girl with RS or anyone else) is unable to express herself through speech does not mean that she does not have a need or a desire to communicate. In fact, repeated contact with girls with RS shows that they have a rich inner world, and a strong need and desire to communicate. They frequently use natural communication strategies as their means of interacting; as indicated above these include vocalizations, laughter, crying, eye gaze, facial expression, and hand and body movement. Several studies have looked at the intentionality and patterns of communication in girls with RS [10,12-18] with varying results. Overall there appears to be a consensus that girls with RS demonstrate some level of communicative intent through the use of a variety of nonverbal strategies. In our interactions with girls with RS it is essential that these strategies be recognized and acknowledged at all times. If a girl shows with her eyes that she is indicating a "yes" response, then we must acknowledge what she has told us, for example by saying "great, I see you want to eat now, so let's eat" or something similar, specific to the situation at hand. It is also essential that everyone interacting with the girl understands the signal that she is giving in the same way. Take, for example, the girl who would suddenly stand up during mealtime. The staff in her classroom interpreted this behavior as meaning that she had had enough to eat – and acted accordingly - while her family interpreted it as meaning that she had to go to the toilet - and also acted accordingly. How confusing for the girl!

Table VIII-1. _xxxx 's Personal Communication Dictionary
Prepared by (names of family members, caregivers, staff, etc who were involved)
Date of preparation: Date of update: _____

What I do	What I mean	What you should do
Stand up during mealtime	I need to go to the toilet	Take me to the toilet, accompanied by verbal input "good, you told me you need to go to the toilet, lets go"
Turn my head to the left	I have had enough	Stop the activity, accompanied by verbal input "you are telling me that you have had enough – okay we will stop"
		OR say: I see you are telling me that you have had enough –but we need to continue, we will stop in a short while"
Etc.		

Frequently, the first step in developing a communication program for a girl with RS is the preparation of a personal communication dictionary. A personal communication dictionary is a document that helps to outline the ways in which an individual communicates. This is important for people who don't communicate using speech. For people who are non-speaking it is important that their communication partners recognize and understand their communication behaviors. A communication dictionary can help to ensure that all family members, classroom staff, and anyone else interacting with the girl with RS are aware of her communication behaviors and agree on how to respond. It assists communication partners to respond in a predictable manner so that any and all communication attempts are understood and responded to appropriately. To create a personal communication dictionary, people who know the girl well need to observe and describe her behaviors, determine what these behaviors mean, and then agree on an appropriate response [19]. It is important that all the persons involved come to an agreement as to the meaning of each behavior, as often these communication behaviors are interpreted differently by different people.. As an example, the use of a personal dictionary would have ensured that the situation described above where the girl's communication attempts were interpreted differently by her family and her classroom staff would not have occurred; as a basic premise preparation and use of the dictionary would have required open channels of communication between school and home. It is best for the personal communication dictionary to be prepared as a large wall poster, so that it can be hung prominently in one or more places which the girl frequents i.e. a girl with RS will likely have at least two copies of her dictionary, one to be hung in a prominent place at home and the other in her classroom. A personal communication dictionary might look like

Personal communication dictionaries need to be regularly reviewed and updated as an individual's communication behaviors can change. They also need to include the person's name, the date it was created, and by whom it was created.

Aided communication

As with all persons, these informal communication strategies are not enough to enable the girl with RS to express everything she might want to say – to tell what happened at school, to ask a question, to say what is hurting, to express emotion, etc. It is thus necessary to identify additional communication strategies which will enable a full range of communicative possibilities, depending on the needs and abilities of each specific girl. The field of augmentative and alternative communication (AAC) provides the strategies for communicative expression which are so essential for girls with RS, to enable social participation, interpersonal interaction, language and cognitive development, development of feelings of self-worth and confidence, increased motivation and reduced frustration, and a multitude of other possibilities. These aided strategies include communication charts/displays, communication passports, voice output communication aids (VOCAS – also referred to as speech generating devices (SGDs), and computers with communication software.

Communication charts/displays are low tech tools which are made up of objects, pictures, and/or the written word to represent vocabulary items to enable communication. The communication chart should contain vocabulary specifically chosen to meet the girl's specific needs and interests – family and friends, kindergarten/school, work setting, likes and dislikes, feelings, activities, holidays, special events, etc. Most girls with RS indicate what they want to say on their communication charts through the use of eye gaze; for them it is the fastest, motorically easiest, and most accurate way to indicate what they want to say. Some girls do try to point with their hand to what they want to say; it appears that at times this is easier to do than at other times. At those times when hand pointing is effective, we naturally accept what the girl has communicated to us in this way. It should be noted that temporarily holding the less active hand (generally the less dominant one), often enables the girl to point more freely and more accurately with her more active hand. At those times when hand pointing is slow or there is a discrepancy between the eye gaze and the message indicated through hand pointing, a gentle reminder of "let's talk with our eyes" often helps. The method of indicating what one wants to say is referred to as her means of access. It is important to understand that using her eyes as a girl's means of access during communication does not mean that we have given up on hand function, but rather that hand function should be encouraged in other situations. In most instances, the communication chart should be gradually developed, consisting of pages according to topics, with the pages being housed together in some form of ringed binder. Frequently we start with two to four pictures per page, with each picture in a corner of the page so that we can easily follow the eye pointing and thus understand which concept the girl is intending to express. With time the number of pictures per page can generally gradually be increased, according to the girl's ability to deal with a larger number of concepts, taking into account factors related to language, cognition, and means of access. Gradually it will also likely be possible to expand the number of pages and topics in the communication chart. Topics for pages can include:

- family members, including the extended family – grandparents, etc (this will likely need more than one page)
- her classmates
- other important people in her life – therapists, teacher, babysitter, etc
- birthday, and specific holidays
- pages for specific games
- activities that she likes and does not like to do
- activities that she takes part in on a regular basis – playground, physio, occupational and communication therapy, horseback riding, swimming, etc
- places where she likes to go
- feelings
- opinions
- people, places and things that she does NOT like
- speech acts – yes, no, more, enough, etc
- social phrases – hello, goodbye, thanks, wow, yucky, etc
- topics being discussed in class
- special events – a family wedding, etc.
- any other topic area that is specifically relevant for the girl for whom the chart is being constructed

It must be remembered that a communication chart is forever evolving as new vocabulary items are added at all times, based on the new experiences and changes which continually take place in the life of the girl. Figure VIII-1 is an example of a "feelings" page on communication chart.

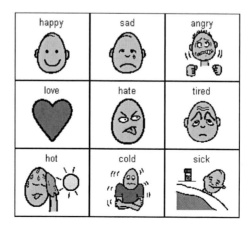

Figure VIII-1. Example of a "feelings" page on communication chart.

Another form of communication display which is being used more and more with girls with RS is what is referred to as a pragmatically organized dynamic display - PODD [20-22]. PODDs are low tech communication charts which are based on the concept of a Windows program on the computer. The choice of a concept on the menu page indicates to what page to turn in order to continue to speak on the selected topic (see figure VIII-2).

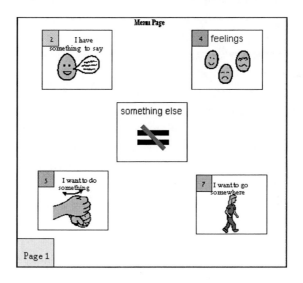

Figure VIII-2. Pragmatically organized dynamic display – an example.

For example, if the girl chooses the concept "I want to go somewhere, included in the square of "I want to go somewhere" on her communication chart will be the number 7 enclosed in an olive green square, which means that we should turn to page 7 (which will say "page 7" with an olive green tab at the bottom) to continue talking on that topic. On page 7 we will find a selection of places to which the child might want to go i.e. shopping mall, playground, grandmother's house, and school (see figure VIII-3).

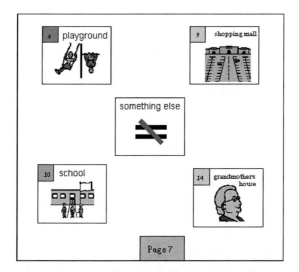

Figure VIII-3. a selection of places to which the child might want to go to.

Each of these items might then also have a number, leading us to another page for further expansion of the topic. Using a PODD enables the girl to have a large and relevant vocabulary while limiting the number of items per page (this could be 4, 6, 10 or whatever number is appropriate for the girl in question),. This approach is particularly suited for girls with RS where the means of selection is through eye gaze, thus necessitating a relatively small number of concepts per page, while at the same time enabling a wide and varied vocabulary to meet their communication needs. Later, as the vocabulary gets larger and more items are included per page (thus making it difficult to rely on eye gaze as the only form of access), a combination of partner assisted visual and auditory scanning can be used to provide the means of access. Partner assisted scanning (PAS) [23] is a method of accessing a low tech communication chart which requires no technology. The person with whom the communicator is communicating (i.e. the communication partner – also sometimes referred to as the listener) identifies, either by naming or pointing or a combination of both, the vocabulary items from which the choice is to be made and waits for the user to indicate (via a sound or a movement) the item he/she wishes to communicate (UWAugCom, http://depts.washington.edu/augcomm/00_general/glossary.htm.)

Communication passports are something like an identification card; their purpose is to provide an introduction about the girl to the people with whom she is interacting. They are used in addition to the communication chart; not in place of it. The communication passport can be in the form of a single page, or, as is more often the case, in the form of a small booklet with attractive and colorful pages arranged according to topic. The passport provides background information about the person, including name, age, and method of communication. It can also include information about the girl's family – with pictures of everyone including the family dog. Creating a passport is a process; it is strongly suggested that it be prepared together with and with input from the girl for whom it is being made. She can decide what she wants to tell about herself and what she does not; she should be entitled to the option of saying "I don't want that in my passport!" The aim of the passport is to present the person as an individual, not as a set of 'problems' or disabilities. It can include pages relating to "Things I like to do", "Things I don't like to do", "my favorite TV programs", "Music I do and don't like to listen to", etc. – all information which will let others who are interacting with the girl know who she is, to provide a basis for communication [24]. Furthermore, if specific instructions need to be given with regard to seating, feeding, medications, the swimming pool, the handling of seizures, etc., they can be included here. Further information on communication passports can be found at http://www. communicationpassports.org.uk/html/introduction.html

Voice output is a powerful tool for persons who are non-speaking as it enables them to be heard by others and makes the communication more concrete for them. Some girls with RS are able to communicate using the computer with voice output; however the greatest number use voice output communication aids (VOCAS – also referred to as speech generating devices SGDs) as their tool for voice output. VOCAS come in a variety of different forms, with differences in their shape, the number of messages they can contain at a given time, the type of speech (digitized versus synthetic), the method of access (direct selection versus scanning), the amount of recorded message time available, the number of levels (different pages of messages) which can be recorded and saved in the device at a given time, etc. Most girls start by using a single message device; these are known by different names depending on the company which manufactures them – BigMack, Clicker, Partner One, etc. They may use either one or two single message devices, depending on the purpose of the communication – a single message device for the purpose of saying a greeting, singing a song, participating in the reading of a story (where the girl can "read" the line that occurs repetitively in the story), relaying information, etc. or two devices for the purpose of "yes" and "no" responses, choice-making, answering questions, etc. Whereas it is possible to use a two message device in these situations, it is often preferable to use two separate single message devices, as it is then possible to determine and control the space between the two, which will enable optimal access for the girl using them. Girls with RS may access these devices by hitting them with their hand; more frequently we see them accessing them through the use of their forehead, chin, or nose. Access using the head is generally much faster and motorically easier for them and is perfectly acceptable; our purpose is communication and to attain this we must use the quickest and most efficient means of access.

Another type of VOCA which is frequently used with girls with RS is a device in which messages can be recorded sequentially (called a Step by Step, Sequencer, etc. again depending on the company of manufacture). Ideas for using a device with sequenced messages include:

- giving instructions in sequence such as in baking a cake,
- making juice, etc.,
- singing interactively (taking turns singing alternate lines of a song),
- telling a sequenced story or a joke,
- social scripts [25].

In addition, there are girls who communicate using VOCAS with four, eight, nine, twenty or thirty-two messages. The choice of VOCA is determined through an AAC assessment, in which factors such as access, cognition, and language ability are taken into account. There are girls who have several kinds of VOCAs within their communication systems, such as two single message devices and a device with sequenced messages, to address their communicative needs and abilities in a variety of situations. Moreover, a girl may start with a single message device, move on to a device with four messages, then to a nine message device, etc – the process is dynamic depending on the needs and abilities of the girl in question. VOCAS can be used in a great variety of situations of social interaction; only bounded by the imagination of the person with whom the girl is interacting. Because the size of the vocabulary is limited, based on the number of messages which can be recorded into the device (as opposed to a computer where the number of vocabulary items is unlimited), VOCAS based on digitized speech should always be used in addition to the communication chart, not in place of it. As much as possible the picture representing the verbal message should be attached to the VOCA (this can be done using velchro). This is important as it helps the girl to understand the relationship between the visual and auditory aspects of the message and so that the device does not just randomly say different utterances. It is suggested that a supply of pictures (with velchro already attached to their backs) be prepared to have readily available at all times, representing as many as possible of the messages which are regularly used by the girl both at school and at home throughout the day. However it must be remembered that it is more important that the device be used spontaneously in unexpected situations than not used because the corresponding picture is not available (see figures VIII-4-6).

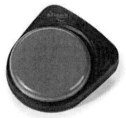

Figure VIII-4. Big Mack: single message device.

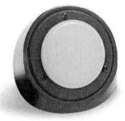

Figure VIII-5. Step by Step: sequenced.

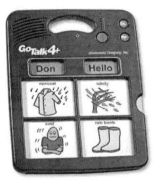

Figure VIII-6. Go Talk 4+. 4 messages device messages on each of 5 different levels.

It is also possible to use a laptop computer with an appropriate communication program and speech output for the purpose of communication. There is communication software available in various languages in which the communication displays are available as separate pages on the computer screen and it is possible to navigate easily between pages. Here too the number of items per page will be specific to each girl, depending on her language, cognitive, communication, and access abilities. The method of access is one of the more critical issues with regard to including the computer as a tool for communication with girls with RS. Some computers can be operated through the use of touch screens; while very few girls with RS have the motor coordination ability to operate a touch screen by touching it with their hand/finger, one girl was known to indicate her choices by hitting the touch screen with her nose. The ideal form of access to the computer for girls with RS would be through the use of an eye gaze system, in which the girl can make her selection by simply looking at the item which represents what she wants to say. There are a number of eye gaze systems currently available, some of which are more easily operated than others. Unfortunately, for the most part these systems are currently available commercially at prices, which are unaffordable for many families, particularly in countries in which there is no insurance coverage or government funding for the purchase of communication equipment. Hopefully these eye gaze systems will become more commercially affordable in the near future. For girls who do not have access to eye gaze access technology, the computer can be operated through visual and/or auditory scanning systems using one or more single switches i.e. a marker moves from item to item until it reaches what the girl wants to say; she then hits the switch attached to the computer in order to make her selection, and the computer "says" the item put loud.

As can be ascertained, the critical point in using all these aided strategies is to determine the means of access most effective for each girl, whether it be pointing with her hand, forehead or nose, or eye gazing, always taking into account the slow response time typical of these girls. This slow response time of girls with RS, due to the strong apraxic element of the syndrome, is a critical element to be taken into consideration in the execution of their communicative interactions. It is essential that we WAIT! WAIT! WAIT! in order to give the girl time to organize herself motorically and then respond. Our repeated commands/requests for a response only serve to delay the response time even further as they cause the girl to stop and listen – and then the whole process of motor organization starts all over again. When the girl with RS is breathing intensively, gazing up or to the sides, moving her body back and forth, and/or engaging in intense hand mannerisms, it is her way of organizing her body to give you the answer you requested…. Wait for her, don't think she has forgotten. Don't move to a different topic or to another child. Wait patiently and quietly for her to respond.

AAC strategies can and MUST be used by girls with RS in a great variety of activities throughout the day. A partial list of activities in which AAC can be used includes:

- Choice-making – clothes, food, play, feelings, people, etc
- Speech acts - "yes"/no", "more"/enough", "my turn/your turn", etc.
- Imaginative play
- Interactive singing
- Literacy
- Participation in school/work place where relevant
- Relaying information
- Talking about emotions
- Asking questions
- Participation in general conversation
- Etc. etc. etc.

For a more detailed discussion of developing programs to meet the communication needs of girls with RS, see [26].

Case study c

C is a girl of 15 years of age who has been diagnosed with Rett Syndrome. At the time that this case report was written she was 14 years old. One of the biggest challenges and learning experiences of this author's professional career has been C; both C and her foster mother N, who have repeatedly made me question some of my most basic assumptions and the clinical reasoning process regarding AAC intervention; C who I have had to defend before other professionals, C who at the age of 14 years has completed 6th grade in a regular school, whose therapy sessions now dwell on discussions of topics such as C's concerns about her peer relationships. C who recently told me "you are annoying me", using her pragmatically organized dynamic display (PODD) [20-22], accessed through partner assisted visual and auditory scanning. In this situation, further discussion revealed that my sitting silently and waiting while she was accessing a message on her computer made her nervous and that she preferred me to talk with N. during this preparation time. And I thought that I was being polite!

Despite C being one of my greatest professional challenges to date, I have learned a great deal from her and from N. Working together with them has put me to the test of not only listening to the parent but of also letting her take the lead, of truly working together as a team.

I first met C, when she was 8 years old. She arrived at the center where I was working for an AAC assessment together with N. and the staff from the school for children with severe developmental challenges which she was attending. C had a diagnosis of significant developmental delay of unknown origin, together with severe cognitive disability. N. was working as a teacher's assistant in the school, which C was attending and had developed a strong interest in communication and AAC intervention. The request for the assessment came from N, who explained her purpose as being the identification of a tool to enable C. to initiate communication, taking into account her motor difficulties. As the assessment progressed it became clear that there was a secondary agenda in requesting the assessment, which was the resolution of the differences of opinion between N and the school staff regarding C's general cognitive ability and her communication potential. Much of the discussion during the assessment focused on this issue, with obvious differences of opinion between those attending the assessment. Observation and interaction with C at that time did not provide the information to help resolve the conflict; on the one hand C was easily distracted, seemingly uninterested in the materials with which she was presented, and very involved in self-stimulation activities. On the other hand she certainly seemed to understand what was being said and was definitely responding appropriately to yes/no questions and using the communication chart with home drawn pictures which N. had prepared for her. I myself came out of the situation conflicted in my thoughts and impressions.

Several months later I was approached by N to work with C in my private practice, to assist in the on-going development of C's AAC system. I reluctantly agreed; if I myself was in conflict regarding C's abilities how could I ethically work with her along the lines that N was requesting of me? But N was persuasive so I agreed to give it a try! And so our six year working relationship began. Therapy was initiated once weekly. N accompanied C to all therapy sessions. At that time C was communicating at home with a communication chart consisting of pictures hand drawn by N which she used to respond to questions; she did not use it to initiate communication. C indicated her responses at that time through a combination of gross hand pointing and eye gaze. She was able to express the concepts of "yes" and "no" consistently, by pressing on N's hand to indicate "yes", and the absence of "yes" meaning "no". N reported that C was also able to let her know what she wanted through her actions, for example going to the sink to show that she wanted to drink. The school staff was certain that C did not have the understanding and ability to express the concepts contained on her chart. The communication chart was not used at school. In therapy it was observed that while C rarely engaged in eye contact, her general behavior indicated that she was aware and attentive to what was going on around her. She was frequently observed to be watching what was happening out of the corner of her eye. She had a severe problem of motor planning, and there was frequently a considerable lapse of time between when she was asked to do something and her response. When given sufficient time, she was often able to respond using the AAC tools that were placed before her; these tools included a communication chart, a single message voice output communication device (VOCA), and a VOCA in which messages could be recorded in sequence. In addition, C had "sensory problems" which greatly interfered with her functioning. Her hands were constantly in her mouth; this was a serious source of distraction as it was difficult for her to function once she began the hands in mouth ritual. In terms of her understanding of language C was an enigma. While she gave the impression of not understanding what was said to her, with on-going interaction and the building of a good rapport, it was possible to see that she did in fact understand much, if not all, of what was being said. At this point the diagnosis of Rett Syndrome had not yet been made, although it became increasingly evident that her clinical manifestations were those that are typical of girls with RS. A video was prepared and presented to the staff of the Israel Rett Syndrome Center, and arrangements were made for C's diagnosis to be investigated. While blood tests were not conclusive, a medical diagnosis was made of atypical Rett syndrome, based on C's clinical features.

At the end of the first year of working with C, she changed schools and began to attend a school for children with moderate cognitive disabilities – she attended this school for two years and then, with the intervention of N, she began to attend a school for girls within the religious educational system; although she had no prior experience in a regular learning environment, she began at the 3rd grade level with her peer group.

To go back to the beginning, the focus of therapy was on the development of C's communicative skills. Initially the tools of therapy were primarily single pictures and single message voice output devices; C understood the use of these tools and used them effectively to respond to and later, to also initiate, interactions. At this stage N traveled abroad and purchased a double message VOCA; I felt that this was a totally inappropriate tool for C, because of the proximity of the two buttons one to another – how would she operate it with her very poor hand function? However, within one week there she was using it – N was changing the messages constantly according to the situation and conversational topic – C was watching out of the corner of her eye and listening intently and responding appropriately. My feeling was "Is she really doing this?" "Maybe any message she hits will be appropriate to the situation. However with time it has become increasingly certain that C is in fact using her own abilities and skills to communicate in this way.

The focus was then expanded to include the use of communication charts on which were displayed six or eight concepts per page. Access to these charts was through partner assisted scanning. It was my intention to construct the chart using primarily PCS (picture communication symbols) to represent the concepts to be included; N. insisted that she would take the construction of the chart upon herself, including choosing the vocabulary items, etc. Several weeks later C and N arrived for the therapy session with C's chart in hand – a multi-page chart with about 100 concepts per page – all represented by the written word. C started to use the chart – with N doing the auditory scanning ("Column A, Column B, Etc; Row 1; Row 2; etc;) and C barely looking at the chart except out of the corner of her eye (in fact typical of many girls with RS) and then tapping "yes" on N's hand to indicate when N had reached the item she wanted to say, with utterances that were appropriate and made sense.

ד	ג	ב	א	
People	I'm thinking	Something happened	Turn the page	1
I want	I have a question ?	If only ….	I feel	2
I remember	Do you want to hear a story?	I'm complaining	Places	3
Something else		I have an idea	Judaism	4

Figure VIII-7. Example of C."s communication chart - Menu page.

ה	ד	ג	ב	א	B
					1
					2
					3
					4

ה	ד	ג	ב	א	A
					1
					2
					3
					4

ה	ד	ג	ב	א	D
					1
					2
					3
					4

ה	ד	ג	ב	א	C
					1
					2
					3
					4

ה	ד	ג	ב	א	F
					1
					2
					3
					4

ה	ד	ג	ב	א	E
					1
					2
					3
					4

Figure VIII-8. Layout of following pages (each square contains a written word or phrase).

I kept watching N closely, certain that she was assisting C or giving hints in some way but just could not see any way that this could be happening. And then one day after C's double message VOCA had been lost and a new one was purchased, I asked C. what steps could be taken to make sure that doesn't happen again. She answered me "to pray". Given the religious community to which she belongs, this was a most appropriate response and I was convinced!

Together with the chart, C began to use a 10 message VOCA with visual scanning for messages with voice output. Despite N's prediction that she would never be able to use a switch, C began to use one and then two single switches with step scanning which she operated one on either side of her head. Use of the switches took months and months of practice due to the severe apraxic aspect of C's difficulty, but her determination enabled her to master this skill. The device was programmed for messages which were social and interactive, and included the message "I want to say something with my chart".

Persons less familiar with C have questioned her ability to read and understand this large number of written words and have tried to explain her ability to communicate in this way as being a function of the familiarity of her communication partner with what she wants to say; however repeated interaction with C has proven her ability to express innovative and complex messages with a variety of communication partners and with content unknown to those communicating with her. However, when an attempt was made to use a writing program on the computer, it was discovered that C does not have the phonological or analytic skills necessary to break down the word into its component sounds, thus indicating that her reading, even of this vast number of words, is somehow global in nature.

Today C's communication system consists of a word-based partner assisted scanning PODD which is available at all times and a tablet computer consisting of written words and phrases representing socially interactive messages, accessed with two switches. C has just completed 6th grade class in a regular school; she has a personal aide to assist her in school who also serves as her communication partner. She does homework as do all the rest of the students, although she does not always finish it. She takes exams which are adapted to enable "yes/no" responses and is able to pass them within the class standard. All is not easy; social relationships are difficult for her and she has instances of volatile behavior and screaming, which necessitate her leaving the classroom for a time. Current therapy sessions are focused on working out a set of personal communication rules, to improve the communication process for both her and her partners. For example, as indicated above, C does not like the persons with whom she is communicating to sit silently while she is preparing her messages on her tablet as it makes her nervous – she would prefer they chat between themselves or do other tasks during this time.

In one of our recent conversations I told C that I had arranged to come to her school (not the first time). It must be explained that C attends a religious school where women do not wear pants. She told me, using her chart: Kiryat Sefer (where she lives in an Orthodox community where women wears dresses and not pants) principle pants don't want. I verified that she was telling me that she did not want me to wear pants when I came to her school; I asked if she was worried I would embarrass her and she excitedly indicated "yes", the relief on her face that I had understood this important message was evident. This led into a long conversation regarding mutual respect and acceptance of individual differences. And this with a girl diagnosed as having a severe cognitive disability!

Today's accomplishments with C have not been the result of a progression along a defined path of development; at every point there have been challenges and doubts, which in retrospect have been basically related to a belief (or lack of belief) in C's capabilities. N and I have challenged each other at every step along the way – the type of communication chart, the form of graphic representation, the means of access, the type of VOCA, etc, etc. Each time a new step was considered, C went home and several weeks/months later came back, again proving her abilities and ready to meet the next challenge. Working with C. has been a challenge; there is always more to learn about her abilities, with many questions always to be answered.

Conclusions

There are a significant number of barriers and challenges to communication intervention for girls with RS. These include the lack of speech which typifies most of the girls, the difficulty in ascertaining their cognitive and language comprehension levels, the severe dyspraxia which typifies the syndrome, their very severe hand dysfunction, a very slow response time, and – perhaps the greatest barrier of all – a lack of belief regarding their ability to communicate on the part of many professionals (doctors, therapists, educators) and family members. However, when these elements are recognized and taken into account in the planning and implementation of the AAC program then very significant gains can be made in each girl's communicative output. They have the ability, as well as the right, to let their voices be heard.

References

[1]   International Rett Syndrome Association. What is Rett syndrome? Clinton, MD: Int Rett Syndr Assoc, 1998.

[2]   Ayres JA. Sensory integration and the child, 5th ed. Los Angeles, CA: Western Psychol Serv, 1982.

[3]   Ayres JA. Developmental dispraxia and adult-onset apraxia. Torrance CA: Sensory Integr Int, 1985.

[4]   Kerr AM. The future for Rett syndrome girls. Int Rett Syndr Assoc Newsletter 1992;13-14.

[5]   Lindberg B. Understanding Rett syndrome: A practical guide for parents, teachers, and therapists. Cambridge, MA: Hogrefe Huber, 2006.

[6]   Zappella M, Mari F, Renieri A. Should a syndrome be called by its correct name? The example of the preserved speech variant of Rett syndrome. Eur J Pediatr 2005;164(11):710;

[7]   Zappella M. The preserved speech variant of the Rett complex: a report of 8 cases. Eur Child Adolesc Psychiatry 1997;6(Suppl 1):23-5.

[8]   Hetzroni O, Rubin C, Konkol O. The use of assistive technology for symbol identification by children with Rett syndrome. J Intellect Dev Disabil 2002;27:57-71.

[9]   Elefant C. Enhancing communication in girls with Rett syndrome through songs in music therapy. Unpublished dissertation. Aalborg, DK: Aalborg Univ, 2002.

[10]   Hetzroni OE, Rubin C. Identifying patterns of communicative behaviors in girls with Rett Syndrome, Augment Altern Commun 2006;22:48-61.

[11]   Lariviere J. ACCESS: The key to communication and learning for girls with Rett syndrome. Presentation, 22nd Ann CSUN Conf, Los Angeles, CA, 2007.

[12]   Skotko BG, Koppenhaver DA, Erickson KA. Parent reading behaviors and communication outcomes in girls with Rett syndrome. Council Except Child 2004;70:145-66.

[13]   Elati R, Gershenowich I. What are the language comprehension abilities of 6 to 8 year old girls with Rett Syndrome? Unpublished BA research project. Jerusalem: Hadassah Acad Coll, 2009.

[14]   Bartolotta T. The effects of communication intervention during mealtime in Rett syndrome. Presentation, Am Speech Language Hearing Ann Conf, Miami, FL, 2006.

[15]   Elefant C, Wigram T. Learning ability in children with Rett syndrome. Brain Dev 2005;27: S97-S101.

[16]   Sigafoos J, Laurie S, Pennell D. Teaching children with Rett syndrome to request preferred objects using aided communication: Two preliminary studies. Augment Altern Commun1996;12:88-96.

[17]   Sigafoos J, Woodyatt G, Tucker M, Roberts-Pennell D, Pittendreigh N. Assessment of potential communicative acts in three individuals with Rett syndrome. J Dev Phys Disabil 2000;12:203-16.

[18]   Von Tetzchner S. Communication skills among females with Rett syndrome. Eur Child Adoles Psychol 1997;6:33-7.

[19]   Doyle BT. New Horizons for Learning. 2003. Site: http://www.newhorizons.org. Accessed 2009 Sep 09.

[20]   Burkhart L, Porter G. Partner-assisted communication strategies for children who face multiple challenges. Handout, ISAAC conf, Düsseldorf (also available at: www.lburkhart.com), 2006.

[21]   Porter G. Ideas for the design of light- tech dynamic displays: User friendly, multi-level communication books. In: Porter G, ed. Students with physical impairment: Augmentative and alternative communication. Brisbane, QLD: Dept Educ Brisbane, 2001.

[22]   Porter G. Low-Tech dynamic displays: User friendly multi-level communication books. Presentation, Ninth Biennial Conf Int Soc Augment Altern Comm, Washington, DC, 2000.

[23]   Partner assisted scanning. See: http://www.actwmids.nhs.uk/AAC/resources/partner-assisted-scanning-1/

[24]   Millar S. Personal communication passports: Guidelines for good practice. Edinburgh: CALL Centre, 2003.

[25]   Musselwhite C, Burkhart L. Can we chat? Co-planned sequenced social scripts, CD, 2004.

[26]   Wine J. Resource for the development of a communication program for girls with Rett Syndrome. Ramat Gan, IL: Israel Rett Syndr Center, 2009.

In: Rett Syndrome: Therapeutic Interventions   ISBN: 978-1-61728-080-1
Editors: Meir Lotan and Joav Merrick   ©2011 Nova Science Publishers, Inc.

Chapter IX

Rett Syndrome: Physical Therapy Intervention

Meir Lotan, BPT, MScPT, PhD[*]

National Evaluation Team, Israeli Rett Center, National Evaluation Team, Chaim Sheba
Medical Center, Tel HaShomer, Ramat Gan, Zvi Quittman Residential Centers,
Elwyn, Jerusalem and Department of Physical Therapy,
Ariel University Center of Samaria, Ariel, Israel

Individuals with Rett syndrome (RS) present a vast array of orthopedic and neurological challenges. Typical problems, which may need to be addressed when treating this population, are functional limitations, low cardiovascular capacity, hypotonia, ataxia, apraxia, loss of transitional movement, spasticity, scoliosis and/or kyphosis, loss of ambulation, loss of hand function, foot deformities and spatial disorientation. Coping with such difficulties and overcoming the associated limitations are wearisome tasks for the individual with Rett as well as for her family. An informed and intensely applied physical therapy regime can help the child and her family to cope and even overcome the above- mentioned limitations. The present chapter presents some insights into the intervention with individuals with RS, an overview of typical neuromuscular problems associated with RS and appropriate suggestions pertaining to clinical intervention, that have been found to contribute to this population's well-being. The information offered is mainly based on the clinical knowledge of the author.

Introduction

Rett Syndrome (RS) is a genetic disorder that primarily affects females [1,2]. The disorder causes a neurological and developmental arrest that manifests itself in a variety of disabilities, such as loss of functional hand use, loss of acquired speech, apraxia, ataxia, autonomic system dysfunction, epilepsy, breathing abnormalities, failure to thrive and muscle tone irregularities [3-5]. In order for the children and women with RS and their families to live life to the fullest, proper intervention should be applied. The present chapter addresses the physical difficulties typically exhibited by individuals with RS and suggests possible intervention techniques according to the scarcely existing literature and mainly based on the experience of the author for the past 18 years as part of the RS Israeli national evaluation team and also as a therapist managing about 10 individuals with RS on a weekly basis.

Physical therapy for rett syndrome

Due to the longevity of individuals with RS [6] and the complex nature of the RS disability, physical therapy is an important part of the management of the disorder. Individuals with RS show a considerable functional diversity. Some girls might never achieve independent sitting or standing, while others may gain high functional abilities such as running, skiing and trampoline jumping [7]. Due to such versatility, a thorough evaluation should be performed of each child entering an intervention program. After such an evaluation, preferably by a multi-disciplinary team [8,9], an intervention program should be drawn up, specifically tailored for each client. In many cases, the child with RS is treated by a team of therapists, from such fields of expertise as: physical therapy, occupational therapy, speech therapy, music therapy, hydrotherapy and hippotherapy (horseback riding). Each of the disciplines involved in the therapeutic program uses a combination of different techniques intended to maintain and maximize physical functions of the individual with RS. While these therapies do not cure RS, they can help the client by lessening the difficulties experienced by her, thus helping her and her family cope with the above-mentioned limitations [10].

It is vital for the success of the intervention program that different members of the team co-ordinate their therapeutic efforts into a combined management approach, in accordance with all team members' agreement (including that of the parents and the child with RS). A well-planned intervention is of great importance to individuals with RS [11,12]. Such a program may maintain or improve function, prevent deformities and provide positioning and mobility [12], thereby contributing to the social accessibility of the client. It is important to remember that while individuals with RS share many similarities, their problems and responses to intervention may vary dramatically. The basic goal of the PT intervention program is to enhance the quality of life and functional abilities of the client with RS. These goals might be achieved if the intervention is aimed at:

- Maintaining or increasing motor skills
- Developing or maintaining transitional skills
- Preventing or reducing deformities
- Alleviating discomfort and irritability
- Improving independence.

* Correspondence: Meir Lotan, BPT, MScPT, PhD, Department of Physical Therapy, Ariel University Center of Samaria, IL-40700 Ariel, Israel. E-mail: ml_pt_rs@netvision.net.il

On top of the "hands on" intervention, the physical therapist may assess and then improve walking and sitting patterns, monitor changes over time, support other members of the education/habilitation team and parents on topics such as adapted seating systems, assistive technology and mobility devices.

Regarding the physical therapy program, however, the therapist is in a dilemma. On one hand, it is known that functional and clinical advancements of individuals with RS have been reported several times by different intervention teams, during childhood as well as in adulthood [12-17]. On the other hand, it is important to understand that each individual with RS has limits of achievement, which are determined by her underlying neurological situation. Therefore, the physical therapist should advise parents regarding that which is reasonable to expect from a child or adult with RS. Much as all professionals want their clients to achieve a high level of function, it is also important to respect what is possible and not spend time and resources on goals which cannot be met at the expense of other aspects of school and family life. This type of understanding may require time and input from the parents, pediatrician, orthopedic surgeon, neurologist and therapist.

Due to the fluctuating nature of RS [12,18] and to external influencing factors (such as surgery or fracture), the child might be occasionally exposed to periods of inactivity. Enhanced physical therapy intervention is warranted after illness, fractures or surgery or whenever special effort is made to regain all the skills that the individual previously possessed [19].

Despite the above-mentioned variability in physical abilities among individuals with RS, there are some neuro-motor problems typical of many with this disorder. Such common occurrences should be taken into account when treating the individual with RS. This chapter will describe such common characteristics and suggest appropriate intervention approaches.

Basic steps when approaching a child with RS

When considering intervention for an individual diagnosed with RS, therapists must have an understanding of the complex problems associated with the four stages of the condition, in order to develop appropriate management plans. A variety of treatment strategies can be applied at a given stage and may be helpful in achieving or maintaining a level of independence in a particular functional area. The therapist must assume a key role in instructing parents and teachers in the handling of a child with RS.

Andreas Rett (1924-1997) himself [20] reminded professionals of the responsibility to care for, nurture and advance these special children. For the therapist involved in the child and family, such responsibility carries with it a commitment to develop practical solutions to daily problems in caring for the child with RS. This approach, however true it is for most children with disabilities, is greatly emphasized for individuals with RS. The daily and periodical fluctuations in mood and function and the constantly evolving nature of this syndrome (development of scoliosis, loss of mobility and eruption of epileptic seizures) can sometimes discourage even the experienced physical therapist. Thus, the intervention plan should be flexible and constantly adjusted to the child's state. Furthermore, the therapist should always be sensitive to the needs of the family and give appropriate advice and support when needed.

Individuals with RS usually show age-appropriate emotional abilities [21,22] and those abilities should be addressed by the therapist while treating the child and even before intervention initiation [23]. Before the beginning of any intervention, the person with RS should be verbally prepared for the up-coming session. The physical therapist as well should familiarize him/herself with the current state of the child and a short opening ritual is recommended at the beginning of each therapeutic session [22]. During therapy sessions it is advisable to enable the child to gain control over the sessions by letting her choose her preferred activity via an appropriate communication device (see figure IX-1).

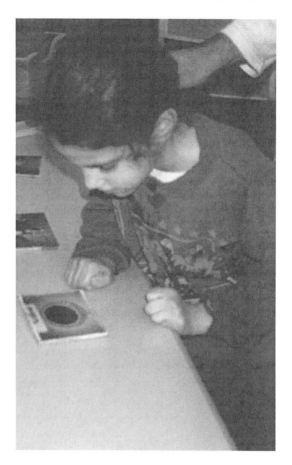

Figure IX-1. Empowering the child by enabling choice between different parts of the session.

The intensity of activities should be adjusted according to the reaction of the child. Some girls with RS show fear of movement and strongly resist external facilitation. If the child is having a difficult time adjusting to physical activity, the pace of the intervention should be altered and motivational factors such as: music, switch-operated games, video tapes, pets [24] and/or the involvement of family members/caregivers should be included in the session.

Guidelines for physical intervention

Over many years of working with females with Rett syndrome the following guidelines have been developed:

- The individual with RS is essentially controlled by her body instead of controlling it. Therefore, in most cases, physical activity by an external facilitator will not be greatly enjoyed by individuals with RS. The therapist should approach the child by initiating interpersonal bonding. They should try and pace themselves with the child, conveying serenity and security. It is preferable to commence with physical exercise only after establishing basic trust.
- The sensory system of the child with RS is usually disorganized and incoming information (especially proprioceptive input) shows difficulties in being received and processed (personal experience of the author). Therefore throughout physical experiences, sensory input should be intensified to register, thereby establishing improved body scheme by the person with RS.
- In physical intervention necessitating manipulation, the therapist should apply caution, since individuals with RS have been reported to have low bone mineral density (i.e. "fragile bones") [25,26,27] and a delayed reaction to pain due to high pain threshold [10,28] or long reaction time to pain [29]. For this reason the therapist might not be aware if the child is in pain.
- The major functional setback of the client with RS is apraxia. Therefore, verbal guidance should precede and accompany the performance of a specific task. The therapist's hands should gently but decisively direct the child's body to the requested goal and do all this without altering the client's personal pace; trying to rush the individual with RS will most likely lead to her stagnation.
- Eighty seven percent of individuals with RS display difficulties in coping with external facilitation [30]. This fear of movement must be addressed by the therapist and his approach must be holistic, despite his engagement in physical intervention. The discomfort of the client and the tension her body presents should be eased before active participation is demanded.
- Music, especially familiar songs, is an excellent motivational factor [31]. Using live or recorded songs can relax the client with RS, easing the intervention for child and therapist alike [22].
- The progression of RS has a tendency towards dynamic fluctuations [18]. During one week, the child may walk and constantly advance in her ambulation abilities and by the next week she might refuse even to stand on her feet. The attentive physical therapist should learn to become flexible and flow with the unexplained changes, updating the goals to address new issues, while constantly evaluating the child's state and abilities and trying to maximize them.
- Physical intervention was found to improve the concentration of individuals with RS [18]. Therefore, it is recommended that educational tasks are planned, closely following physical interventions (hydrotherapy, physical therapy, occupational therapy).
- Enhancing the child's desire to move and explore her surroundings can be achieved by stimulating her in varies ways, such as:
    - Talking to her (most individuals with RS are extremely fond of soft whispering)

- o Diverting her attention to peers and events in her vicinity
- o Surrounding the person with interesting objects (such as those that shine or flicker in a dark room – Snoezelen, big mirrors on the walls)
- o Giving ample opportunities for tactile experiences
- o Using interesting gadgets (like voice or hand operated communication devices and household appliances, computer programs)
- o Supplying switch-operated toys
- o Suggesting water-games
- Children with RS, who have learned how to walk at advanced ages, have been described by parents, in the past, on several occasions. A few studied have reported several individuals with RS who have regained "lost" walking abilities [13,14]. In some cases, adult women with RS have regained walking abilities after 15 or 20 years of wheelchair usage [12,15]. Some children with RS exhibit a marked distortion of their orientation in space and have been reported to regain walking abilities, in several instances due to intensive "over-correction" intervention [13,32]. In regard to the previous data, the connection between walking ability and severity of scoliosis has been frequently reported by differing authors [3,33,34]. Furthermore, the disadvantages of a sedentary life-style for all populations have been constantly reported in medical literature [16,35]. Therefore, individuals with RS should always be encouraged to walk.
- When walking with the individual with RS, the client should always be given the minimal amount of support required for her safety, since, in most cases, she will try to lean on the person holding her, in order to ease her efforts [36].
- Losing the ability to walk can originate from: the development of scoliosis, deformed feet [3,12], general medical deterioration, muscle tone changes, muscle shortening and the loss of mid-line orientation [13]. Conscious of secondary dangers of long-lasting immobility such as loss of function, reduction in muscle strength, reduction in body and limbs range of motion, the development of contractures and reduction in cardio-pulmonary fitness [37-39], the therapist should be alert to changes affecting ambulation. When such changes are observed, interventional goals should change accordingly and enhanced efforts should be invested in walking programs throughout the day.
- When the child is non-ambulatory, a daily program in a standing frame is mandatory [34]. Such a program can assist in the maturation of the hip joints, thereby reducing the risks of hip dislocation, osteoporosis and other associated problems [40-42]. Such a program can also increase the child's postural control and introduce her to healthier alternatives than sitting [4]. Standing should always challenge the child's postural abilities suggesting the minimal support needed for each client and, therefore, the use of the most active systems should be encouraged (see figures IX-2 and IX-3).

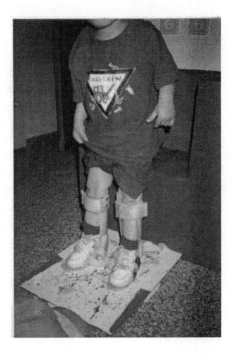

Figure IX-2. A "splint standing frame".

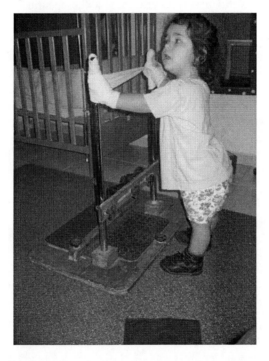

Figure IX-3. An active standing frame.

- Due to developmental dispraxia (see chapter on occupational therapy in this book), the functional abilities of individuals with RS improve with continuous practice; The emphasis of practice should be placed on chores that the individual with RS finds rewording (e.g. putting rings in a box has no purpose but taking cookies out of a jar does, at least for the child, and is an action which demands planning and the execution of a motor act, fine motor abilities and hand-eye coordination).

- Developmental dispraxia may lead to a situation in which an individual with RS is able to perform a functional task, such as getting up from the floor to a standing position, in a very specific manner and even only in one familiar place [12]. It is therefore important to identify such conditions and use them as a fulcrum for further generalization and development.
- Some individuals with RS demonstrate agitation when confined to small or crowded rooms with no opportunity for free movement. Such situations are better avoided.
- Due to the difficulty of some individuals with RS to adjust to changes in routine [23], it is advised to keep the structure of the intervention stable. When changes are due, the child should be informed in advance and the planned adjustments gradually implemented.
- In many developmental diseases, intervention is gradually reduced as the child gets older. As individuals with RS grow older, their bodies stiffen and muscle tone increases, their risk of developing scoliosis becomes essentially higher. In such circumstances, as well as taking in to account the longevity of individuals with RS, it would be logical to preserve or increase intervention intensity[19] rather than reducing it.
- Intervention for individuals with RS should be implemented through a complete and comprehensive program that accompanies the child throughout her daily routine – a total program [12]. Such a program casts a therapeutic net around the child and constantly combats the difficulties caused by RS (i.e. a total program means that the child is properly seated while at home, at school and on the way to and from these places; every care-giver will always demand of the child that she performs at her highest capacity; feeding habits of the child are known and similarly addressed by the parents, grand-parents, siblings, school facilitators and anyone who might contribute to the child's care, etc'). The author however would assert that any such program, however helpful for the child, can only be performed within the capacity of the human environment in which care of the individual with RS is being taken. Therefore, the physical therapist should be aware of such limitations when aiming at establishing such a program, keeping it within realistic boundaries.

Suggested physical therapy goals

The goals set out below should be specified for each child after a thorough individual evaluation during which the therapist should carefully evaluate the person's abilities, in order to detect obstacles impairing her functions. These obstacles can be modified through facilitation of movement, tone reduction activities and balancing responses. It is reiterated that an intensive therapeutic program should envelop the client's daily activities and surroundings as well as set clear intervention tasks for anyone taking care of the child. Regardless of the importance of such a program, the client's tolerance must at all times be considered, expecting that she will probably resist being moved or manipulated [43].

In spite of the phenotypic variability of individuals with RS, our experience suggests that the following physical therapy goals may be appropriate for many of them:

- Normalize muscle tone
- Advance or at least preserve articular range of motion
- Reduce dyspraxia by repetitive functional experiences
- Increase and improve cardio-vascular fitness by applying an appropriate program
- Stimulate hand use by challenging the child to climb, swing and/or support herself
- Achieve better balance reactions through exercises and daily activities
- Promote better co-ordination and balance through practice in various situations and environments
- Reduce setbacks cast by ataxia by training the child through different, gradually increasing postural challenges
- Improve body awareness by deep proprioceptive input and active motion
- Reverse progression of scoliosis through proper intervention (see below)
- Maintain and improve mobility
- Increase protective responses.

Intervention according to rett syndrome stage

Stage I: Onset - most children at this stage are not yet diagnosed as having Rett syndrome. Most often, they are diagnosed as having hypotonia, cerebral palsy, autism or both [44]. The child will display characteristics such as: delayed developmental milestones, reduced hand function, play skills and communication and the child may appear easy to handle and quiet. Since physical therapy intervention is symptomatic, the therapeutic program will address the problems the child presents. Usually, the response to stage I typical stagnation is to enroll the child in a therapy program. In many cases, some improvement will be noted during this stage, although the ultimate gradual deterioration is undeniable. Specifically, it is realistic to work toward independent standing and even ambulation, since many of the girls appear to maintain ambulation, attained in stage I over a long period of time. On the other hand, the outcome of therapy aimed at developing other functional skills may be found to be less positive, yet it should not be avoided.

Stage II: The rapid destructive phase - The loss of acquired developmental milestones is the significant characteristic of stage II. This rapid deterioration may pose a difficult management problem for the family and the specialist team involved. The child may still not be diagnosed as having RS or a final diagnosis may still be pending. The child who is involved in a therapy or educational program is not making progress or is losing ground. The stereotypical hand movements are fully present at this time. Additional medical problems may become apparent. These can include seizures, deceleration of head growth, irregular breathing or hyperventilation and initiation of spinal asymmetry. In order to alleviate the chaotic nature of this short stage [18], relaxing techniques in different environments have been suggested [23,45]. Gentle handling of the child at this stage has been recommended as a means of reducing sensory intake; this approach was hypothesized to benefit brain development [46,47] at this stage. Such an approach can also enhance bonding between the therapist and child and will yield positive results in future therapeutic interventions.

Stage III: Plateau - Stage III is a lengthy one in RS, characterized by a relatively calm period wherein intervention aimed at advancement is advised. Nevertheless, during this stage, most of the individuals with RS develop significant problems, such as deformities and contractures (which require shoe inserts, orthoses and a daily intervention program - see below for more information) [12]. If scoliosis is present, it can progress rapidly and might require surgery in 25% of mobile females with Rett Syndrome and in 61% of non-mobile females [33]. Stereotypical hand mannerisms are obvious and are usually accompanied by minimal hand function. The use of splinting and the intensity of splints usage is controversial among different practitioners. Some will generally refrain from splinting the child's hands as a regular intervention (ML), while others believe that splinting often improves the child's function and enhances her awareness of the environment. Nevertheless, splinting or arm restraints have been found helpful in the following cases:

- Situations in which skin problems develop as a result of constant hand-to-mouth behavior.
- When restraining the less active hand, it was found that the individual with RS increases control over her other hand.
- When the stereotypical movements prevent the child from being properly fed (i.e. if the child is constantly putting her hand in her mouth throughout meal-times)
- When it disrupts the child's social interactions (e.g. a child with RS that was integrated into a mainstream school and was not approached by non-disabled peers due to constant drooling and spiting over her hands. The use of splints, preventing her from putting her hand in her mouth, thereby diminishing the accompanied smell, has turned things around and the child was immediately accepted by her peers).

Stage IV: Late motor deterioration - Significant decrease and lack of mobility is characteristic of stage IV. Many of the individuals with RS, although non-ambulatory, may still be able to participate in a supported transfer (e.g. moving from a wheel-chair to a bed). Individuals who constantly use a wheel-chair will typically present a worse phenotypic expression, consequentially requiring more care. Individuals with RS at this stage are often described as having improved emotional contact and better-controlled epilepsy. In some cases, however, additional medical issues are encountered. Such problems may include worsening scoliosis and contractures, lower extremity atrophic changes [4], circulatory (cold extremities) and feeding problems (e.g. dependent eating, reflux, constipation) may become worse [48,49]. Growth retardation will usually be more apparent since most individuals with RS are of short stature and are slim[50]. At this point, the physical therapist should provide extended therapeutic support and support involved individuals (i.e. therapists, care-givers, available family members) with regard to a daily exercise routine aimed at improving: mobility, range of motion, transfer skills, positioning and lifting of the child. If it is within the professional expertise of the therapist, he/she should evaluate and customize a properly supported seating system. The physical therapist's role should be favorably considered in pre- and post-surgical follow-up and management [12,19].

Specific motor problems in Rett syndrome

RS is a disorder which presents an array of neuromuscular limitations that need proper therapeutic intervention. Specific motor problems associated with RS, which may need to be addressed by the physical therapist are, changing (over time) and fluctuating muscle tone (hypotonia, spasticity, dystonia) [51], ataxia, motor apraxia, loss of transitional movements, scoliosis and/or kyphosis, loss of ambulation, reduced hand function, foot deformities and spatial disorientation. In this section of the chapter, the development of most of these difficulties will be highlighted and intervention techniques and hints will be suggested.

Muscle tone

As with other characteristics of RS, variability among individuals is the norm. The infant with RS will typically show hypotonia or the muscle tone might be within the norm. With age, most individuals with RS change from being hypotonic to becoming hypertonic (mostly rigidity, usually starting from lower extremities). 30% of adults with RS remain hypotonic, 40% show rigidity as their main tonal characteristic and 30% become dystonic [51]. These changes influence the handling of the child and therefore necessitate ongoing evaluation of muscle tone by the therapist. When tonal changes are observed, the physical therapist should alert other team members involved in caring for the child, while at the same time initiating the proper handling instructions for the educational team and for the parents.

When muscle tone of the individual with RS gradually changes from low to high, the change might cause a unique phenomenon. In contrast to children with cerebral palsy (toe walking), the child with RS might present an asymmetrical reaction, causing her to side-tilt the trunk, leading to initial development of asymmetry of the spine, eventually resulting in scoliosis. Another unique reaction of individuals with RS to the shortening of the Achilles tendon could be the tilting of the pelvis backwards, causing the child to lose the ability to walk independently. Such events should be expected and dealt with in order to prevent their severe consequences. If rigidity/spasticity is severe and becomes a constant disruption to function, other physical interventions such as hydrotherapy (with emphasize on slow movement in the water), serial casting, daily muscle stretching and deep pressure stimulus could all be found helpful in the management of high muscle tone. Continuous intrathecal baclofen infusion was found to enhance functional benefits among various populations with high muscular spasticity [52], not including individuals with RS. This type of intervention may be considered in severe cases, yet it is reiterated that in most cases individuals with RS show rigidity (rather than spasticity), which is impervious to Baclofen.

Deformities

Because of the abnormal muscle coordination and hypertonicity typical of RS, some muscles are over-active and pull certain joints out of balance. This happens most commonly about the ankle and hip, especially when the child lacks the ability to ambulate [53]. Over the ankle, the excessive pulling of muscles (gastrocnemius and tibialis anterior) may cause severe plantar flexion with supination.

In some cases, where the adult with RS is ambulatory and shows fixed deformities that neither interfere with balance nor cause calluses, these deformities may be left un managed. However, since such deformity may interfere with the future standing and walking abilities of the child, making her completely dependent on her care-givers, preventive intervention is usually advised [12]. Regularly implemented standing and walking programs are also recommended [12,34] in order to prevent osteopnia and osteoporosis due to low bone mineral density, typical of individuals with RS [25-27]. When imbalance of muscle action around the ankles starts to cause muscle shortening or even joint deformation, a daily prevention program should be introduced. Such a program should include preventive splinting, daily standing in a standing frame or on a wedge so that the toes are higher then the heels (see figure IX-4).

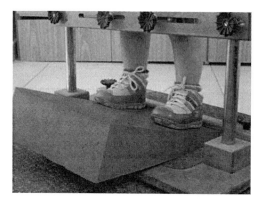

Figure IX-4. Stretching the gastrocnemius muscle while standing.

Daily manual stretching exercises can be beneficial in this situation and the use of active splinting is recommended (see figure IX-5).

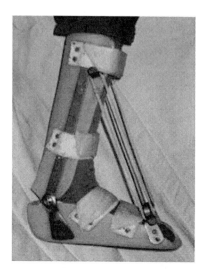

Figure IX-5. An active stretching splint.

If all those preventive measures fail, serial casting can be suggested. In severe cases the orthopedic surgeon may suggest Botox (Botulinum toxin) injections or even surgery [53]. It is mandatory that such intervention programs be followed by intensive physical therapy [12].

In the hip joint, the adductor or flexor muscles are occasionally pulled excessively tight. This can impede walking or even prevent the child from resting the hip in an extended position. Such a process, left untreated over time, may end up as dislocation of the hip. The tightness in these muscles should be noted, and the physical therapist should advise the parents to consult with an orthopedic surgeon in order to follow the development of such tension over time and make sure there is no development of dislocation. In the case of such muscle tightness, the physical therapist should institute a daily positioning program carried out by the educational team and/or the parents, including prone-lying and positioning that will maintain hip abduction (seating on a roll). Hyppotherapy, beside its other advantages, is beneficial in maintaining hip abduction [54].

Spinal deformities

The most common deformities seen in RS involve the spine. Such predicaments can be found in 80%-85% of adults with RS [3,33]. Due to its frequency, all girls with RS should be checked for spinal curvature during their yearly physical examination. Another problem involving scoliosis is its rapid progression, averaging on a 14 degree annual rate [3,33]. Moreover, due to the high incidence of scoliosis it is recommended that each child with RS be involved in a scoliosis prevention program from a young age. The prognosis of scoliosis development in RS is worse, when the scoliosis appears before age five, when severe hypotonia exists from childhood, when there is an inability to walk or when walking was gained but lost at an early age [3]. When such circumstances occur, follow-ups on the spinal curvature should be intensified, the frequency of child's visitations to the orthopedic surgeon increased and therapeutic intervention applied accordingly [4].

It has been reported that 25% of mobile females with Rett Syndrome and 61% of non-mobile females presenting scoliosis will eventually require surgical intervention [33].

Scoliosis and kyphosis often begin with muscle tone problems, which are brought on by the child's inability to correctly process her body scheme (orientation in space). Active exercise and passive range of movement routines are helpful. Maintaining spinal alignment is important and can be facilitated by activities designed to provide proprioceptive (alignment of the body), kinesthetic (sensations received from joints and muscles) and tactile (sensations received from receptors over the skin) input, thereby enhancing the individual's awareness [43]. The common intervention approach for treating scoliosis is usually a combination of the following techniques:

- Intensive physical and hydro-therapy treatments were reported to yield maximal benefits, according to the results of a questionnaire completed by 107 parents and care-givers in the United States [33].
- Aggressive treatment starting as soon as the first spinal asymmetry is noticed, was suggested by McClure et al [55], who found a close correlation between the primary

asymmetry of the trunk and the later developing scoliosis, according to 262 responses to a questionnaire completed by families.

- Intensive walking or standing if the individual is non-mobile, was suggested by Lyn Weeks [34], for at least half an hour a day. This element of the program is also supported by the findings by other authors indicating a correlation between walking and reduced percentage of spinal corrective operations [33].
- "Over-correction" treatment, suggested by Hanks [13,32], is applied in order to re-adjust the skewed mid-line perception of females manifesting scoliosis dominated by their skewed sensory system. There are reports of 4-5 cases where the progression of scoliosis was arrested using this method [48].
- Active anti-scoliosis regime – this intervention has managed to reverse the scoliosis from 30 to 20 degrees in a child with RS. Within a year from intervention cessation (due to transfer of the child to a different educational facility), the spinal curvature deteriorated from 20^0 to 40^0 and the child was administered a corset [17]. This intervention is based on the following principles:
  - o Visits to an orthopedic surgeon (at least twice a year; more if the child is showing initial signs of scoliosis and is younger than five years of age) [4,56]
  - o Commencing treatment as soon as asymmetry of the spine is detected [55]
  - o Intensive implementation of the program throughout sleeping and waking hours
  - o Opposing (to the natural scoliosis curve) asymmetry postures (see figures 6-10)
  - o Walking and/or standing for at least two hours a day [34]
  - o Maintaining spinal mobility through passive manual manipulation
  - o Parental and staff guidance [17].

This intervention regime addresses the sensory and musculature deviations associated with scoliosis in RS and tries to balance the child's asymmetrical activity through use of various positioning equipment (see figures IX-6-10).

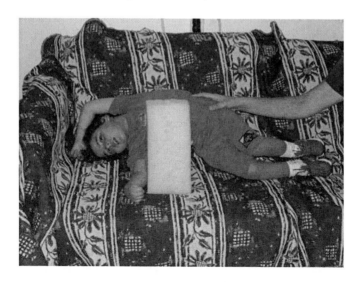

Figure IX-6.

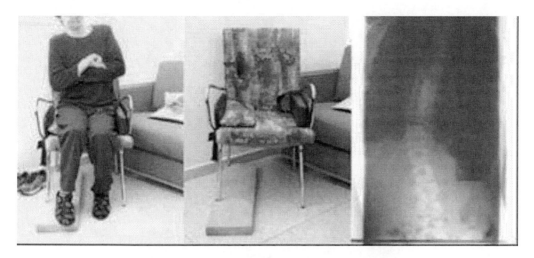

Figure IX-7.

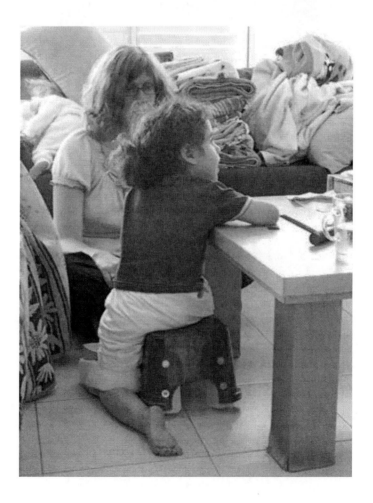

Figure IX-8.

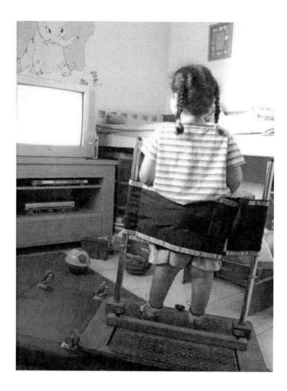

Figure IX-9.

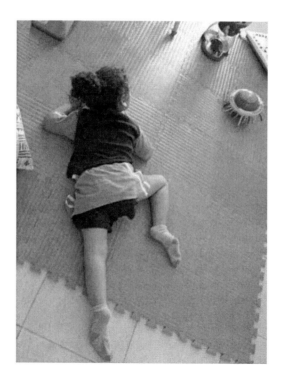

Figure IX-10.

Figures IX-6-10. Different positioning equipment for management of scoliosis in RS.

- Corsets and temporary casting, when used, were mostly reported as unsuccessful in slowing the progression of scoliosis in people with neuromuscular scoliosis in general and in females with Rett syndrome in particular [33,57]. Nevertheless, corsets may be used on occasion in order to align the child when functional performance is called for.
- Surgical intervention - when everything else fails, a surgical solution may be proposed. It should be noted that the success of the surgical intervention depends on the spine's flexibility and also that the post- surgical spinal curves can range from 40% to 60% of the pre-surgical curves [33], meaning that, regardless of the scoliosis management approach chosen, it is the responsibility of the physical therapist to maintain spinal mobility and flexibility.

Improving functional ability and physical fitness

Ambulation, or walking, is a skill which requires a certain level of coordination. 50%-85% of all children with RS achieve the ability to walk [3]; some lose this ability later in life; some never gain it. Walking helps to prevent osteoporosis and strengthen lower extremities muscles, activates the heart and lungs and keeps the child in shape. It is good to encourage walking in those who are able to do so [34], but it is sometimes impossible to teach a child to walk if the required co-ordination is not present [53]. Generally, it is a good idea to establish routine daily walks as a preventative measure against inactivity and a sedentary life-style. It should be reiterated that a correlation between ambulation ability (specifically stair-climbing) and milder cases of scoliosis was found [33]. In accordance with this view, a daily training program on a treadmill was designed for females with RS. The participants were four girls with Rett Syndrome, aged 8½-11 years (mean: 10 years) attending an educational facility at the center of Israel. All the girls showed independent mobility and had the typical characteristics of stage III RS.

The intervention was executed in order to improve the physical fitness of these children and to evaluate the contribution of such an exercise program on the functional abilities of the participants. The training was conducted on an analogue treadmill (1400 model produced by Trimline), capable of very low speeds <0.5k/h, with very long side rails. Special low-side rails were added to the treadmill in order to fit the height of the children and Velcro straps were added to assist in the safe placing of the hands (see figure IX-11).

Pulse was constantly monitored during each exercise using an A3 polar pulse transmitter belt. Since only four participants were involved and no control group was available, three tests were taken to evaluate the change derived from the intervention (test 1 was conducted two months before intervention was initiated, test 2 at intervention initiation and test 3 after the completion of the intervention program). The time between tests 1 and 2 enabled detection of spontaneous changes occurring in this group of participants without the treadmill intervention.

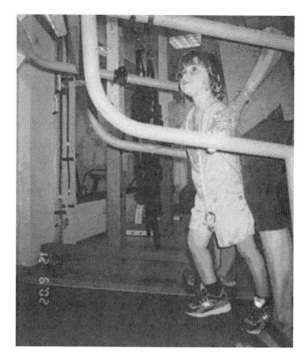

Figure IX-11. Treadmill training.

The intervention program was executed daily for half-hour sessions for the duration of two months. The results of the above mentioned program showed that:

- Results of a two-tailed paired student T-tests on heart rate changes between tests 1 and 2 (before intervention) showed no significant change. Heart rate reduction between tests 2 and 3 (intervention period) was found to be statistically significant $p < 0.005$ (see figure IX-12 and IX-13). The results suggested that aerobic fitness was improved according to reduction in pulse measurements at rest and during training.

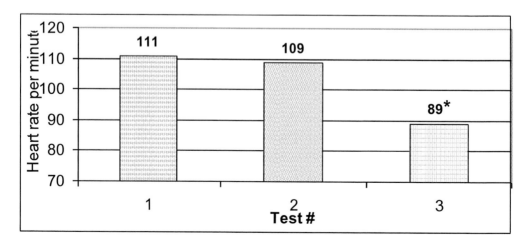

Figure IX-12. Change in heart-rate at rest before and after a treadmill intervention program, all participants.

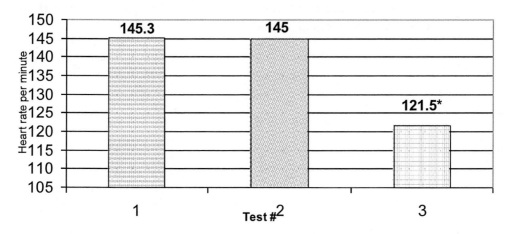

Figure IX-13. Change in heart-rate during exercise before and after a treadmill intervention program, all participants.

- Functional abilities were measured in the same manner, tests 1and 2 before intervention in order to estimate spontaneous functional improvement. Tests 2 and 3 at the beginning and end of the intervention period. Results show that despite lack of change in functional abilities between tests 1and 2, functional abilities of the four participants have shown statistically significant improvement ($p<0.0001$) between tests 2 and 3 (intervention period). Specific functional changes were observed in the ability to get up from a kneeling position to standing, walking a given distance, walking up and down stairs and the ability to knee walk (see figure IX-14 and IX-15).

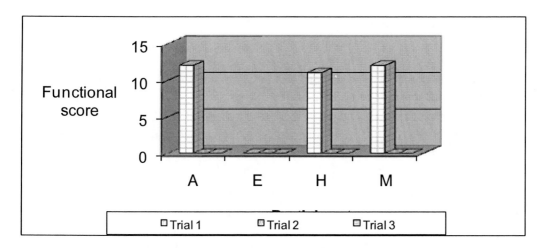

Figure IX-14. Change in stair-ascending ability tests 1-3, all participants.

- When comparing the change in activity heart-rate and the change in functional improvement during the treadmill intervention period, (tests 2 and 3) a high (-0.76) negative and significant ($P<0.05$) correlation was found between functional improvement and changes in heart-rate. The results suggested that as heart-rate levels are reduced (due to improvement in aerobic fitness), functional ability of individuals with RS improves (see figure IX-15).

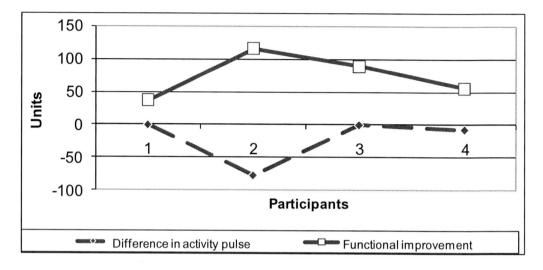

Figure IX-15. Correlation between reduction of heart rate during activity to change in functional activity due to a treadmill intervention programs (tests 2-3).

The conclusions that can be drawn from the above-mentioned physical fitness program were that a daily intervention program could change the fitness level of individuals with RS and that the resulting change may improve the functional abilities of this population. The program was also found to be attainable by non-professional personnel under the supervision of a qualified physical therapist [16] and therefore could be implemented even under strict budgetary limitations.

It is restated here that information from parents disclosed that in some cases, individuals with RS have gained walking ability at the age of six and even at the age of sixteen. In two different cases (studies from Sweden and Norway), two women with RS who had not walked for 15-20 years, have resumed walking ability due to an intensive program [12,15] Similar result was also reported by the author of the present chapter [58]. Due to the importance of ambulation on health and quality of life issues, it is believed that the pursuit of walking should be constantly maintained for persons with RS [4].

Ways of walking

Walking stimulates the joints and muscles and improves functional abilities and aerobic capacity [16] as well as helping the child explore her environment. Walking with a person with RS takes patience and experience. The individual with RS will usually walk slowly and often stops or abruptly changes directions and speeds. The person with RS also has a tendency to lean on the person aiding her and, therefore, it is better to stabilize the child through her shoulder, or through the use of a transfer belt, while avoiding massive support

[10]. Kerr and Budford have defined it as "the art of supporting the child without harming her independence" [36].

Loss of transitional abilities

Loss of transitional movements – due to apraxia, ataxia and sensory abnormalities, the individual with RS may find that performing what we perceive as the simplest actions, such as sitting down or lowering from kneeling to heel sitting, impossible for her. Since loss of transitional skills is frequently seen in individuals with RS [13,32,58], daily use of all these skills should be practiced. Performing the activities indicated below lying on her back, rolling from supine to prone and back, then moving to a hands-and-knees posture and then standing up, can prolong or maintain the ability to perform these skills. Through proper instruction to the family and educational staff on functional abilities, for instance, standing up from sitting in a chair, can be actively practiced throughout the day, each time the child is in transit. Due to Apraxia, the individual with RS might appear unable to perform transitions unless tested in a specific place and using her individual technique. In a case study, a person with RS regained transitional ability from floor to chair when the clues to her memory and motivation were found (i.e. she exercised in the same place and manner that she had done in the past and when it was successful under those conditions, her ability was later generalized) [12].

Osteoporosis

Haas et al [25] have established the fact that individuals with RS are at risk of developing Osteoporosis. This group of researchers has found bone mineral density, mineral bone content and mineral density of the spine compared among 20 young females with RS, 11 females with CP and 25 controls with no pathology to be lacking. Their findings were supported by other groups [26]. Budden and Gunness [27] found similar results in a study of five children with RS. They suggested that slow bone creation at a young age in individuals with RS eventually causes low bone density in this population. They hypothesized that the influence of MECP2 (the gene responsible for RS) is not restricted to damage to brain tissues and that these abnormal findings in bone development are an influence of the RS gene [27].

Osteoporosis is a multi-factorial problem requiring proper diagnosis and organized intervention. In order to achieve appropriate therapeutic intervention, suitable experts should be consulted (physician, dietitian and physical therapist). The basic steps for an anti-osteoporotic regime should include:

- Thorough evaluation of the child in order to sustain or eliminate a diagnosis of osteoporosis and if the osteoporosis is found present, then
- Introduction of appropriate dietetic changes.
- Application of programs aimed at increased mobility, movement and strengthening, according to the child's limitations (if the child is not mobile, an intensive daily standing exercise program should be applied – see below).

- Exposure to sunlight.
- Walking has been discussed at length within the content of the present chapter; for non-ambulant individuals, standing can be used to:
  - Achieve positional changes from continuous sitting
  - Prevent the appearance of pressure sores
  - Align lower extremity joints in extension
  - Maintain and increase bone calcium levels
  - Enhance circulation to internal organs
  - Provide an improved point of view on the individual's social and physical environments
  - Improve function by doing standing transfers, reducing the need to lift the person.

For the prevention, or at least reduction of osteoporosis, and for all the above-mentioned reasons, individuals who do not walk independently should be encouraged to bear weight and practice aided-walking. Children who cannot walk should be situated daily in a standing frame supported just sufficiently to reach their highest ability [4].

Special consideration

Fractures

Individuals with RS show low levels of bone density [25-27] and are at higher risk of receiving fractures than non-RS girls of similar age. Special care should be taken by patients who do not walk at all, are not menstruating despite their maturity or have just come out of a cast. If the child has had several fractures, a specialist should be consulted about some of the newer medications, which are moderately helpful in decreasing the risk of fractures. The measurement of bone density can help in the decision-making regarding appropriate intervention [53]. Management of the child's condition should include fall-prevention strategies [59], proprioceptive dynamic posture training (PDPT) [60] and proper nutritional changes [61].

Manual management for the child, especially one who has already shown pathological fractures, should only be introduced after receiving permission from her family, with careful considerations of the "pros and cons" of activation versus non-activation. The intervention it self should always be initiated after a calming explanation intended to prepare the client for the forthcoming actions.

Surgery

In cases when surgical intervention is needed (e.g. heel-cord lengthening, scoliosis), the therapist should provide support for the family in the pre- and post-surgical management phases and enhance the intensity of the physical therapy program[12]. The surgeon should be aware of the specific challenges facing and techniques developed for this population by referring to appropriate articles[62,63] and consulting with experienced surgeons. Follow-up instructions include recommending appropriate adaptive equipment and intervention regimes.

Sensory problems

Sensory problems in individuals with RS have never been investigated. Nevertheless, parents and clinicians across the world have reported different sensory abnormalities in this population [10,18]. These abnormalities should be considered when treating the individual with RS. Reduced reaction to pain was reported on numerous occasions [10] and should be taken into consideration when applying passive physical manipulations to a child with RS. In fact, a case study suggests that an intense sensory diet implemented both at the educational center and the house of the client with RS might bear positive results. In the above mentioned intervention the individual with RS have shown a reduction in hand mouthing (and therefore reduction in wounds over the palms and around the mouth), enhanced attention span, a slight improvement in hand function and a reduction of a delay in reaching during play activities [64].

Depth perception

It seems that depth perception in this population is faulty, making stair climbing, especially descending stairs extremely difficult. This should be taken in to consideration when working on stair-climbing, stair-descending in particular (at such instances the therapist should stand in front of the child, blocking her line of sight). With one child whom we treated, crossing over on/off the end of a carpet was extremely difficult for her to perform and was achieved only after many hours of training and repetition.

Tactile hyper-sensitivity

Most individuals with RS present some form of hyper-sensitivity of the facial area, especially around the mouth [10,18]. Such sensations may put up barriers on proper oral hygiene and eating habits and should be dealt with using appropriate sensory desensitization. In addition to such reports of hyper-sensitivity around the mouth and face, in several cases the author noticed a rejection reaction when touching the forearms of individuals with RS.

Proprioceptive mechanism

Due to the abnormal central sensory processing of individuals with RS and due to the fact that their body achieves different milestones and than losses them again (stages II and IV of RS), it is logical to assume that the child's body scheme is quite distorted in this group of clients and the person with RS has no confidence in her body. Moreover it is the author's experience that many with RS suffer from an extreme fright of movement that may be defined as Proprioceptive Defensiveness (PD). Therefore it is suggested that the person with RS should receive deep proprioceptive input, on a regular bases, and especially prior to educational experiences were we expect the child to be focused. Such an intervention will assemble the child and enhance her sense of security from her body. Evidence suggests that swaddling is extremely southing for individuals with neurological impairments [65] and we recommend trying swaddling within a flexible material such as lycra (enabling movement through constant resistance), with the person with RS (more information on this topic is available in chapter 10). Improving physical activity through enhanced sensory input could be achieved when using rubber bands across the child's body while performing physical activity (figure IX-16).

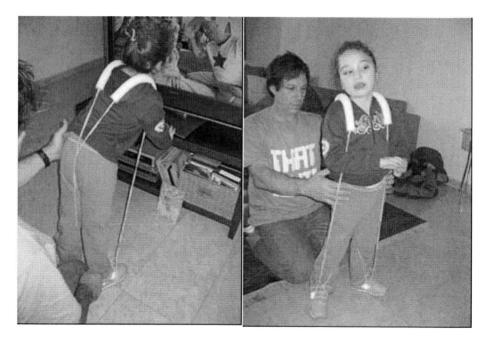

Figure IX-16. Enhanced sensory input during physical activity.

Fear of movement

87% of children with RS display a fear of movement[30], some of them even to an extreme extent. Such fear prevents them from enjoying different activities involving movement, such as physical therapy. This fear should be handled by a sensory program applied on a regular basis. A verbal warning should be given to the child when the therapist is planning on moving her. When motion is applied, it should be done in slow movements while constantly reacting to the child's facial expression and verbally reassuring her. It is advisable to create a movement-stimulating environment around the child. The recommendation is to raise attention to peers, introduce water games and various switches, suggest toys and sensorial stimulation or place mirrors on the walls [4].

Concentration

Lindberg [18] in her book, expressed the view that physical activity improves concentration in children with RS. This assumption should be investigated for each individual with RS under the management of the physical therapist. If found to be correct, appropriate changes in curriculum, such as individual educational intervention after physical sessions, should be made.

Rett syndrome extreme

Most individuals with RS show severe mobility problems, nevertheless, some have displayed extreme physical abilities. Therefore giving in to the disabilities of RS should not be done without a struggle. This part of the chapter describes anecdotal cases of very active individuals with RS in the hope that such examples will inspire others involved in RS.

Motion by individuals with RS can be achieved by using a bicycle. According to parental reports, most children will have a hard time controlling the handle-bars and the pedals and because of this the full function of riding a cycle will be achieved with the aid of a facilitator. Although riding a cycle is a normative skill, it enables the non-mobile person to experience motion and join family trips, even if "just" in a towed trailer. Mutual riding trips can be very positive joint experiences for both the child and her family (Figures IX-17-18).

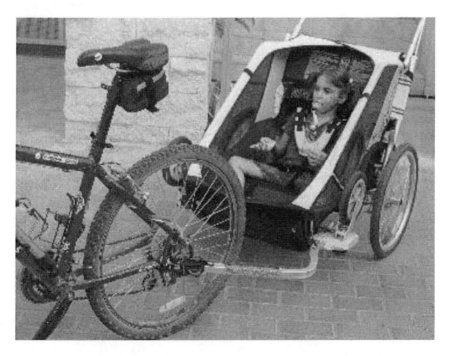

Figure IX-17.

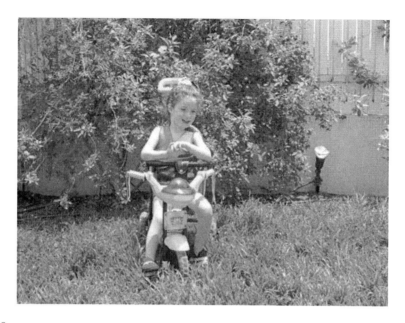

Figure IX-18.

Figures IX-17-18. Using a cycle both as a recreational and physical activity.

There are several known cases of individuals with RS mastering the art of skiing (see figure IX-19). The ability to master such a skill cannot be easily achieved by a child with RS but nonetheless, any form of activity is recommended and advised for this population

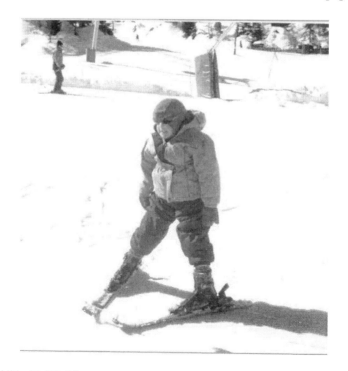

Figure IX-19. A child with RS skiing.

A trampoline is a unique tool for individuals with RS, since it facilitates extremely good muscular and postural control. An account from Australia reports of a child who practices on the trampoline on a daily basis [7]. An active daily practice routine (not necessarily on a trampoline) can improve the body scheme, fitness levels, circulation and muscle strength of the individual and, therefore, is highly recommended.

Conclusions

The present chapter was written with the intention of introducing Rett Syndrome (RS) to the physical therapist familiarizing her/himself with this population and in order to offer some of the author's clinical experience in applying physical therapy intervention programs for these individuals.

Some basic guidelines are drawn up in order to help initiate a physical intervention with this population. Due to the variety of phenotypic manifestation of this syndrome, individual evaluation of each client is advised and treatment should be conducted in accordance with the findings of such an evaluation and with the available knowledge regarding RS prognosis.

The proper intervention for the individual with RS should create a net of human support in which everyone caring for her is familiarized with the client's needs. The authors, as well as others who are acquainted with this disorder [12], believe that the physical therapist should be well informed regarding RS, in order to apply the proper intervention program. Such a program should be conducted through well-communicated teamwork, this being the basic step towards answering the complex therapeutic needs of the individual with RS.

Due to the emotional sensitivity of this population, each individual with RS should be approached with care after a positive rapport is established with the child and specific motivational factors have been established. Due to possible changes in the child's functional and medical levels, the physical therapist is advised to make routine follow-ups as to the client's state and adjust the intervention program in accordance with such changes.

Acknowledgments

Children and parents of individual with RS, the Israeli Rett Center, National Evaluation Team, Chaim Sheba Medical Center, Tel Hashomer, Ramat Gan, Israel, Beit Issie Shapiro, Raanana, colleagues and collaborator are thanked for their input and contributions.

References

[1]   Amir RE, Van den Bellver IB, Wan M, Tran CQ, Francke U, Zoghbi HY. Rett Syndrome is caused by mutations in X-linked MECP2, encoding methyl-CpG-binding protein 2. Nat Genet 1999;23(2): 185-8.

[2] Amir RE, Van Den Veyve IB, Schultz R, Malicki DM, Tran CQ, Dahle EJ, et al. Influence of mutation type and X chromosome inactivation on Rett Syndrome phenotypes. Ann Neurol 2000;47: 670-9.

[3] Hagberg B. Rett syndrome: Clinical and biological aspects. London: Mac Keith Press, 1993.

[4] Lotan M. Management for Rett syndrome. Tel Aviv: Israel Rett Syndrome Center, 2006. [Hebrew]

[5] Kerr AM, Julu PO. Recent insights into hyperventilation from the study of Rett Syndrome. Arch Dis Child 1999;80:384-7.

[6] Percy AK. International research review. Presentation, IRSA 12th Ann Conf, Boston MA, 1996 May 24-27, tape 622-15.

[7] Rett Syndrome Association of Australia Newsletter. October, 1996.

[8] Lotan M, Wein J, Elefant C, Sharf A, Yoshei Y. The Rett syndrome evaluation center in Israel. A play based assessment model. Presentation, Ann Isr Phys Ther Assoc Conf, Dead Sea, March 2005.

[9] Ellaway C, Christodoulou J. Rett Syndrome: Clinical characteristics and recent genetic advances. Disabil Rehabil 2001;23:98-106.

[10] Hunter K. The Rett syndrome handbook. Washington, DC: Int Rett Syndr Assoc, 1999.

[11] Cass H, Reilly S, Owen L, Wisbeach A, Weekes L, Slonims V, et al. Findings from a multidisciplinary clinical case series of females with Rett Syndrome. Dev Med Child Neurol 2003;45(5):325-37.

[12] Larsson G, Engerstrom IW. Gross motor ability in Rett Syndrome-the power of expectation, motivation and planning. Brain Dev 2001;23(Suppl 1):S77-81.

[13] Hanks SB. Physical therapy strategies. Presentation, IRSA 12th Ann Conf, Boston, MA, 1996 May 24-27, tape 622-08.

[14] Budden SS. Rett syndrome: Habilitation and management reviewed. Eur Child Adolesc Psychiatry 1997;6(Suppl 1):103-7.

[15] Jacobsen K, Viken A, Von Tetchner S. Rett syndrome and aging: A case study. Disabil Rehabil 2001;23(3/4):160-6.

[16] Lotan M, Isakov E, Merrick J. Improving functional skills and physical fitness in children with Rett Syndrome. J Intellect Disabil Res 2004;48(8):730-5.

[17] Lotan M, Merrick J, Carmeli E. Scoliosis management in Rett syndrome. A case study. ScientificWorldJournal 2005;5:264-73.

[18] Lindberg B. Understanding Rett syndrome: A practice guide for parents, teachers and therapists. Toronto, Hognefe Huber, 1991.

[19] Beuchel K. Physical therapy and gross motor skills in Rett Syndrome. Handout, IRSA Ann Conf, Washington, DC, May 2001.

[20] Rett A. Grundlagen der Musiktherapie und Music-Psychologie. Stuttgart: Fischer, 1982. [German]

[21] Elefant C. Emotional/musical communication of children with RS. Presentation, Ann Conf Rett Syndr, Sheba Hospital, Ramat-Gan, Israel, 2005.

[22] Elefant C, Lotan M. Rett syndrome: Dual intervention – music and physical therapy. Nord J Music Ther 2004;13(2):172-82.

[23] Lotan M, Hadar-Frumer M. Aquatic rehabilitation for individuals with Rett syndrome. A guidebook for hydro-therapists and parents. Washington, DC: IRSA, 2003.

[24] Gammonley J, Howie AR, Kirwin S, Zapf SA, Frye J, Freeman G, Stuart-Russell R. Animal-assisted therapy: Therapeutic interventions. Renton, WA; Delta Society, 1997.

[25] Haas RH, Dixon SD, Sartoris DJ, Hennessy MJ. Osteopenia in Rett syndrome. J Pediatr 1997;131(5):771-4.

[26] Leonard H, Thomso M, Glasson E, Fyfe S, Leonard S, Ellaway C, et al. Metacarpophalangeal pattern profile and bone age in Rett Syndrome: Further radiological clues to the diagnosis. Am J Med Gen 1999;12(83:88-95.

[27] Budden SS, Gunness ME. Possible mechanisms of osteopenia in Rett syndrome: bone histomorphometric studies. J Child Neurol 2003;18(10):698-702.

[28]   Coleman M, Brubaker J, Hunter K, Smith G. Rett syndrome: A survey of North American patients. J Ment Defic Res 1988;32:117-24.

[29]   Defrin R, Pick H. Pain sensation of individuals with mental retardation. A research report. Tel Aviv: Shalem Foundation, 2006.

[30]   Mount RH, Hastings RP, Reilly S, Cass H, Charman T. Behavioral and emotional features in Rett Syndrome. Disabil Rehabil 2001;23: 129-38.

[31]   Elefant C. Speechless yet communicative: Revealing the person behind the disability of Rett Syndrome through clinical research on songs in music therapy.In: Aldridge D, di Franco G, Ruud E, Wigram T, eds. Music therapy in Europe. Rome: ISMEZ, 2001.

[32]   Hanks SB. Motor disabilities in the Rett Syndrome and physical therapy strategies. Brain Dev 1990;12:157-61.

[33]   Rossin L. Effectiveness of therapeutic and surgical intervention in the treatment of scoliosis in Rett Syndrome. A seminar work. Pittsburgh, PA: Univ Duquesne, 1997.

[34]   Weeks L. Rett syndrome. Presentation, Sydney, Feb 1997.

[35]   Erikssen G. Physical fitness and changes in mortality: the survival of the fittest. Sports Med 2001;31(8):571-6.

[36]   Kerr AM, Burford B. Towards a full life with Rett disorder. Pediatr Rehabil 2001;4(4):157-68.

[37]   Rittweger J, Frost HM, Schiessl H, Ohshima H, Alkner B, Tesch P, et al. Muscle atrophy and bone loss after 90 days' bed rest and the effects of flywheel resistive exercise and pamidronate: results from the LTBR study. Bone 2005;36(6):1019-29.

[38]   Spaak J, Montmerle S, Sundblad P, Linnarsson D. Long-term bed rest-induced reductions in stroke volume during rest and exercise: cardiac dysfunction vs. volume depletion. J Appl Physiol 2005;98(2):648-54.

[39]   Belozerova I, Shenkma B, Mazin M, Leblanc A. Effects of long-duration bed rest on structural compartments of m. soleus in man. J Gravit Physiol 2001;8(1):P71-2.

[40]   Pfeifer M, Sinaki M, Geusens P, Boonen S, Preisinge E, Minne HW. ASBMR Working Group on Musculoskeletal Rehabilitation Musculoskeletal rehabilitation in osteoporosis: A review. J Bone Miner Res 2004;19(8):1208-14.

[41]   Ward K, Alsop C, Caulton J, Rubin C, Adams J, Mughal Z. Low magnitude mechanical loading is osteogenic in children with disabling conditions. J Bone Miner Res 2001;19(3):360-9.

[42]   Caulton JM, Ward KA, Alsop CW, Dunn G, Adams JE, Mughal MZ. A randomised controlled trial of standing programme on bone mineral density in non-ambulant children with cerebral palsy. Arch Dis Child 2004;89(2):131-5.

[43]   Lieb-Lundell C. The therapist's role in the management of girls with Rett Syndrome. J Child Neurol 1998;3(Suppl):S31-4.

[44]   Leonard H, Bower C, English D. The prevalence and incidence of Rett syndrome in Australia. Eur Child Adolesc Psychol 1997;1:8–10.

[45]   Lotan M, Shapiro M. Management of young children with Rett disorder in the controlled multi-sensory (Snoezelen) environment. Brain Dev 2005;27(Suppl 1):S88-94.

[46]   Kaufmann WE, Johnston MV, Blue ME. MeCP2 expression and function during brain development: implications for Rett Syndrome's pathogenesis and clinical evolution. Brain Dev 2005;27(Suppl 1): S77-87.

[47]   Johnston M. Neurobiology of Rett syndrome. A disorder of synaptic development. Presentation, Int Course Rett Syndr, Ostersund, Sweden, 2003 Jun16-18.

[48]   Budden SS. Management of Rett syndrome: A ten-year experience. Neuropediatrics 1995;26(2):75-7.

[49]   Motil KJ, Schultz RJ, Browning K, Trautwein L, Glaze DG. Oropharyngeal dysfunction and gastroesophageal dysmotility are present in girls and women with Rett Syndrome. J Pediatr Gastroenterol Nutr 1999;29(1):31-7.

[50]   Motil KJ, Schultz RJ, Wong WW, Glaze DG. Increased energy expenditure associated with repetitive involuntary movement does not contribute to growth failure in girls with Rett Syndrome. J Pediatr 1998;132(2):228-33.

[51]   Kerr AM. The future for Rett syndrome girls. Int Rett Syndr Assoc Newsletter 1992;Winter:13-4.

[52]   Sampson FC, Hayward A, Evans G, Morton R, Collett B. Functional benefits and cost/benefit analysis of continuous intrathecal baclofen infusion for the management of severe spasticity. J Neurosurg 2002;96:1052-7.

[53]   Sponseller P. Orthopaedic update in Rett syndrome. Rett Gazette 2001;1:4-5.

[54]   Graffman J. Hippotherapy: never heard of it. Rett Gazette 2002;Winter:3-5.

[55]   McClure MK, Battaglia C, McClure RJ. The relationship of cumulative motor asymmetries to scoliosis in Rett Syndrome. Am J Occup Ther 1998;52:196-204.

[56]   Downs J , Bergman A, Carter P, Anderson A, Palmer GM, Roye DP, et al. Guidelines for management of scoliosis in Rett syndrome patients based on expert consensus and clinical evidence, Spine 2009;34(17):E607-17.

[57]   Percy A. Introduction to Rett syndrome. Presentation, IRSA Ann Conf, Las Vegas, NV, tape RS 1, 2000.

[58]   Lotan M. Regaining waking ability in individuals with RS – A case study. Isr J Health Intellect Disabil 2008;1(1):32-43. [Hebrew].

[59]   Dargent-Molina P, Favier F, Grandjean H, Baudoin C, Schott AM, Hausherr E, et al. Fall-related factors and risk of hip fracture: The EPIDOS prospective study. Lancet 1996;348:145-9.

[60]   Sinaki M, Lynn SG. Reducing the risk of falls through proprioceptive dynamic posture training in osteoporotic women with kyphotic posturing: A randomized pilot study. Am J Phys Med Rehabil 2002;81:241-6.

[61]   Heaney RP. Advances in therapy for osteoporosis. Clin Med Res 2003;1(2):93-9.

[62]   Dearlove UR, Walker RW. Anasthesis for Rett Syndrome. Peadiatric Anasthesia 1996;6:55-8.

[63]   Konarzewski WH, Misso S. Rett Syndrome and delayed recovery from anesthesia. Anaesthesia 1994;49(4):357.

[64]   Cantor A, Vizel E, Lotan M. Successful sensory integration intervention with a child with Rett Syndrome. Isr J Health Intellect Disabil 2009;2(3):154-62. [Hebrew]

[65]   Ohgi S, Akiyama T, Arisawa K, Shigemori K. Randomised controlled trial of swaddling versus massage in the management of excessive crying in infants with cerebral injuries. Arch Dis Child 2004 89(3):212-6.

In: Rett Syndrome: Therapeutic Interventions
Editors: Meir Lotan and Joav Merrick

ISBN: 978-1-61728-080-1
©2011 Nova Science Publishers, Inc.

Chapter X

Rett syndrome: Occupational Therapy Intervention

Yael Yoshei, OT, HT and Meir Lotan, BPT, MScPT, PhD[*]

Israel Rett Center, National Evaluation Team, Chaim Sheba Medical Center, Tel HaShomer, Ramat Gan and Department of Physical Therapy, Ariel University Center of Samaria, Ariel, Israel

Some of the difficulties presented by individuals with Rett syndrome (RS) are limited hand function, stereotypic hand movements, a chaotic dysfunctional sensory system, and difficulties in planning and executing motor acts (apraxia). In order to successfully handle such a multitude of difficulties and to suggest a sensible individually adapted intervention for the person with RS, the occupational therapist should be familiar with commonalities characterizing this population. Since the life expectancy of individuals with RS is about 50 years it is essential that the therapeutic environment be constantly adapted and presented in an age appropriate manner in accordance to the changing needs of the child, the girl, and the woman with RS. Moreover, the individual phenotypic expression of each person with RS necessitates a thorough evaluation followed by an individually tailored intervention program for each person with this disorder.

In this chapter we discuss clinical commonalities of individuals with RS and suggest some possible directions for intervention with this population. The chapter is based on the limited literature and our clinical experience working with this population.

Introduction

Rett syndrome (RS) is a genetic disorder mainly affecting females [1,2] characterized by an arrest of brain development [3]. A person presenting the symptoms associated with RS will present an array of functional limitations such as dysfunctional hand usage, stereotypic hand

---

[*] Correspondence: Meir Lotan, BPT, MScPT, PhD, Department of Physical Therapy, Ariel University Center of Samaria, IL-40700 Ariel, Israel. E-mail: ml_pt_rs@netvision.net.il

mannerisms, limitations in sensory perception, and difficulties in initiating and executing motor acts, known as apraxia [4]. In order for the occupational therapist (OT) to successfully handle the diversity of these functional limitations he/she needs to familiarize him/herself with the commonalities of this disorder. Since the life span of individuals with RS is estimated today to be in the area of 50 years [5] it is important for the OT to adapt the therapeutic environment in accordance with the changing needs of the child, the girl, and then the woman with RS, thus making the intervention age appropriate.

In many cases, individuals with RS present changes in mood and functional level. Such changes can sometimes be linked to change in the person's medical state or they may be completely unexplainable. Such changes may appear abruptly or gradually; they may be present for a few month or change within the time frame of hours [6]. These changes obligate the therapist (in this case the OT) to practice understanding and flexibility in regards to both the level of difficulty of the immediate goals, and the handling of the client, while at the same time keeping the individual in the same general path of progression and achievement.

Another clinical characteristic of RS is the phenotypic diversity of individuals within this population [7], necessitating appropriate evaluation and the construction of an individually adapted therapeutic intervention for each client [8]. In general, due to the many challenges presented by the person with RS to her caregivers and therapists and the long time it takes some individuals with RS to acclimate to new places and people, it is imperative that the staff working with the person with RS be familiar with her individual preferences. Time should be provided for care personnel to acquire as much information as possible from the person's parents and her former educational facility. Time should also by available and planned in advance for non-stressful bonding of staff members with the person with RS.

The present chapter will discuss challenges in the life of the person with RS which might be alleviated by the skilled intervention of an OT. The chapter is based on the very limited literature available on the topic of therapeutic intervention with RS, and, to a greater extent, on the clinical experience of both authors (over 16 years each), both as therapists working with this population on a daily basis, and as members of the national Israeli Rett syndrome multidisciplinary evaluation team [9], which has to date evaluated over 140 individuals with RS.

The role of the OT changes according to the facilities and settings in which she\he meets the individual with RS. Yet we believe that in most cases the OT will focus on one or more of the following areas:

- evaluating, improving, and maintaining hand function
- improving sensory processing and dealing with sensory processing issues
- adapting the environment
- therapeutically relating to the apraxic elements of the person with RS
- enhancing independent and age appropriate play and interactions

Hand function and hand stereotypical movements

Limited hand function is one of the main characteristics of RS and the stereotypical hand movements are one of the trade marks of RS, considered as one of the main clinical diagnostic elements of this syndrome. These hand mannerisms typically appear at chest level and in body midline; they mostly include hand washing, hand wringing, and hand clapping but can also be observed as hand mouthing, hands behind the back, pulling on clothes, object banging, hands over head [6] and more. These movements appear gradually starting from a young age; they increasingly develop until they form a constant movement pattern, individually typical for each child. In older ages these movements gradually decrease (probably due to increased rigidity) and might only be observed as slight finger movements. Due to the intense nature of these movements there have been numerous attempts at stopping or at list minimizing them, as well as an ongoing debate as to whether these movements should be controlled or disregarded [10].

The InterRett Output Database [11], dedicated to collecting data from around the globe, suggests that stereotypical hand movements increase as the young child with RS grows up (table X-1).

Table X-1. Change in hand mannerisms in RS according to age of child

Age of child	Hand mannerisms (percentage of appearance among persons at this age)
Up to age 6 month	1.67
7-10 month of age	3.19
12 month	23.21
2-3 years of age	61.73
Adults with RS	100

Very young individuals with RS may perform minute hand movements; yet these movements are fully developed at around two years of age. This might be connected with the maturing process at the cerebellar cortex level [12].

Mount et al [11] found that hand mannerisms are apparent in 100% of the adult RS population. Lindberg [6] pointed out that these hand movements are different from the ones exhibited by autistic children. When you observe the autistic child you see that some of the hand movements are specifically meant for visual stimuli, while other movements involve object manipulation. Individuals with RS rarely use the hand movement for visual stimulation and\or for object manipulation. In fact, one sometimes gets the feeling that the person with RS cannot stop her hand movement even when she is motivated to do so. The actual cause for the hand stereotypical movements is unknown. No connection has been found between enhancing sensory stimuli to the hands and reduction of hand mannerisms, therefore the basic assumption is that the hand movements are not performed to provide a sensory need [13].

The intensity of hand movements might change according to different situations. Wehmeyer, Bourland and Ingram]14] observed stereotypical hand movements in individuals with RS under four different conditions: spontaneous (no demand); when encouraged to perform certain activities (verbal instructions and physical encouragement); attention (no demand but with physical contact); and leisure time (physical proximity to preferred objects with no demand). The researchers found that the attention time and leisure time were the most effective in reducing stereotypical hand movements. Often we might see the hand movement's intensity increases in situations where the person with RS is agitated, exited, upset or angry. On the other hand we can observe a reduction in hand movements when there is an external cause that draws her attention.

The combination of ataxia, apraxia, and muscle tonal changes (hypo/hypertonicity), highly reduces hand function and makes it very hard for the person with RS to accurately perform functional movement. Therefore, most individuals with RS are in need of full support in most areas of ADL. But there are apparent differences between individuals with RS, as some can use their hands only to perform a basic pushing\shoving action, while others might reach out and grab or even hold objects, perform a simple manipulation, or even show functional abilities. More advanced manual abilities can be found in the mildly affected individuals and in the "Angleman type" RS [4].

Despite such limitations in hand function, it is known that when the person with RS is presented with a powerful motivating factor an impressive change from her "usual" abilities can be observed. In one incidence a girl who presented with a very poor ability to manipulate objects, let alone hold them for prolonged periods of time, was able to completely empty a glass of Coca-Cola (pick the glass up from the table, press it against her lips, and hold it until the glass was completely empty) but only when the glass was filled with Coca-Cola. When she was done the glass fell to the floor. This same girl was also able to hold, without dropping it for the whole duration of time it took to completely eat a sandwich with chocolate spread (only chocolate spread) that was put in her hands, and to use a teaspoon to completely demolish a cone of chocolate pudding (only when it was chocolate flavored). The importance of a motivating factor in improving hand use in individuals with RS was demonstrated by Elefant [15] and Elfant and Wigram [16,17]. In this case seven participants in a research project were encouraged to select a preferred song from a list. The results of that intervention indicate that both experience (repetition) and song preference had a positive influence on the ability of the participants to indicate their choice with their hands. Similar results were found in a research examining the ability of individuals with RS to use a computer program through the use of a touch screen [18]. Achieving manual function is extremely important for the person with RS. Such an achievement might enable the person with RS to gain control in many aspects of her life: pointing at signs and/or objects, enhancing communication through augmentative and alternative communication (AAC), activating an array of household equipment through the use of switches, operating a computer, using food utensils, playing games, and more. The more the person with RS will be able to improve her manual capabilities, the more she will be able to gain independence and control over her daily life. Such successes might encourage her to keep trying and improving her abilities.

Evaluating hand function

When our therapeutic aim is to encourage hand function it would be wise to begin with a precise evaluation of the client's initial hand function and potential. This evaluation should be thorough and the therapist should take the needed time for a full evaluation. An analysis of the child's initial hand function can also be achieved by video-capturing during common daily situations, and through the use of functional charts [13]. Taking the first few sessions to fully acquaint yourself with the child with RS is also advised due to the fact that individuals with RS are extremely motivated by emotional bonding. Therefore a therapist who takes her/his time to achieve good rapport with the client with RS will be able to achieve fuller cooperation when the going gets tough (and it will). When evaluating functional hand usage of the person with RS the therapist should take into account:

- The existence of stereotypical hand movements
- How is the movement performed, does it involve two hands or one, is there a dominant hand, is the mouth involved?
- At what times and situations do they increase and when do they lessen
- What is the muscle tone of the trunk and of the shoulder girdle? Is the person hypotonic or rigid\spastic?
- Is there a scoliosis that might influence the client's posture in a seating\standing position? And how does it influence the child's manual function?
- Is the person with RS mobile and is she able to ambulate independently from one place to the other?
- Is she able to hold objects in her hands? What are the size, shape and texture of those objects?
- How long can the client with RS hold an object in her hands?
- Can she independently release a held object from her hand?
- If an object (a spoon for example) is held in her hand, can she bring it to her mouth?
- Can she manipulate different objects (move, push, hit, or transfer from hand to hand)?
- Are there some functional abilities that are performed better than others? How long is her reaction time in a task requiring manual function?
- Can she cross midline?
- Can she separate her hands and can she function with each one separately or activate both hands as one unit?
- Can she regulate her movements and force and to what extant?
- Does she show any sensory processing difficulties in her hands? In what areas of the hands? What substances and textures increase her sensitivity?

The information gathered from such an assessment should later be used to construct an appropriate intervention program with the aim of advancing hand function.

Splint usage

Some incongruence exists in regard to the use of arm and elbow splints. Some research findings suggest that the use of elbow splints reduces spasticity and stereotypic hand movements while at the same time enhancing object usage [19,20], other research studies do not find a significant influence [21]. According to Dr. Rett's statements [22,23], and also in accordance to our experience, the use of splints might divert the stereotypical movements from the hands to other body parts (leg swaying, body movements, tilting the body to the side). Other disadvantages of splinting the hands of individuals with RS might be presented as discomfort and even frustration. When splints are used it seems that the person with RS is trying to "compensate" for the time in the splints with excessive hand mannerisms when the splints are removed. Therefore it is our belief, that as rule, splints should not be used with individuals with RS. Yet when it comes to individuals with RS, each is a unique individual presenting a specific set of challenges for the therapist and therefore there are some exceptions to this guideline. These include:

- When the stereotypic hand movements cause self abuse or medical problems
  - On occasion, especially when the hand movements involve mouthing, the constant repeated movements can cause skin breakdown on the hands and around the mouth. The wetness can also provoke the growth of fungi
  - When the movements are continuously performed in the same position muscle shortening may later appear, leading to reduction in joint range of motion and contractures usually at the elbow.
  - When the movements are continuously performed in the same position the continuous thumping can cause skin breakdown both to the hands as well as at the place where the hands are constantly banging
- When the hand movements cause social isolation by her peers
  - If the child with RS has social contact with her peer group and the hand mannerisms include mouthing with excessive salivation, the use of splints might prevent the child from being rejected by her peers. In this case as well the use of other measures less conspicuous than splints are preferred (these options will be discussed later)
- When the use of splints clearly improves the hand function of the non-splinted hand. In this case, the use of splints should be limited to individual intervention sessions during which the child is expected to perform manual tasks.
- When the stereotypical hand movements harm the child's functional abilities.
  - When the child is in need of a walker for ambulation, yet is unable to use the walker due to her hand movements [12].
  - In some instances it can be determined that the child is "trapped" within her hand movements and is unable to separate one hand from the other in order to perform a manual task
  - In some cases it appears that the manual movements completely engulf the child's attention, thereby preventing her from taking part in any other functional/social/creative activity. In such cases periodic prevention of hand stereotypical movements through the use of splints at appropriate times might be implemented. Such intermissions should be carried out only if the child agrees with such actions and does not become unduly stressed [12].
  - If during meal times the child with RS is putting her hand in her mouth preventing feeding and removing food items from the mouth, thereby preventing proper feeding; a discontinuation of hand mannerism should be considered.

To date, hand splints have been tried both uni- and bi-laterally, with a variety of sizes and materials. The most effective splints have been found to be elbow splints, with lesser success attributed to finger and wrist splints. In other words, the influence of splints has been found to directly relate to their size; the bigger the splint the more effective it is [24]. In any case, splints should always be used as functional and health enhancers and not as movement blockers per se. When splints are considered, it is advised that their use be periodical rather than constant, that the use be directed towards achieving specific goals (such as educational, self-feeding, mobility through the use of a walker, and communication goals) and not as a constant way of being. We also advise that the initial intervention be kept to the minimum (the smallest splints; the use of soft materials) and only if such interventions are unsuccessful in achieving the desired goal should other more intense measures be considered (harder materials; longer splints; longer duration of wear). The use of splints should always be considered with the aim of achieving the maximal results with the minimal harm to the child's daily activities and quality of life. Despite the abnormality and weird appearance of the stereotypical movements they are, whether we like it or not, a part of who the person with RS is [6].

Reducing stereotypical hand movements

Techniques described in the literature to negate the stereotypical movements of individuals with RS include:

- Oppressing bilateral stereotypical movements
  - o Rigid splints have been found to improve the ability of children with RS to participate in play and A.D.L activities [25, 26].
  - o Splints made out of soft materials (rubber products) attached to the elbows have been found to slow down and reduce stereotypical movements [27].
  - o The use of a device called TALK BACK (typically used by speech therapists as a sound enhancer) on the mouth area has been reported to prevent a child with RS from inserting her hands into her mouth [27].
  - o Towels wrapped around the palms have been found to be effective in reducing hand mouthing [6]; socks or gloves could be used for the same purpose.
  - o Small inflatable swimming buoys placed over the child's elbows will allow full range of motion in the shoulder girdle and palms, yet stop the child from achieving the last degrees of flexion at the elbows, thereby preventing mouthing.
  - o Thumb abduction splints have been, by chance, found by the authors to reduce stereotypical movements in RS (unpublished data).
- Repressing activity in the non-preferred hand. Preventing stereotypic activity of the less active hand usually "frees" the other hand to become more active and functional. Usually the hand which is more active in performing the manual stereotypical movements will also be the child's more functional hand [28].
  - o Putting a soft splint (i.e. neoprene) on the non-preferred hand.
  - o Side sitting with weight bearing on the non-preferred hand [6].
  - o Placing the less active hand under the table during mealtimes and during individual intervention.

  o   Placing a small weight on the wrist of the less active hand [27].
  o   A "hand over hand" technique is widely used during individual intervention
      and meal times; this technique is reported by many caregivers to be an
      effective method for enhancing the manual abilities of the child with RS.
- Physical activity that necessitates hand use [6]
  o   Ascending and descending stairs with the use of the rails
  o   Horseback riding
  o   Use of a seesaw or a merry-go-round
  o   Taking a walk with the child's favorite dolls, while grasping the dolls'
      stroller
  o   Jumping on the trampoline while holding the rails.
  o   Wheelbarrow walking
  o   Riding a bike
  o   Holding flotation devices in a swimming pool
- Improving functional abilities
  o   In order to prevent wiggly movements of the palm and fingers during meal-
      times, fingers III and IV were tied together. Later it was accidentally found
      that this maneuver enabled the child to achieve finger-thumb grasping [27].
  o   Placing objects in a tank of water sometimes makes it easier for the person
      with RS to capture them [6].
  o   Velcro strips over the palms can help the child maintain her grasp on an
      object for long durations (this technique should be cautiously applied as it
      might achieve the opposite; thus causing the child to completely abandon
      independent grasping).
  o   Improving grasp and holding for long durations might be achieved through
      covering different utensils by materials that are pleasant to touch (fur, silk)
      or interesting to look at (shiny, colorful).
  o   Constant practice of a single movement over a long period of time may
      enable the child to overcome her apraxia and perform the movement
      automatically (this method may requires a long duration of practice and the
      use of motivators will enhance the learning process).
  o   The use of switch operated toys is a motivating factor for the young child
      with RS to initiate hand movement. Attaching the switches to a tape playing
      the child's favorite songs will shorten the time required for the acquisition of
      such a task.
- Sensory stimulation. The use of sensory stimulation is reported to be effective in
  reducing hand stereotypical movements [29]. For example, the use of motivating
  sensory elements in a sensory room that combine several sensory modalities such as
  the bubble pole (light, vibration, sound) or audio-visual games (touch, sound, light)
  have been found to be effective. However, in a trial held with two girls with RS it
  was found that a sustained vibratory intervention to the palms and hands had an
  inconsistent effect in reducing hand mannerisms [13]. Nevertheless, there is a variety
  of suggestions that might be found useful in reducing stereotypical hand movements
  of the child with RS (these modes of intervention have not been specifically
  investigated in individuals with RS), as well as improve hand function.
- Verbal Feedback
  o   Verbal suppression as a form of behavioral modification can also be used to
      ask the person with RS to stop her hand mannerisms. However care should

be taken not to turn this feedback to the person with RS into a game, where the child is doing her stereotypical hand movements just to get more attention [6]. It should be mentioned however that this type of behavioral approach was not found extremely useful in reducing stereotypical hand movements [31].

- o Verbal support might be used as an opposite method for verbal suppression. If this method is used the child is constantly praised when she stops doing the stereotypical hand movements. The two methods suggested in this section could be used simultaneously.

- Improving hand function in RS
    - o Brushing the child's hands with brushes of different textures. At the beginning of the brushing experience the child can be offered an array of brushes; later she should be given the opportunity to choose her favorite brushes (the type of brush selected by the child can give the OT a clue regarding the child's sensitivities or lack thereof).
    - o Massaging the arms, hands, and palms with cream. This experience can also be used to enhance body awareness and acknowledgment of body parts, for example if the clinician sings to the child, describing each different body part being touched, while massaging her hands.
    - o Deep proprioceptive massage compressing the upper extremity joints. These compressions should be performed by the OT or by the prime caregiver following instructions given by the OT. They should be performed slowly and rhythmically. The caregiver\therapist performing this intervention should be constantly aware of the child's reaction, making sure it is not causing any discomfort or aggravation to the child, and maintaining her privacy.
    - o Introducing a variety of sensory experiences through the use of different materials such as foam, sand, beans, hand paints, or water.
    - o Bearing weight on the hands while the child is seating on a role or a ball, or is standing on all fours. When introducing a weight bearing activity the facilitator should bear in mind the sensitivity of the person with RS to movement, particularly movement of the limbs and body, mainly attributed to sensitivity of the proprioceptive system.
    - o Heavy vests filled with sand, beans or lentils can be used to organize the child's body schema, thereby enhancing body awareness and preventing some forms of hand mannerisms.
    - o Heavy bracelets can be used to prevent hand stereotypic movements. The size, weight, and duration of use for each bracelet should be individually assigned to each client. During the time the bracelets are in use, the child's reaction for irritation and aggression should be monitored; the duration of use should be determined based on the child's reaction. In some cases the wearing of a bracelet on one hand organizes the child, reduces hand mannerisms, and enhances function while in other children it might cause aggravation and thus the use of the bracelet should be suspended or reconsidered.
    - o A single study reports on the successful use of Transcutaneous Electrical Neural Stimulation (TENS) in reducing hand mannerisms with two girls with RS [30]. A retest of the effectiveness of this approach has found no

correlation between the use of the TENS and occurrence of hand mannerisms (unpublished data).

o   Our past experience with two girls with RS has suggested that through full immersion of the child's body and hands in a ball pool, with a peaceful background music and a serene atmosphere, it was possible to cause the stereotypical hand movements to stop, for the duration of the time the children stayed in the pool. Moreover, once outside the ball pool a carryover effect was observed for a duration of time equal to the time when she was in the pool (if the child stayed in the ball pool for half an hour she did not do any hand movement for that duration and for the next half hour after exiting the ball pool). This phenomenon was found inconsist [12].

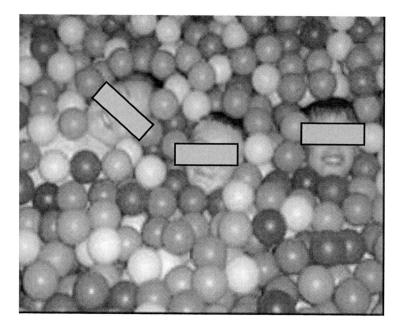

Figure X-1. Immersion in a ball pool.

o   Different games that involve weight bearing on the upper extremities while moving, such as standing on all fours on a vestibular plate, wheelbarrow walking, climbing a ladder, holding the ropes of a swing, walking with a doll buggy etc. all help to improve hand function.

o   Identifying a factor of interest for the person with RS could temporarily reduce hand mannerisms [13]. Introducing a preferred song, a video or a favorite food item might capture the child's attention and do the trick. The excitement might, on the other hand, produce the opposite effect by enhancing hand movement.

o   Distracting the child's attention might also be found useful in reducing stereotypical hand movements. This could be achieved through: A connection with other people, a flashlight, candles, shadows, soap bubbles, dancing, looking at photographs, listening to a story or a person playing an instrument, watching TV, taking a ride in a car or taking a walk

- o   Auditory reward such as attaching rattles to the child's hands was found successful in preventing the child with RS from putting her hands in her mouth due to the fact it made a noise every time the child moved her hands.
- o   Voluntary control can be tried if the child shows a high level of understanding and can control her stereotypical hand movements. It might help to ask her to stop doing the repetitive movements.

We reiterate that each person with RS reacts differently to different approaches and that a variety of approaches should be tried with each person until the method that best suits the specific child is determined. When the caregiver\therapist is applying different approaches, he\she must be flexible and attuned to the girl, since fluctuations in mood, behavior, and function are very common for the person with RS. We would also suggest that the therapist bears in mind that the child with RS finds it hard to adapt to new experiences and therefore the implementation of a new program should be gradual.

The good news is that when intensive consistent programs aimed at improving hand function and reducing stereotypical hand movements were implemented under the supervision of OT, the participants were able to show good functional abilities [32]. If one method of intervention is decided upon it should be consistently implemented until we are sure that the child has adapted to the program and only then should we decide if the program should be continued or withdrawn, also taking the child's reaction into account.

Sensory intervention

The sensory system is our perception system, through which we receive, process, and imbed our daily experiences, and react accordingly. Our sensory channels can relax our body or stimulate it; therefore this important route should be used for the benefit of the person with RS. Happy music, bright colors, and a supportive atmosphere will encourage and enhance function and mood, while a dark room, slow quiet music, and close rhythmical physical contact will contain and reduce the crying and irritability of most children. To date no scientific evaluation has explored the sensory system of individuals with RS and therefore it is extremely difficult to assess the magnitude of the deficiency with which these individuals are struggling, yet it is believed that the person with RS has to struggle with severe impairment in sensory modulation.

Despite the fact that we cannot physically alter and control the way the world is perceived by the sensory system of children with RS, we can however mold their daily surroundings to adapt to their being so that it would feel right for them. An adapted environment would enable the child with RS to achieve education, joy, and functional improvements, and would reduce discomfort. It is obvious that the complex nature and the uniqueness of each RS client place a heavy burden on the caregiving and therapeutic staff, yet they can use their knowledge within daily situations to make every experience a learning one and every day functionally and educationally fruitful.

Elements of the sensory system

We will begin addressing the sensory issue by briefly presenting the different elements of the multi-modal sensory system.

Tactile system

The tactile system operates through sensory receptors scattered over our skin. These receptors transfer the information about temperature, texture, pain and touch of the external world to our brain. The tactile system is especially sensitive around the mouth and palms as these are the primary areas through which the small baby explores his surroundings. This system, in combination with the proprioceptive system, is responsible for constructing our body scheme. A complete, mature and intact body scheme is essential for proper propulsion of our bodies through our daily surroundings [33]. A dysfunctional processing of the tactile information may be expressed in "over sensitivity". In this case, referred to in the literature as tactile defensiveness (TD), many ordinary daily stimuli are perceived by the person with TD as threatening. In severe cases the person will reject any physical contact and will resent being held or touched or even feel uncomfortable with certain clothes over her body. Our experience with children with RS has shown that there are certain areas that are more sensitive to touch than others. For instance, individuals with RS commonly present high sensitivity around the face especially around the mouth [6]. This type of sensitivity might cause difficulties during mealtimes and when oral hygiene is pursued. The difficulty in correctly assessing the external world will prevent the development of a mature and intact body scheme which is necessary for the person to properly relate to her physical surrounding. One of the major problems resulting from a difficulty to properly address external challenges is the inability to learn and\or execute motor acts which is defined as apraxia. Apraxia is typical for most persons with RS.

Proprioceptive system

This system sends information from the deep tissues of our body, and it enables the person to evaluate the position of different body structures in relation to one another. The sensors of this system are scattered within the muscles, joints and deep tissues. Our brain uses the information supplied by the proprioceptive afferent pathways in conjunction with information coming from the vestibular system to enable us to decipher the way our body moves through space, how different organs are moving in relation to the trunk and to one another. This system is the basis for smooth rhythmic and coordinated movement. Despite the scarcity of knowledge in relation to this system, it is our experience that many persons with RS suffer from an extreme fright of movement that may be defined as proprioceptive defensiveness (PD). This situation can be observed in individuals with RS more commonly than in others with developmental disabilities and should be suggested as a unique characteristic typical for individuals with this syndrome. When PD is presented at an extreme, the person with RS refrains from movement and reacts with extreme distress, to the point of crying, to movement of the body and limbs, especially if such movement is not initiated by the person but rather by an external facilitator. When the child is immobilized for long durations (for a few weeks – in cases of a trauma or casting) the situation is aggravated; in three different cases we have seen that the children were able to regain their previous movement abilities only after more than two years of intensive, but gentle intervention and the use of sedatives (in one child) and anxiety reducers (in a second child).

Vestibular system

This system is the foundation of our equilibrium system, and is based in the inner ear. The receptors of this system send messages to the brain regarding the movement and position of the head in space. Through the process of sensory integration our balance perception and reaction is assembled, utilizing the combined information from the vestibular, visual and proprioceptive systems.

Visual system

The visual system reports the details of our physical world to the brain. It enables us to enjoy a variety of colors and visual experiences as well as grasp the height and depth of objects. The connections between the visual system and the other (proprioceptive and vestibular) systems which constitute our balance system enable us to maintain our equilibrium, to handle obstacles and stairs, and to avoid being hurt by the hectic constantly moving and changing world around us. When this system is malfunctioning, for instance when the person is crossed eyed, he will have an extremely hard time evaluating the height of objects (How high is the stair I am descending from? How high is that carpet? Can I go over this doorstep?) thus making a line drawn on the floor an impassable barrier. Most individuals with RS can only be diagnosed with mild visual impairments [6,34], therefore their eye sight is considered to function within the norm. In some cases the processing of incoming information is lacking for this population. In an interview with a person with RS with the preserved speech variant (PSV) she said that walking down the stairs is the most difficult and frightening task for her to do (unpublished data).

Auditory system

The receiving part of the auditory system is situated within the middle and inner ear. The sensors are sensitive to airwave vibrations that are being deciphered by the brain as sounds. The majority of individuals with RS present an undisturbed functioning of their audio system [35]. When comparing the normally functioning audio sensory channel to all other sensory modalities of the person with RS, one might understand why songs and sounds are the most motivational elements in the world of the person with RS.

Taste

The receptors of this system are situated on the tongue and enable us to distinguish between different types and tastes of food items.

Smell

This system receives its input from the outer world through sensors situated at the base of the nose. The sensors transmit the smells around us to the brain. This system is not very developed in most humans and this is no different in individuals with RS. However, in a study taking place in the United States it was found that the smell receptors in individuals with RS do not develop properly. [36]. Since the smell sensors are an extension of the brain tissue, these findings suggest that the rate of development of neurons in the brain of individuals with RS is somewhat different, but the full impact of these findings in regard to both the smell abilities of individuals with RS and brain nerve cells maturation is unclear as yet.

Dysfunctions of the sensory system

A dysfunctional sensory system is a most baffling state. This situation of uncontrolled unexplained incoming messages leaves the child in a state of chaos that is very typical of stage II of RS [6], and might explain why most individuals with RS withdraw into what is usually perceived by the outside observer as an "autistic like" behavior. If your own sensory system has crushed and can no longer be trusted, than the most logic thing to do would be to separate your self from the outer world to reduce the number of stimuli. In fact experts in the field of RS have suggested that sensory input should be controlled and sensory stimuli to the brain minimized during the second stage of RS [29].

Considerable work in the area of sensory processing was done in the late 1960s by Jane Ayres. In order to develop an appropriate sensory intervention program for the child with RS, it is essential for an OT experienced in the field of sensory integration to evaluate her client in this area. In the next part of this chapter we will present some principles/suggestions regarding sensory intervention in individuals with RS. Some of the following suggestions have been made by parents, some by OT's, and some by the authors in light of their experience with this group of clients. However, we would like to reiterate that the dissimilarities between individuals with RS necessitate the therapist to individually construct his intervention for each child in light of her unique set of difficulties. We suggest that the OT refrain from absolute generalization of our suggestions to every individual with RS.

- Many with RS encounter difficulties in reception, deciphering, processing, and integrating of sensory stimuli. An OT experienced with sensory integration should evaluate the sensory difficulties that the child faces, and adjust her sensory surrounding to fit the child's needs.

- During stage II of RS, the child experiences total sensory chaos. Therefore we will find the child at that stage mostly touchy and irritable or distant. In this stage it is advised to reduce the amount of incoming stimuli. Therapeutic interventions should be relaxing in nature, with slow, deep rhythmic touch accompanied by dimmed lights [29,37].
- Individuals with RS sometimes display a delayed reaction to pain [38]. It is assumed that the delayed reaction is not caused by reduced sensation to pain, but rather by a long reaction time generated from slow central sensory processing. Since a child with RS who has been hurt might only show evidence of this sometime later, it is essential that care should be taken when physically handling the child with RS.
- Many persons with RS show hypersensitivity around the mouth. Therefore when approaching the mouth of the child with RS (during mealtimes or when oral hygiene is being kept) it should be done slowly, with accompanying verbal preparation, and with close attunement to the child's reaction. We suggest using the NUK primary dental kit when working in the oral area, as preparation for both teeth brushing and eating.
- The oral hypersensitivity of the child with RS might necessitate that mealtimes start with an oral desensitization program and accompanying verbal preparation. The child should be allowed ample time to acclimate her mouth to the taste, temperature and texture of the food items. If new food items are introduced they should be presented slowly and gradually.
- The oral hypersensitivity of the child with RS might also express itself as a reaction towards food temperatures. Therefore we might find that the child, despite being hungry, will refuse food in her mouth. This possibility necessitates that the staff working with the child be familiar with her personal preferences and act accordingly. If the child prefers colder temperatures the food should be cooled while if the child likes the food warm then special utensils that keep the food warm even through long mealtimes should be used (see figure X-2).

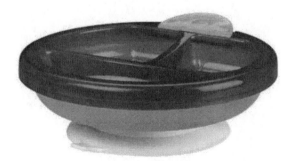

Figure X-2. Baby warming dish.

- It is probable to assume that the person with RS will not tolerate metal utensils in her mouth and plastic ones are preferred. Due to the ataxic characteristic of RS, the girl's bite might not be controlled and therefore we suggest the use of thick plastic food utensils, which will not break under force.
- Some parents report that their child is also sensitive to touch under the palmar side of her feet. Such hypersensitivity might escalate to a point where the child refrains from walking to avoid unpleasant sensory input. Deep sensory massage and feet

movements, as well as the use of different materials on the feet (preferably with the child setting the pace and choosing the type of materials) are advised in such cases.

- It is probable that the constant movements of the hands together with abnormal sensory processing cause the child to receive unclear messages from her surroundings. Therefore, stabilizing the child's less active hand (with a splint or through the caregiver\therapist's hand) will reduce the constant flow of incoming irrelevant information and make the control over the more functional hand easier for the child, thereby enhancing functional hand use. We would like to highlight the fact that individuals with RS react differently to external manipulation of their hands. For most girls with RS, separation of the hands enables function of the dominant hand; however, for others, the hand movements are used as an organizational strategy and as a preparation for movement - in such cases separating the hands only cause inhibition to functional usage.

Due to the abnormal central sensory processing of individuals with RS, coupled with the fact that their bodies achieve different milestones and then lose them again (stages II and IV of RS), it is logical to assume that their body schemes are quite distorted and that they have no confidence in their bodies. Therefore, it is suggested that the person with RS should receive deep proprioceptive input on a regular basis, and especially prior to educational and other experiences where we expect the child to be focused. Input of this sort will organize the child and enhance her sense of security from her body. Evidence suggests that swaddling is extremely soothing for individuals with neurological impairments [39] and we recommend trying this technique with the person with RS, preferably with elastic, lycra type, materials.

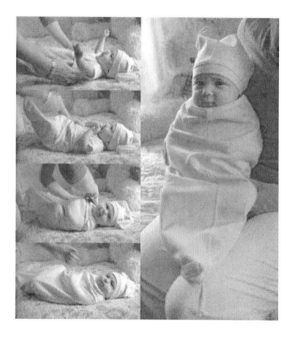

Figure X-3. Swaddling.

- Most individuals with RS will be diagnosed with scoliosis [34,40] with an occurrence of 85%-100% [34,41]. It is believed to be caused by skewed body mid perception [42], meaning that the child perceives her body to tilt to the side and as a result she will try and restore her mid perception by tilting her body to the side. In extreme cases this might deteriorate to the point of the child losing her ability to walk and even to - sit unsupported and later to the development of severe scoliosis. Since individuals with this syndrome show such high occurrence of scoliosis it is recommended that a proprioceptive\vestibular daily intensive program be implemented for children with RS from a young age to maintain mid body perception.

- It seems that the abnormal sensory processing, and especially that received through the proprioceptive system, which is experienced by the person with RS causes every movement, especially if provided by an external facilitator (such as in physical and occupational therapy), to be perceived as threatening. This causes the child to become anxious and to strongly fixate her body. In some cases this deliberate rigidity might be misdiagnosed, and treated as if it was spasticity. This fixation can harm the child's motor development and thus it would be wise to prepare her for movement. This could be achieved by verbal preparation, by slow movement in a safe situation such as in an elastic hammock or on a water bed [29] or during hydrotherapy. The desired outcome is the enhancement of the child's confidence in movement, thereby reducing her fear of movement by supplying a constant flow of non-threatening sensory motion experiences.

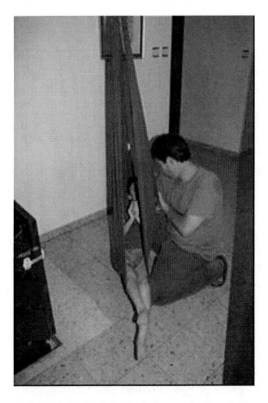

Figure X-4. Working with a child inside an elastic hammock.

- Most individuals with RS better perceive or react to auditory input when it is conveyed through singing. Therefore, if we sing the request to the child rather than ask her to act, we might achieve better results.

- Some parents report that their child with RS is sensitive to specific sounds. When this situation is suspected, especially if it interferes with the child's daily activities, a speech therapist should be consulted to suggest a proper intervention program.
- Some individuals with RS positively react to fast high pitch sounds (such as a shriek, a shout, laughter, and/or cartoon type voices), and others to animal sounds (the bark of a dog), while others are very responsive to quite low deep male voices (whispers). Such preferred sounds should be identified and used with specific reference to each person with RS, to enhance enjoyment, motivation, and participation in different activities.
- Mild to moderate hearing impairment has been found in 17.3% of individuals with RS, while no persons with RS were found to have a severe hearing impairment [35]. These mild to moderate impairments were found to be connected to anticonvulsive drug use. Since reduction in convulsive activity has been noticed with age in RS [43], the person with epileptic condition should be constantly monitored as she grows old. Due to the many side effects related to convulsive medication cessation of anti-convulsive medication should be considered, if the child condition improves and convulsion free over a long period of time (years).
- Since the visual and auditory inputs are relatively intact sensory tracts, they help the person with RS to cope with the external world. Therefore they are extremely enthusiastic when familiar sounds are presented [17] and familiar books and photographs are shown. These forms of familiar safe experiences should be used to enhance educational and functional activities.
- Findings show that 50%-80% of individuals with RS are diagnosed with mild visual impairments [6,34]. Therefore it is recommended that an optometrist or an ophthalmologist specializing in children with developmental disabilities be consulted to evaluate the child's eyesight and to adjust visual aids if such support is necessary.
- Many individuals with RS can be found to have depth perception issues. These persons find it very hard to cope with going down stairs. As indicated previously, a person diagnosed with the preserved speech variant (SPV) of RS enlightened us with the fact that going down stairs is her "biggest fright" despite the fact that she is able to go up and down stairs unaided (unpublished data). In some cases parents reported that irlen lenses have been found useful in these situations, in other cases there were positive reports by parents regarding "prism lenses".
- In an evaluation of the visual abilities of five girls with RS aged 5-10 years in Israel by an optometrist who specializes in children with special needs, 80% of the girls were diagnosed with strabismus (crossed eyes) (unpublished data). With strabismus the brain receives a blurred double image of the visual field; in order to solve this problem it starts relating only to information received by one of the eyes. This solution enables a clear visual perception of the world but prevents the child from constructing the three dimensional world that enables depth perception. In this situation the child is not able to estimate distances and the height of obstacles; she will feel unsafe in unknown places and uneven terrains which might lead to anxiety, fixation of the body, and unwillingness to ambulate which is common to so many girls with this syndrome. This predicament should be evaluated since it could be easily avoided through professional counseling.
- Individuals with RS show clear preferences for specific colors. Such preferences should be recognized when using communication, when choosing clothing, or

deciding upon the colors for the child bedroom. The therapist can use such preferences as motivational factors when intervening with the person with RS.

- We assume that individuals with RS have better peripheral than direct vision [6]; therefore when presented with a new visual stimulus (a toy) the person with RS will start with a series of quick gazes towards the object and then appear to look away. It might be confusing to the inexperienced therapist since the child is looking as if she is uninterested in the object. Barbro Lindberg [6], an experienced educator from Sweden, suggested that an object should first be placed at the corner of the eye of the child with RS and then gradually transferred into the center of the child's visual field, after the child has had the time to familiarize herself with the new object.

- It has been suggested that the olfactory sense be developed so as to be able to distinguish between desired and unwanted smells, get further information regarding food items, and revive memories. We can then utilize this skill to enable the child with RS to identify food items, thus enabling her to be able to smell food items and in so doing prepare herself for having the food put in her mouth [32]. This act of food recognition might serve as a preparation for eating and thus lessen the length of mealtimes typical of so many girls with RS.

- It is possible to implement a sensory intervention program that presents the child with "pure" sensory experiences, but we suggest that the child also be exposed to complex sensory experiences through accidental learning as these are very common in everyday situations. We cook for lunch by cutting the vegetables which have different colors and tactile textures, we might also hear the sound of the blender or the sounds of cooking and frying, we season the food with different spices and then we smell the food when it is done, and finally we eat and feel the temperature, the texture, and the taste of the food.

The next section of the chapter will deal with apraxia. We will discuss the topic in a few words and suggest some principles that could be applied, when the OT is individually working with the child with RS.

Apraxia in Rett syndrome

The person with RS is defined as apraxic, yet this definition does not stand well with the fact that apraxia is usually associated with some form of head trauma and no damage can be found in the brains of individuals with RS. This chapter will try to amalgamate two different terms "apraxia" and "developmental dyspraxia" in order to characterize the type of difficulty experienced by individuals with RS, and thereby suggest an appropriate form of therapy through sensory integration intervention as suggested by Jane Ayers. The term praxis refers to the ability to plan and execute a motor task [44] and is originated from the Greek words doing, action, and performance.

Definitions of apraxia:

- Apraxia: Inability to carry out a complex or skilled movement; not due to paralysis, sensory changes, or deficiencies in understanding [45].

- Apraxia: impaired planning/sequencing of movement that is not due to weakness, incoordination, or sensory loss. Apraxia mostly results from dissociation of parts of the cerebrum and is often associated with parietal lobe lesions [46].

Both the above mentioned definitions are usually attributed to acquired apraxia, meaning an impact or trauma to the cerebrum or to the parietal lobe causing damage to the brain in a person who was born with intact brain functions. The brain damage that causes apraxic symptoms might occur in the frontal and or parietal lobes as well as in the connection between the associative motor area and the inferior parietal lobe. Other areas that might be injured to cause apraxia are the basal ganglia and the junction between the parietal and occipital lobes. Since those areas are not physically offended in individuals with RS the inability of this group of clients to perform motor tasks should be explained through different sources. Explanations that might shed some light over the inability of children with RS to perform motor acts can be found within the frame of sensory integration theories developed by Jane Ayers during the 60's of the previous century. When Ayers first related to this issue in 1972 she referred to it as developmental dyspraxia (DD). To distinguish this term from the term "apraxia", associated with head injured clients [47] Ayers claimed that the term apraxic is more suitable for someone who can learn to perform a task yet both the learning period as well as his task performance are slow and do not reach high efficiency [47]. In Ayers' terminology, the term DD means a problem in brain function that stems from the child's difficulty in processing sensory information from the tactile, proprioceptive and vestibular systems, thereby harming motor planning. The term "developmental" points to the fact that the problem is initiated at the early stages of the child's life, and affects his development [48].

Since learning is a process in which we cognitively internalize repeated information until it becomes automated, a child with an impaired body scheme will be unable to transfer motor patterns from the cortical level to an automated level. This inability will require long and repeated planning by the child for each task she is asked to perform. Since no motor patterns are being built, the child will relate to each new action as it has never happened before and with every new task the child will have to assess her position and the way she is requested to act. These types of difficulties are very consistent with the description of the dyspractic child by Fisher et al [33]:

- Extreme difficulty in performing new motor tasks which usually end in a failure in performance.
- A transition from one position to the next is a huge challenge.
- There are difficulties in timing, sequencing, and rhythm of motor activities and motor tasks.
- Difficulties in relating the body to physical objects in the space around the child.
- Difficulties in mimicking unfamiliar body positions.
- Difficulties in directionality and movement. For instance a toy that needs to be pushed or lifted will be thrown or pushed.
- Difficulties in regards to oro-motor planning (oral apraxia) which will affect eating abilities and speech.
- When the child is asked to play she will not initiate any activity or her actions will appear aimless.
- The child will appear to move aimlessly and directionless in space.

- The child will perform repetitive movements such as beating objects or pushing them.

Since there is no damage to those brain areas usually connected with apraxia in the brains of individuals with RS, since this behavior is apparent from a young age, since the strong resemblance between Fisher's description of the dyspractic child and the typical behavior of individuals with RS can be observed by all working with individuals with RS, we believe that the definition of the disability of child with RS should be changed from apraxia to developmental dyspraxia (DD). This change will enable us to recommend an adaptation of Fisher's guidelines for intervention with children with DD as suitable for OT intervention also for individuals with RS.

Guidelines for ot intervention

Based on, and adapted from principles of treatment for the dyspractic child by Fisher and Ayres [33,48-50]. Apply judgment before selecting new educational tasks for the dyspractic child. It is important to apply a small and consistent number of tasks, focusing on the ones that are most important and are imbedded in the child's daily situations and experiences. The tasks that are chosen to be performed should be practiced regularly. The environment should be structured so as to invite interaction, rewarding, and easy to manipulate. An appropriate organization of the surroundings helps the child function better.

Intervention guidelines:

- The child with RS will present a problem in her ability to predict an action that will be needed in the future – therefore, after presenting the child with RS with a task, she should be given ample time to plan, process and then perform the requested action.
- The dyspractic person with RS experiences many failures during her day, therefore it is of utmost importance that the level of demands be adapted to the child's ability so that during intervention she will be able to achieve a high level of success (one should aim at achieving at least an 80% level of success). We should bear in mind that a demanding performance at levels that are much higher than the child's personal ability will put off the child, prevent initiation, and provoke avoidance of function [32].
- The activities of the child with RS should be multi-modal, meaning that the sensory stimuli applied during intervention should activate a number of sensory systems which in turn will stimulate the child into action.
- It is essential that the child with RS be activated against resistance. Active movement stimulates proprioceptive sensory receptors that help the child build her body scheme.
- During an activity the therapist should give the child with RS verbal cues which will help her to organize herself. The verbal cues should not be repeated (after the child has been asked to perform a task the therapist should refrain from repeating his request since it will cause the child to re-initiate her reorganization process).

- Physical contact with the child's body is extremely helpful and should be done skillfully in order to support the verbal request. The tactile stimulus gives the child the sensory cues she needs to complete her organization.
- Singing helps the child with RS get organized. Singing supports the activity while giving it structure and rhythm, and therefore a sense of security.
- In order for the child with RS to internalize the action and its consequences outcome, feedback should be given (for instance, if the child is holding the swing with her hands to prevent herself from falling, the therapist might say "good for you, you are holding the swing"; If she is climbing the ladder "wow you have lifted one leg, now lift the other one" – and give physical stimulation to back up the verbal cue).
- In order to achieve improvement in a selected function it should be implemented in all the daily settings of the child in a similar manner by all. (For example, if the task to be improved is eating with a spoon then the OT will practice eating with a spoon in the therapy room, the caregiver in the classroom will practice the same task, and the parent as well will practice eating with a spoon). Since the child has problems generalizing different performances into one task, everybody working with her should perform in an identical manner (videos could be made at school and transferred to the home environment – or vice versa).
- When the child with RS has acquired a new task and its quality gradually improves, a new slightly different element can be added to the function to get some generalization (For example, a child who has acquired the ability to sit on a stool with no support can now try to sit on a T chair to enhance her equilibrium abilities; If a child has mastered the ability to go up or down stairs it will make it a bit different and more interesting if we put a colored strip at the end of each step). The task has not changed but for the child with RS these changes necessitate building up more motor patterns; it makes the drill a bit more interesting and it makes the child handle a known yet slightly different challenge (a slightly different motor plan in the brain).
- When the activity is changed, the similarity to the known\previous activity and the change from what she can already do should be verbally emphasized to the child with RS. This is done with the aim of directing her mind to the fact that there's an already existing motor pattern in her brain that will help her initiate and perform the task.
- If the person with RS has only minimal movement the therapist can construct an array that will react to the slightest movement (for example, surround the child with plastic bowling pins so that every movement she makes will cause them to fall).
- When a new experience is presented to the person with RS the therapist must make sure that the level of difficulty assures a high level of success. If the child succeeds it is likely that she will happily repeat the experience, making it possible to gradually enhance the level of difficulty.
- It should be taken into consideration that the therapeutic equipment might be found strange\threatening to the person with RS; therefore if we see that the person is hesitating we should:
  o Take the time to acquaint the child with the therapeutic environment (if needed, a few meetings should be spent to go through this process)
  o Time should be spent for the child to move or be moved from one side of the therapy room to the other.
  o Start the intervention with known objects such as mattresses, dolls, and small balls, rather than with crawling tunnels, vestibular plates, or physio-

balls. The latter might be perceived by the client with RS as an unknown object which needs gradual introduction.

    o   A small group of two therapists and two clients might be a good start for the child with RS. In such a setting she can observe the therapist demonstrating the requested task, as well as the other child performing it, while she takes the time she needs to organize herself. Further along the road we aspire to gradually reduce the introduction time and the physical support, and suffice with verbal encouragement.

- It goes without saying that any activity performed by the child in the therapy room should be transferred to all her other daily settings.

Age appropriate activity

The following section will address different adaptations in play and daily activity across the life span of the client with RS.

Playing is vital for child development as it enables children to develop creativity, imagination, and physical abilities and skills, and to enhance their cognitive and emotional abilities [51]. Through play the child can interact with the world, to explore it and control it. Controlling the world through game playing enhances the development of confidence and flexible thinking necessary for the child when encountering future challenges. Free play teaches children how to work in a team, share, negotiate, resolve conflicts, and acquire self defense strategies. During game playing the child learns how to make decisions and discover his fields of interest [51].

It stands to reason that the play abilities of children with special needs will be limited due to motor and language difficulties, lack of initiative, scarce opportunities, and/or difficulty in grasping the roles of objects and individuals. When we reflect on the state of the child with RS, we find a huge gap between her ability to play independently and with mediation. Since most games necessitate some level of manual function, the possibilities available for the child with RS are extremely limited, and many parents and educators are faced with a dilemma since the child's independent ability enables only games that are below both her age and comprehension levels. Adapting games for the child with RS definitely necessitates imagination and creativity; yet, since game playing plays such an important role in her development while providing her with a path towards discovering her surrounding world, it is important that we dedicate the time needed for this chore. Playing has many advantages for the therapist. Through game playing we can not only provide opportunities for enjoyment and learning but can also provide motivation for participating in an activity thus enabling repetition and skill learning. In order for the game to be purposeful and achieve its goal, we must first define the purpose of the game or the activity. Is our main goal to achieve hand function? Or learning? Or do we prefer to focus on and achieve balance, range of motion, or muscle tone reduction?

In this context it is important to note that the motivation of the person with RS to participate in an activity is significantly higher if it is connected to her inner emotional world, or is given some personal significance or functional meaning. For instance, motivation will be higher if the activity is connected with a story that has been learned in class, or to television programs that the child likes, or when the picture we create is destined to be hung in her bedroom. Motivational factors can also be related to factors such as the person she likes being present in the therapy room or the greeting card that she makes being intended for a sibling.

Games according to age and development

As any child, individuals with RS have the desire and the need to explore the world around them, yet, in contrast to other children, that desire is usually restricted due to their physical disabilities. Their ability to experience the world around them by operating, manipulating, and touching objects is limited and it is our responsibility as therapists to enable them access to such experiences. This could be done by mediating the world for them, by suggesting appropriate games and activities, by adapting un-achievable games to the abilities of our clients with RS and by encouraging the people in their immediate environments to support and assist in such interventions. One of the basic skills acquired at a young age is the understanding of the relationship between action and reactions. This skill is an essential basis for learning throughout life. When the child learns her ability to influence her surrounding by action on her part, she gains a sense of empowerment and control [52]. At this stage it is advisable to choose simple and easily manipulated games, so that a slight push or movement will result in an immediate and obvious reaction, thereby enhancing a sense of success and encouraging the child to keep trying.

Games intended for toddlers are suitable for this stage, since the majority of those games are easily operated and those which are harder to control might be operated through the use of switches. When deciding on a switch one might choose between a simple switch where one touch operates the game for as long as the switch is being pressed, or a timer operated switch, where any touch starts the activity for a pre-determined duration. The use of purchased toys is always possible, but the therapist can also improvise or construct different games using existing and familiar household objects – the same ones that any child with unaffected abilities would experiment with most naturally while exploring within the house.

- Plastic bottles of different sizes can be filled with colored water or with different objects (small bells, rice, chick peas, etc.) and then rolled on the ground or pushed over.
- Simple musical instruments such as rattles or bells can be held and shaken to make music. If the limited functional hand use of the child prevents independent holding of the toy, one can use Velcro tapes and/or gloves to attach the toy to the child's hand or turn the musical instrument into a bracelet, thereby creating interesting sounds with every movement of the child's hand.
- Soap bubbles make a cheap, simple, and extremely enjoyable game. They can be used to encourage hand function or to improve hand-eye coordination. If the child with RS operates the bubble making toy with a switch, she can choose to send the stream of bubbles towards other children, thereby changing a simple game into an opportunity for social interaction.

- Building blocks can be used to build a tower (with mediation by either the therapist or another child), and destroying the tower is also a lot of fun. Such activities ensure a high level of success while requiring simple manual abilities.
- Pic-a-boo games can be played by placing a thin scarf over the child's face, and encouraging the girl with RS to pull the scarf away. Having the scarf over the therapist's face or over the face of other classmates is also a possibility.
- Playing with different materials (sand, foam, water, finger-paints, clay, and dough) can be used to encourage hand function. Games using these materials can be experienced through touching, pushing, rolling, flattening, poking, and even through making different shapes. One of the advantages of using games of this nature lies in the fact that they can be played without involving elements of failure and success. These types of games can be used to encourage hand function and the opening and closing of palms and fingers, to give varied sensory experiences to the palms and upper extremities, and to work on bilateral hand coordination and separation of fingers. Hiding objects of varies sizes within a bowl with sand, foam, water, or beans and asking the child to search for the hidden items is a game that stimulates the palms with different sensations. It is also a way to learn spatial orientation through expressions and experiences that address concepts such as within, under, and above.
- Playing in front of a mirror is another option. When in front of the mirror we can stimulate different body parts as well as having the child look at those body parts in the mirror, thereby helping the child to build her body scheme and enhance body awareness. Other games\activities in front of the mirror could include covering the mirror with a cloth and having the child taking it off, or playing with foam across the glass covering or discovering our selves in the mirror.
- Getting objects in and out of boxes can be used to learn spatial concepts such as "on" versus "under" or "inside" versus "outside", while at the same time enhancing manual function. We can use the boxes with or without the cover, with a narrow or wide opening, to make the activity different, challenging and interesting. We reiterate that the activity should have a personal interest for the child with RS, for instance the objects in the box could be snacks that the child can enjoy, books we can jointly read, or objects and characters that will afterwards be used to illustrate the book we are reading together.
- Adhering figures\pictures\symbols to a board is a good method for stimulating hand function. Such figures might be made from thick cardboard attached to the board with Velcro strips or magnets. Pulling these pictures away from the board is a marvelous activity, since retraction of the shoulders is a movement almost never performed by children with RS. Again, let it be said that the activity will have more meaning, and therefore be more motivating, if the pictures are from a book that is currently being read in class, or if they are photos of family members or classmates, or that they can be used by the child to send messages/greeting cards/holiday blessings to family members and other people who are important to her.

Kindergarten age

Symbolic play enables the child to reconstruct and process emotional experiences through games and thereby to control events that are taking place in an imaginary world, which might eventually lead into mastering the real world [52]. For the child with RS who usually has very little control over her world symbolic play can enhance a sense of confidence, security, and ability. Through symbolic play the child can learn about different roles, social behaviors, and the way in which the world around her operates.

In that context we would like to suggest once more that if the learning process is connected to known and meaningful happenings in the child's life and not as a separate issue, the child with RS, like all children, will learn much more easily and effectively. For instance, the child will more easily learn to identify colors if she gets to pick a new red ribbon for her hair or to choose between the blue or green shirt which she would like to wear, rather than through the frontal formal teaching of colors.

As the age of the child advances, age appropriate games become increasingly demanding and necessitate more controlled manual skills. The parents\caregivers\therapists are confronted with the problem that was mentioned earlier; the level of games which the child can play independently is much lower than the games that might be played through mediation. The consequence is that the same games, mostly below her level of ability, are repeatedly being suggested to the child. One solution to this predicament is to use switch operated games. Computer games can also be adapted to operate through the use of a single switch or a touch screen and we can advance and change the software of those games without having to change the operating mode, the switch or touch screen. The use of computers can enrich the child's world and enable her to enjoy independent play.

Software such as "Clicker" (manufactured by Cricksoft) and "PowerPoint" (by Microsoft®) can be used to write and tell personal stories. The personal story can be composed by the child and include pictures of the child and members of her environment (family members, classmates, therapeutic\educational team members), animals that she relates to such as the cat she likes and the dog she is scared of, and objects of special interest to her like her favorite doll. All these can be scanned and inserted into the computer software intertwined with appropriate text; the child can then listen to the story with its accompanying pictures or tell it to her friends and family by simply pushing a button. The same techniques can be used to choose different songs and books. If the child has some basic hand function ability and is able to grasp an object, we can add some clips (or even simple clothes pins) to the pages of a book and the child can use a picture book by independently flipping the pages. The switches mentioned above can be used to operate a CD player thereby enabling the child to independently listen to her favorite music. The switches can be used to either encourage sustained hand pressure (the songs only play during the time that the child is actually pushing on the switch) or repeated movements (the timer necessitates repeated movements each time the music is stopped) in order to listen to the next song.

Mediated play can enable the child to reach richer and more advanced play levels ideas for mediated play include:

- In story telling; the basic action does not change, yet the mediator can increase the cognitive demands and the level of attention required from the child. At this level we can ask the child to identify characters from the story, to match the cardboard figures to the place in the story where they belong, or to ask the child to use her knowledge about the characters from a story and to imagine how those people would react in hypothetical situation (i.e. would you like to invite the wolf [from "little red riding hood"] to your house for lunch? Why not?).

- Some games can be easily adapted to the child's abilities. For instance puzzle parts can be adapted by adding a big handle (made out of a block, a wine bottle cork, or a drawer handle). It is quite probable to assume that most individuals with RS will still need assistance in picking the piece up, moving it to its correct place, and arranging it in relation to the other parts, but she can recognize the right part, grasp it, and put it in proximity to its proper place. A lotto game could be adjusted in a similar manner.

- Motivation can be used to achieve improved hand function while using different materials to create pictures and greeting cards for her favorite people. In situations where the activity can be integrated within a story she knows, a birthday card for a brother or a classmate, or a card for her parents for Valentine's Day, the motivational element becomes increasingly strong. We should always bear in mind that due to dysfunction in sensory integration processing, the child might reject some of the materials offered. In such cases different materials could be suggested such as the use of paint brushes to replace direct hand use. Other children with RS on the other hand, might enjoy the use of the novel materials and be completely involved in the sensory experience (since they are seldom exposed to such experiences), thus paying little attention to the final outcome. In such cases, it is advised to go along with their desire and even take advantage of their new area of interest (tactile sensations) for activities in the future.

- Toy stores supply equipment that can be adapted to the special needs of our clients with RS. These materials include thick and easily grasped paints, brushes and color pens.

- Symbolic play with dolls and objects is a typical activity for this age group. At this age the child learns about her position within the family and about the roles of others, children and adults, by role playing (mother and father; doctor and patient). Playing with a doll provides a sense of control by enabling the child to make decisions as to what the doll should wear or eat, or when she will go to bed. Communication symbols can be used to enable the child to decide whether the doll will take a bath or go to sleep, what types of foods she will eat, or what story should be read to her. If the child takes part in dressing the doll or washing her, this provides an additional opportunity to work on improving hand function and grasp. Taking the doll for a walk in her stroller gives us another situation in which hand function, specifically grasping the bar for an extended period of time, can be practiced. Singing or reading interactively can be done with the child vocally participating through the use of augmentative communication devices such as a "BigMack" or a "Step by Step" device.

- Virtual reality games such as the Sony PLAYSTATION® or Wii™ are constantly developing and are becoming household items. We should introduce these games to the child with RS with the possibility that she might find these games interesting and get involved in playing them, thereby providing yet another opportunity for hand usage.

Activities of daily living

Most persons with RS require considerable assistance in the performance of activities of daily living (ADL); nevertheless there is a constant attempt to transfer responsibility and empower the child to participate and take control to the greatest extent possible. The therapeutic and educational team should constantly convey the message that we are expecting the child to be active and take responsibility; this would contribute to the child's sense of ability and to the amount of involvement she would take in her daily life. The person with RS is constantly coping with minimal manual abilities while coping with the barriers of apraxia, delayed reaction time, and ataxic tremor. Her limitations necessitate that she is for the most part dressed, fed and washed by others. This causes her to gradually become increasingly passive, with the end result of learned helplessness. The easiest way for her to cope is to wait for others to work for her. Nevertheless, we should do our best to invite her to take an active role in her life by making decisions and participating to the maximum of her abilities.

The child can take part in the following activities (the activities can be performed manually with assistance, or the child can take control by verbally declaring the different stages by using a " Step by Step" communication device):

- Choosing the clothes she would like to wear,
- Holding the toothbrush,
- Pushing her leg towards the shoe on demand,
- Putting her hand forward towards the faucet to wash her hands,
- Eating with a spoon or a teaspoon,
- Helping to spread the butter over the piece of bread,
- Helping to cut the vegetables when making a salad,
- Helping to arrange the food utensils on the table before the meal and removing them when mealtime is done,
- Taking part in making a cake, cookies, or pudding
- Operating electrical appliances such as a blender or a food processor through the use of a manually operated switch.

We should always bear in mind that the saying "practice makes perfect" is not only applicable for the general population but is ever so true in the case of the apraxic person with RS. The more the child practices and repeats the action, the more the response becomes automatic, with less and less of a demand on the child for motor planning, thus rendering the movement quicker and more fluent.

Adolescence

We should continue to encourage age appropriate interests when the person with RS reaches adolescence. It is very tempting to hold onto the same games and activities through which she has in the past achieved some success, yet this would mean preserving her low manual and verbal functional levels. By constantly updating her activities we convey the message that we accept her as an adult and relate to her and to her emotional world appropriately. At that age many will show an interest in dressing nicely, in using make-up, in watching specific TV series, in age appropriate books, and more.

A young woman with RS participated in a self care group which the first author facilitated. Her joy from choosing nail-polish, eye shadow, and lipstick was obvious, and she gladly participated throughout the session. At the end of the session, she was delighted with her image in the mirror and she did her best to avoid her stereotypic hand movements in order to prevent the nail polish from rubbing off. Self care activities are a good time to interact and use communication devices which might later be used in other areas of daily activities. It is also a time for achieving intimacy; therefore the activity should take place in a quiet room, with pleasant music in the background, and a table with a nice colored table cloth, supports for the gentle and esthetic nature of the interaction which emulates the real experience of being in a beauty salon.

Within this activity the person with RS can decide on the order of the beautification procedure: what comes first (lipstick or eye shadow) and what colors to use. She can take part in

- Choosing ribbons and hairpins for her hair
- Preparing a decorated hair ribbon and hairpins
- Decorating a frame and inserting her photo (with makeup) into the frame
- Creating different beads and ornaments using Dass, Fimo, paper mache or clay. She can role the materials until she creates a rounded ball and then poke it with a tool to create the hole in the middle.
- Preparing bracelets and necklaces for herself or as a gift to a family member or a classmate (this could be done by inserting beads of different sizes and shapes on a string). In order to ease the task of sliding the beads onto a string a wooden poke can be attached to the string and later (when the task is complete) removed.
- Other age appropriate activities for the adolescent with RS:
- Decorating wooden boxes either for herself or as gifts. Such boxes can be found in arts and crafts shops. Decorating the boxes might involve gluing napkins, coloring, using patches, etc.
- Preparing forms to be used as ornaments or as parts of a mobile. When using materials such as Dass, Fimo, paper mache or clay, a roller can be used to flatten the materials. Then she can use cookie cutters to shape the material into the desired forms.
- Preparing sessions that revolve around her favorite television programs. It is similar to the activities suggested earlier in this chapter regarding books; discussing the events of every episode each week, or the adolescent with RS may look through magazines and locate her favorite actors, collect their pictures, and make a collage for her room at home. Or the theme of the program can be sung, one line by the caregiver ro therapist, the next line by the young woman, etc using the "Step by Step" voice output device.
- Participating in work oriented activities – At this age the person with RS might be prepared to work after graduating school. The activity can be adapted according to the skills and abilities of the person with RS as well as to the needs of the facility that she will be moving to after graduation. An adolescent with RS was for example taught to use her stereotypical movements to feed chickens in the residential setting she lived in and this way be a contributing member in that facility.

Encouraging the person with RS to take responsibility for her needs and wants and to stay active and involved in determining her daily activities and routine should be pursued at all ages. During adolescence such involvement is even more important. The young woman should be able to decide on the food she eats, her timetable during each day, the clothing she wears, and the music she prefers to hear. If her manual abilities at that stage prevent her from doing activities that require fine handedness, she can still be in charge of the music being played on the CD player through the use of a switch, or she can announce the breaks and working sessions throughout the work day through the use of a voice output communication device.

Conclusions

When addressing the needs of the client with RS the OT is involved in a variety of roles designed to improve the function of the child and her family. Empowering the child includes both primary care which involves individual intervention both in the therapy room and in her natural surroundings (classroom, home, playground, community) and secondary intervention aimed at providing guidance to the other staff members and the child's family.

Recognizing the tendency of most girls with RS to give in to their disabilities and to become more and more passive (learned helplessness), the OT must take on the responsibility of encouraging the person with RS to take charge of her life and become as active as possible. The developed emotional status of the person with RS demands that the OT convey her belief in the person, letting her know that we support her abilities and skills that exist despite her limitations. The optimal response from individuals with RS is connected to the bond which they form with their therapists. The clinical diversity of individuals with RS requires state of the art knowledge on the part of the OT with regard to the different phenotypes of RS. There is a need to adapt levels of demands and types of intervention from child to child according to these phenotypes. Moreover, functional fluctuations typical of RS may influence both the child and her family and mandates the OT to adapt her expectations from session to session, sometimes even on a daily basis.

We hope that this chapter will assist the OT in managing the client with RS, while supporting his or her efforts to promote the abilities of his clients.

References

[1]   Amir RE, Van den Veyver IB, Wan M, Tran CQ, Francke U, Zoghbi HY. Rett syndrome is caused by mutations in X-linked MECP2, encoding methyl-CpG-binding protein 2. Nat Gen 1999;23(2):185-8.
[2]   Amir RE, Van Den Veyver IB, Schultz R, Malicki DM, Tran CQ, Dahle EJ, et al. Influence of mutation type and X chromosome inactivation on Rettsyndrome phenotypes. Ann Neurol 2000;47:670-9.
[3]   Armstrong DD. Neuropathology of Rett syndrome. Ment Retard Dev Disabil Res Rev 2002;8:72-6.
[4]   Lotan M, Ben-Zeev B. Rett syndrome. A review with emphasis on clinical characteristics and intervention. ScientificWorldJournal 2006;6:1517-41.
[5]   Percy AK. International research review. Presentation, IRSA 12th Ann Conf, Boston, MA, 1996 May 24-27, tape 622-15.

[6]   Lindberg B. Understanding Rett Syndrome: A practice guide for parents, teachers and therapists, 2nd rev ed. Toronto: Hogrefe Huber, 2006.

[7]   Hagberg B, Hagberg G. Rett syndrome: epidemiology and geographical variability. Eur Child Adolesc Psychiatry 1997;1:5-7.

[8]   Lotan M. Rett Syndrome. Guidelines for Individual Intervention. Scientific WorldJournal 2006;6:1504-16.

[9]   Lotan M, Manor-Binyamini I, Elefant C, Wine J, Saraf E, Yoshei T. The Israeli Rett Syndrome Center. Evaluation according to the transdisciplinary play-based assessment. ScientificWorldJournal 2006;6:1302-13.

[10]   InterRett - IRSA Rett Phenotype Database, Telethon Institute for Child Health Research, Australia. http://www2.ichr.uwa.edu.au/rett/irsa on .

[11]   Mount RH, Hastings RP, Reilly S, Cass H, Charman T. Behavioral And emotional features in Rett syndrome. Disabil Rehabil 2001;23:129-38.

[12]   Lotan M. Angels of silence: Caring for Rett syndrome. Tel Aviv: Rotem, 2006. [Hebrew].

[13]   Lotan M, Roth D. The effect of hand vibrators on the hand stereotypes and function in Rett syndrome - Two case studies. Isr Physiother Quart 1996;52:23-6.[Hebrew].

[14]   Wehmeyer M, Bourland G, Ingram D. An analogue assessment of hand stereotypies in two cases of Rett syndrome. J Intellect Disabil Res 1993;37(Pt 1):95-102.

[15]   Elefant C. Speechless yet communicative: Revealing the person behind the disability of Rett syndrome through clinical research on songs in music therapy. In: Aldridge D, Di Franco G, Ruud E, Wigram T, eds. Music therapy in Europe. Rome: ISMEZ, 2001.

[16]   Wigram T, Elefant C. Nurturing engagement with music for people with PDD: Autistic spectrum disorder and Rett syndrome. In: Malloch S, Trevarthen C, eds. Communicative musicality: Narratives of expressive gesture and being human. Oxford: Oxford Univ Press, 2008.

[17]   Elefant C, Wigram T. Learning ability in children with Rett syndrome. Brain Dev 2005;27: 97-101.

[18]   Hetzroni O, Rubin C. AAC instruction for children with Rett syndrome using assistive technology. Proceedings ISAAC, Dublin, Ireland, 1998:361.

[19]   Zwaigenbaum L, Szatmari P. Psychosocial characteristics of children with pervasive developmental disorders. In: Schwean S, Saklofske D, eds. Handbook of psychosocial characteristics of exceptional children. New York: Plenum, 1999:275-98.

[20]   Jimerson SR. Rett's. Accessed 2009 Nov 08. http://kady.education.ucsb.edu/jimerson/rett.html

[21]   Naganuma G, Billingsley F. Effect of hand splints of stereotypic hand behavior in three girls with Rett syndrome. Phys Ther 1988;68:664-71.

[22]   Rett A. Rett syndrome. Presentation, United Kingdom Rett Syndr Assoc Conf, Coleshill, 1985.

[23]   Rett A. Rett syndrome. Presentation, Presentation, Yorkhill Hosp Conf, Coleshill, 1986.

[24]   Weiss M. Intervention and assessment of hand behavior. Presentation, IRSA 12th Annual Conf, Boston, MA, 1996 May 24-27, tape 622-07.

[25]   Kubas ES. Use of splints to develop hand skills in a woman with Rett Syndrome. Am J Occup Ther 1992;46:358-64.

[26]   Sharp PA. Comparative effects of bilateral hand splints and an elbow orthosis on stereotypic hand movements and play in two children with Rett Syndrome. Am J Occup Ther 1992;46:134-40.

[27]   International Rett Syndrome Association Parent idea book. Washington, DC: Int Rett Syndr Assoc, undated.

[28]   Elian M, De M, Rudolf N. Observations on hand movement in Rett Syndrome: A Pilot Study. Acta Neurol Scand 1996;94:212-4.

[29]   Lotan M, Shapiro M Management of young children with Rett disorder in the controlled multi-sensory (Snoezelen) environment. Brain Dev 2005;27 (Suppl 1):S88-94.

[30]   Hanks SB. Personal communication, IRSA 12th Ann Conf, Boston, MA, 1996 May 24-27.

[31]   Department of Education and Science. Special educational needs: Report of the committee of inquiry into the education of handicapped children and young people. London: HMSO, 1978.

[32]   Lewis JE, Wilson CD. Pathways to learning in Rett Syndrome. Teleford, Shropshire: Wozencroft Printers, 1996.

[33]   Fisher AG, Murray EA, Bundy AC. Sensory Integration theory and practice. Philadelphia, PA: FA Davis Company, 1991.

[34]   Hagberg B. Rett Syndrome clinical and biological aspects. London: Mac Keith Press, 1993.

[35]   Pillion JP, Rawool VW, Bibat G, Naidu S. Prevalence of hearing loss in Rett syndrome. Dev Med Child Neurol 2003;45(5):338-43.

[36]   Naidu S. Research findings on Rett syndrome. Presentation, IRSA Ann Conf, Las Vegas, NV, 2000 May 18-21, Tape RS 9.

[37]   Johnston M. Neurobiology of Rett syndrome, a disorder of synaptic development. Presentation, Int Course Rett Syndr, Ostersund Sweden; 2003 Jun 16-18.

[38]   Hunter K. The Rett syndrome handbook. Washington, DC: Int Rett Syndr Assoc, 1999.

[39]   Ohgi S, Akiyama T, Arisawa K, Shigemori K. Randomised controlled trial of swaddling versus massage in the management of excessive crying in infants with cerebral injuries. Arch Dis Child 2004;89(3):212-6.

[40]   Rossin L. Effectiveness of therapeutic and surgical intervention in the treatment of scoliosis in Rett syndrome. A seminar work. Pittsburgh, PA: Univ Duquesne, 1997:1-19.

[41]   Kerr AM, Burford B. Towards a full life with Rett disorder. Pediatr Rehabil 2001;4(4):157-68.

[42]   Hanks SB. Physical therapy strategies. Presentation, IRSA 12th Ann Conf, Boston, MA, 1996 May 24-27, tape 622-08.

[43]   Glaze DG, Schultz RJ, Frost JD. Rett syndrome: characterization of seizures versus non-seizures. Electroencephalogr Clin Neurophysiol 1998;106:79-83.

[44]   Sanger TD, Chen D, Delgado MR, Gaebler-Spira D, Hallett M, Mink JW, et al. Definition and classification of negative motor signs in childhood. Pediatrics 2006;118(5):2159-67.

[45]   Neurological trauma glossary. Accessed 2009 Nov 18. URL: http://www.ssgfx.com/CP2020/medtech/glossary/neuro.htm

[46]   Glossary of neurological terms and disorders. School of Medicine at the University of St Louis. Accessed 2009 Nov 18. URL: http://www.strokecenter.org/education/glossary.html

[47]   Clark PN, Allen AS. Occupational therapy for children. St Louis, MO: CV Mosby, 1985.

[48]   Ayres JA. Sensory integration and the child. 5th edition. Los Angeles, CA: Western Psychol Serv, 1982.

[49]   Ayres AJ. Sensory integration and learning disorders. Los Angeles, CA: Western Psychol Serv, 1972.

[50]   Ayres JA. Developmental dyspraxia and adult-onset apraxia. Torrance, CA: Sensory Integr Int, 1985.

[51]   Ginsburg KR. The Importance of play in promoting healthy child development and maintaining strong parent-child bonds. Pediatrics 2007;119(1):182-91.

[52]   Wood E, Attfield J. Play, learning and the early childhood curriculum, 2nd ed. London: Paul Chapman, 2005.

In: Rett Syndrome: Therapeutic Interventions
Editors: Meir Lotan and Joav Merrick

ISBN: 978-1-61728-080-1
©2011 Nova Science Publishers, Inc.

Chapter XI

Rett Syndrome: Possibilities through Music Therapy

Cochavit Elefant, RMT, PhD[*]

University of Bergen, Grieg Academy, Department of Music Therapy, Bergen, Norway

Music has been found as a motivating medium for individuals with Rett syndrome (RS) and was recommended as a supportive intervention by Andreas Rett. Music therapy evokes positive responses in girls and adults with RS. It promotes and motivates their desire to interact and communicate with their surroundings as well as develops their cognitive, affective, sensori-motor and physical skills. Since most individuals with RS do not have verbal communication, music can function as a mean for self expression and as a form of communication with their surrounding. This chapter is an amalgamation of existing literature on music therapy for individuals with Rett syndrome shared with 20 years clinical experience with this population .

Introduction

Rett syndrome (RS) is a genetic disorder that primarily affects females [1,2]. The disorder causes a neurological and developmental arrest that manifests itself in a variety of disabilities such as loss of functional hand use, loss of acquired speech, apraxia, ataxia, autonomic system dysfunction, epilepsy, breathing abnormalities, failure to thrive, orthopedic problems and muscle tone irregularities [3-5].

Due to the complexity of the phenotypic manifestation of this syndrome it is suggested that the clinician working with this population should apply intensive and appropriate intervention such as music therapy that will advance the client's abilities and enhance her well-being.

[*] Correspondence: Cochavit Elefant, RMT, PhD. Associate professor in Music Therapy, University of Bergen, Grieg Academy, 5012 Bergen, Norway. E-mail: Cochavit.Elefant@grieg.uib.no

Music therapy was first recommended by Andreas Rett (1924-1997) as early as 1982 as an intervention that evokes positive responses in girls and adults with Rett syndrome (6). Music therapy is a particular helpful medium in developing social relatedness, emotional expressions, cognitive, communication, stimulates movement, functional hand use and learning [7-13]. These will be discussed throughout this chapter.

Through music therapy individuals with RS can express their emotions such as feelings that reflect happiness and enjoyment, while at other times sadness or even melancholy. Having an outlet for different types of feelings provides them with a place and a space where they can feel understood and as a result, they become motivated to communicate with their surroundings. Since motivation is one of the most important key elements in learning, music therapy can provide a pathway to the development of communication and learning. Hill [14] refers to channels that may be discovered and opened by establishing opportunities in which individuals with RS can demonstrate their ability to participate and to succeed. These opportunities to 'succeed' by discovering their resources could be established through music therapy experiences and with each such success they become empowered and driven to attempt new challenges which will enhance their continuous growth.

This chapter is a clinical report presenting some of the existing knowledge on music therapy for individuals with RS supported by the author's years of clinical experience with this population.

There are many different ways of utilising music therapy when working with individuals with RS. In this chapter I will attempt to describe several approaches in music therapy and how these could be used as tools to develop communication and cognition; including musical improvisation (vocal and instrumental) and pre-composed music and songs. In addition, I will discuss how these approaches can be used in individual music therapy, group music therapy, inclusion music programs, co-therapy and working within a multi-disciplinary evaluation team. Before I approach different methods and forms of work in music therapy with the RS population, I would like to emphasize that it isn't the music alone that is accountable for changes and successful growth in individuals with RS; it is the musical interactions that are carried out between a well trained, sensitive and attuned music therapist and the individual with RS. The musical relationship and interaction that is built between the therapist and the client is what will determine her personal growth.

Goals in music therapy

Since music is an extremely motivating medium, so favourable for the person with RS many goals might be achieved through it whether it be individual or group therapy. The following are some of the goals the music therapist could have in mind when working with this population:

- Enhance positive disposition. The person with RS tends to show fluctuating emotions and at times could be smiling while a few seconds later she might be crying in distress. This behaviour was described by Lindberg [15] as "being under a cloud". The cause for this phenomenon is unclear and is sometime attributed to physical problems. Yet through the use of music therapy the therapist can relate to the client's state by verbally reflecting through singing her disposition. This can help her to overcome her distress even if the origin of the distress is not revealed.

- Expose emotional state. The person with RS has experienced normal emotional development over her first years of life prior to the full eruption of the disorder (stage II) and as a result her interpersonal abilities are one of her utmost strengths. The music therapist could use his/her therapeutic skills by connecting to this familiar form of interaction in which the girl conveys comfort. This form of interaction can encourage other team members in addressing the person with RS at her proper level of emotional development.

- Enhance communication. Individuals with RS usually do not have verbal communication, therefore Assistive Augmentative Communication (AAC) is the usual option for them. Through the use of songs and musical instruments the person with RS can have the opportunity to develop independence in choosing and communicating her wishes [9]. Working with the aid of AAC in music therapy could then be generalized in other situations such as her classroom or at home, which in turn could promote communication with her surroundings.

- Promote vocalization. Individuals with RS vocalized, babbled and even had a few words prior to the onset of the disorder. Music therapy can encourage to regain vocalization which is important for self expression.

- Encourage motor abilities. Through various experiences of playing different musical instruments, individuals with RS can enhance functional hand use. This could be done by using their fingers to strum the guitar and by playing the piano, by using their whole palm to beat the drum or by holding a mallet to play the xylophone. Although at times they could be afraid of movement, they do however like moving and dancing when hearing music.

Music therapy assessment and evaluation for individuals with Rett Syndrome

Before appropriate intervention can be carried out, proper evaluation is warranted [16]. This statement is especially true when the clinician is working with a continually changing client such as RS. In this part of the chapter the Israeli RS centre will be described as a model for a holistic assessment and evaluation for individuals with RS.

The Israel Rett Center consists of two assessment teams – a medical and an educational/therapeutic team [17]. The educational/therapeutic team performs assessment to establish suitable intervention program for the person with RS shortly after she had been seen by the medical assessment team.

A team of specialists, including a special education teacher, speech and language therapist, occupational therapist, physiotherapist and a music therapist undertake multi-disciplinary assessment for the purpose of advising at tertiary level on the therapeutic management of RS. The educational/therapeutic team meets 3-5 individuals with RS per month. The model of operation of the Israeli evaluation team was described elsewhere [17] and the present chapter will focus on music therapy and the music therapist who functions as the team's moderator.

The process of assessment is not the same as the process of therapy [13,16]. During the assessment, the team gather information and gain as broad impression as possible of the clients, not only their functional and physical disabilities, but also their resources, motivation, attention, interest in their environment, and readiness and abilities in communication. This will help making educated decisions about future therapeutic and educational interventions for the client.

Individuals with RS tend to be anxious in unfamiliar places, and with unknown people and events. Therefore, the evaluation team tries to perform the evaluation within her most natural environment such as her home, kindergarten or school environment. Still, she could naturally feel "on display" and the centre of attention, while many adults observe her.

The multi-disciplinary team found that it is best for the client and for the therapeutic team if the assessment starts with music therapy. The music therapist begins the assessment by singing a greeting song accompanied by the guitar and invites the client to respond. During the greeting song the therapist introduces the client to some of the people who would engage with her during the assessment. Through the music and personal bonding the music therapist is able to form a 'private' interactive space separating the child and therapist apart from the observing professionals. After the greeting song the therapist prepares by describing to her (through vocal improvisation) what will happen during our shared assessment time. This approach through musical communication usually helps the girl to overcome her anxiety of the unfamiliar people and of the situation, prepares her for what will happen, and gives the team a picture of her as a functional, communicative individual. The music therapist stays throughout the assessment, especially in transitions between one form of therapeutic medium to the other, as well as in aiding other therapists when needed.

The aim of music therapy during the assessment is to build a musical and a personal relationship with the client in order to gain as much as possible information in a very short time. As an evaluator the music therapist is able to find out which instruments or vocal sounds the girl may be responsive to, how they react to changes in melody, rhythm, tempo and volume. The music therapist observes how she reacts to familiar songs, to the therapists mirroring or reflecting to various musical sounds the client is making, to turn taking, and to imitation within the frame of musical improvisation. During the assessments the individual is given many opportunities to direct and interact with the music therapist. This intense short term evaluation also enables an evaluation of the girl's emotional state, as well assisting her in expressing her likes and dislikes, her wants and needs.

Example

The following are examples of the type of communicative interactions that occur during the educational/therapeutic assessment with a girl by the name of Rachel:

I, the music therapist (CE) sing and play a greeting song to Rachel, in which I also introduce other members of the team. At the end of the song I stop singing and ask whether she wants to hear the song again. I inform Rachel that she could indicate it by either looking at me or by looking or touching a BIG MACK (AAC device) with a picture of the guitar and a message saying "I want more music". Once Rachel indicates that she wants more music, I start singing again. After a few phrases of the song, I stop and ask her to indicate whether she wants me to continue and immediately adhere to her wishes.

When she shows her fluency in this procedure, I then provide her a choice of two familiar songs and ask Rachel to choose between the songs. This is done by introducing two picture symbols of familiar songs. I then sing both songs separately while pointing at the pictures one at a time, and let Rachel select between the two songs. Once she makes the selection I begin singing the song of her choice.

After Rachel has had a few chances to select familiar songs, I begin interacting with her through turn taking activity by singing musical phrases of one of the songs she had chosen. For this purpose the 'Step by-Step' communication device is used; I sing one phrase and she 'sings' the next (by pressing the step by step device). This interaction enables the evaluation team (as well as her own team watching the interaction) to evaluate her ability to interact and to learn new concepts, as well as it can reveal that individuals with RS have the capability to learn and can overcome their long reaction time when the incentive is important enough.

From time to time during the assessment I present Rachel with two Big-Mack's with two picture symbols and a statement in one: "I want more music" while the other says: "No more music" or "something else, please".

The type of communication described in the beginning of the assessment when I asked Rachel to show me or to tell me if she wants 'more' music elicits control and empowers her. She becomes more and more engaged in this type of control and independence. The next level gives her even more independence and control when she has had a chance to choose between songs. During this short evaluation process we quickly find out that some experienced clients can select between four or more picture symbols.

During such an evaluation the music therapist is able to observe many aspects in the individual's abilities and needs in the emotional, communicative, cognitive, and fine motor areas while other team members are evaluating the child's abilities each in their own field of expertise.

This evaluation process is the stepping stone for an open discussion with the child's educational team later to be submitted as a holistic elaborated report that suggests a multitude of intervention possibilities for the team working with the individual for future implementation.

Interventions in music therapy

Beginnings

The child with RS could present the music therapist with unexpected challenges, yet it is the responsibility of the music therapist to overcome these hurdles. I recently supervised a young music therapist who had stopped working with a teenager with RS, because she "did not cooperate". I had previously worked with her when she was younger and knew that she was a set minded as well as sensitive in nature; in addition to being in mid puberty. It occurred to me that she may not have felt comfortable musically or personally with the therapist since they hadn't established a close contact. The therapist offered an activity where she was asked to imitate the therapist's drumming, however, this girl may have felt more comfortable with another form of interaction such as melodic/vocal communication. Unfortunately, the few sessions they had been together was interpreted by the music therapist as non-cooperative resulting in the termination of the therapy sessions. Luckily, the therapist returned to work with the teenager after some supervision and is reporting that their relationship has developed and they both can't wait for the next session.

This experience reminded me of my first encounter with a girl with RS. This was more than 20 years ago. I was working in a special education facility and was asked to work with a young child with RS. The girl came always willingly to the music therapy room, yet after a few songs I had sung, she fell asleep and would remain asleep until the end of the session. At that time I could not see what good these sessions did and was considering withdrawing from working with the child.

Yet, after returning from my summer vacation, the special education teacher told me that during my absence, the child had stood day in and day out in front of my picture, touching it while tears running down her cheeks. Only then did I realize the importance of the music therapy sessions, which enabled her refuge from the stressing world a child with RS could experience on a daily basis. This experience taught me that music could be powerful for individuals with RS and that they have hidden emotional abilities, however, perseverance is needed and long lasting bonding needs to be nourished for a successful music therapy treatment.

Improvisation in music therapy

The most common form of working in music therapy is by either improvising or by using pre-composed music, including songs. Music, particularly improvised music making, has the advantage of combining a foundation of structure with measured flexibility and unpredictability. Improvisation in music therapy is a method that provides "intentionally an open or receptive process wherein one tries to create 'interactively meaningful' music that the client can understand..." [18] and react to. During improvisation the music therapist can convey the client's feelings through musical phrases either by playing it or by vocalizing (or both). The therapist tries to be finely attuned to the client in order to establish a meeting point. When the client feels the contact with the therapist, she can then find herself within the musical interaction which could result in developing long and meaningful musical as well as interpersonal interactions. Through this attunement, an interactive communication can be established.

There is usually a structure and order in this type of interactive improvisation with repeated musical patterns, melodic or rhythmic accents and by musical anticipation. This type of 'musical communication' is an interactive play in which both partners are engaged in mutual interaction and emotional involvement [19,20]. Although individuals with RS have limited ways of responding, a sensitive therapist can become aware of and perceive the client's physical and facial gestures or vocalization as indication for her relatedness. The therapist then uses these physical, vocal and facial gestures and expresses them in a musical form. These types of human 'communicative musicality' are evident in parent-child interactions from birth [19,20] and come alive with people of all ages when music is shared as the medium for therapeutic dialogue.

Whether the therapist uses pre-composed or improvised music, the quality of musical engagement and its clinical benefits depend upon the motives of 'communicative musicality' considered to be the foundation for the healing process [18].

Pre-composed songs in music therapy

Listening to pre-composed music, singing songs, or composing songs, is frequently used in music therapy. However, when using pre-composed music or songs it is recommended that it is performed live by the music therapist, in order to attune and accommodate the song to the client's immediate emotional and social needs.

Singing familiar songs was found as an excellent motivator for communicating and for engaging in dialogues with individuals with RS. When the songs are presented in a symbolic form such as pictures or words, the individual can make a selection independently by using her hand, chin, or nose to touch a selected picture or even by pointing at the selected song using her eyes [7,8,21,10].

The songs assist in organising an individual that otherwise could be in a disorganised or chaotic form [8]. Songs that are known to be most appropriate are ones that offer an organised structure; are usually short, predictable and repetitive [8]. This in turn provides security and will help in building their self esteem.

Vocalization

Vocalization is one of the first forms of expression in young infants. Through vocalization the young child communicates with his surroundings. It is an important aspect of the development of the self. Most individuals with RS do not have expressive language and may not always vocalize. It is crucial to help them to regain the vocalization as most of them have previously used and explored their voices and may have even used a few words. Once an individual with RS has established a closer rapport with the music therapist, she may be less inhibited resulting in possibility of the development of vocalization.

Intentional vocal sounds may initially appear in a very gentle and soft quality, while with time they can develop a stronger sound. The sounds become varied and the client seems to have more control over her own vocalization. The development of vocalization can be seen as an extension of her development of self-confidence and follows along the developments in her play [14]. The vocalization becomes interactive between the therapist and the child, a mean of communication. Wigram and Cass [22] describe one girl who during assessment vocalized to a familiar tune with much joy and once the music was stopped the vocalization changed to sounds of dissatisfaction and unhappiness. Once the music began, the girl began to smile and content vocal sounds were heard.

Burford and Trevarthen [23] suggested to encourage and to strengthen vocal interaction with individuals with RS because they believe it helps to promote motivation which in turn could result in better communication.

In one survey, it was described that most of the girls made spontaneous sounds and a few used simple words while hearing music [15]. From my own clinical experience, I have witnessed several girls who not only began to vocalize but who also began expressing single words when interacting vocally; repetitively using the words in musical games These were words the girls had used previously but seemed to have vanished. In many accounts the person with RS would vocalize in an echolalia manner as if trying to repeat a word that had been spoken. These incidences need to be captured by the music therapist and used as a lever to enhance vocal expression and interactive vocal dialogues which can enable the child to express herself and to reflect her more intimate inner emotional feelings [13]. Moreover, the simple act of vocalizing for a silent child enables her to bring herself forth and to become present.

Musical preference

Individuals with RS have musical preferences and favorites [8,9,24,25]. In a survey by Holdsworth [24] music is described as a means to a positive mood change if familiar, and negative reactions are sometimes observed to unfamiliar music. When unfamiliar music was introduced diminishing responsiveness was viewed when one compares levels of responsiveness to those found when familiar music was presented.

Some have reported that individuals with RS prefer simple, bright and energetic music and can show preference for a particular song by smiling and by becoming more animated as these familiar songs are sung [21,10,24,26,27]. Their recognition of favorite songs was also characterized by increasing activity levels and hyperventilation [26,27]. On the other hand, slow music has been found to relax, but in some cases to increase anxiety levels in them [28].

In a study [10], seven girls with RS (ages 4-10) showed clear song preferences. The girls intentionally chose songs through eye pointing or by touching picture symbols of familiar and unfamiliar songs. In this study the therapist asked each girl to make a choice of a song out of either 2- 4 songs represented by picture symbols or orthography. After the intentional choice of a song was made, the song was immediately sung to her. The results indicated that each girl had her own song preference. They preferred familiar songs to unfamiliar ones, which tended to be age appropriate. All the girls who participated in this project preferred songs with faster tempo, with musical elements such as tension and release, rhythmical accents and various vocal plays [7,8,29].

Parents to teen-agers have reported that their girls like to listen to pop or rock music, while others at that age seem to enjoy musicals such as: The Sound of Music, My Fair Lady, Mary Poppins, or Fiddler on the Roof. These could be indication of their understanding as to the content of the story and the music.

Individual music therapy

Persons with RS have many complex physical issues that contribute to their emotional state [18]. Individual music therapy can identify the difficulties the girls might undergo and help her understand them by musical interactions. It can help the client when an empathetic figure (such as a music therapist) can relate to her difficulties, and in turn may be able to build a trusting relationship with that person. There are times when she comes to the session and crying in grief. The therapist can then put words, supported by musical improvisation, into what she sees and feels is happening. The client may usually relate to the content of the improvisation that reflect her emotions. This can partially fulfill her emotional and communicative needs, helping her to sort out and to develop vitality and wellbeing. During such sessions, the therapist tries to help the client to find solutions or acceptance to some of her difficulties. These types of sessions are usually quite profound for both the therapist and the client.

Individual music therapy at times is plain fun and the client is able to express herself by laughing, vocalizing, singing and dancing. It can focus and relate to individual needs of a client. These sessions are typically less structured and tend to change according to individual needs at the time of the session. It is recommended to have music therapy with clients with RS twice a week, or even more frequently when she is in distress.

Music therapy groups for individuals with RS

The next section will address different setting of possible group music therapy for individuals with Rett syndrome. These include: Groups with other children with developmental disabilities, groups with other individuals with RS, and groups with children without disabilities through inclusion.

Individuals with RS are social beings who benefit from the interactions that undergo in group situation. Group music therapy takes into account inter-relationships between individuals in the group. They flourish within such a frame and express their emotions in group music therapy, especially when some of the participants are active and vocal. Because the person with RS can benefit from a group situation, it is highly recommended to integrate her in a music group with verbal children. The child tends to make contact with other children, observe them, imitate and make progress due to their social interest. They show interest in the music group by smiling, swaying back and forth, moving their legs or wringing their hands to the music's tempo. Group music therapy contains typically musical activities that are structured. All children, whether RS or others can benefit from structured activities; they are predictable and give organization, resulting in a feeling of security both on an individual and group basis. The music can function as a container where the children can connect and build relationships.

Individuals with RS are usually quite attentive during music groups, but at times when the attention is not directed towards them or when talking takes place, it could be very easy to 'lose' them during the group activities, or at least it may seem so as they tend to be passive. It is therefore important that the music therapist stays attuned in order to help them engage during the group activities. They also are non-initiators by nature, but with motivating activities they could be encouraged to initiate.

The therapist needs to give them ample time to respond during the activities as their response time is typically delayed. They can participate in almost all activities, choose a song or a game, play an instrument or move to the music similarly to the other participants; however they almost always need this little extra time.

The following is a vignette of a group music therapy session

During group music therapy for children with developmental disabilities the music therapist walked around with her guitar, greeted each child, and invited the child to strum the guitar while singing the child's name. Most children eagerly awaited for their turn and usually managed to strum the guitar with a basic beat. When the therapist approached Hanna, a girl with RS the girl smiled, laughed and swayed her body. The therapist stopped playing the guitar, waited for Hanna to strum the guitar. Hanna stopped swaying, began hand wringing, hyperventilated, pushed her body forwards, brought her face towards the guitar (almost touching the guitar), lifted up her head, looked at the therapist, smiled and swayed her hand forwards and managed to strum the guitar one time.

This is a typical response of a person with RS. Hanna needed ample time to respond but she also needed to have trust in the therapist who waited patiently for her response. An additional way of dealing with this type of delayed response could be to prolong and to slow down the greeting song, thus giving her enough time to organise herself for the task. This whole process could take up to a few minuets if the child is motivated yet inexperienced. Response time could be reduced after she has had many opportunities and has become familiar with the procedure. Another way to shorten reaction time is to start the greeting song with the child with RS thereby getting her in an active mode that could sustain for the rest of the session.

Bringing the girls together is an important experience for them. They seem to identify with one another by physically and emotionally connecting to each other. In such a music therapy group sessions the therapist can identify issues that the girls may be occupied with and aid them in dealing with these issues. It is important to help them realize that they are not 'alone' and that there are other people with the same needs. Different relevant topics to the girls' emotional needs could be explored. These should be age relevant as well as coincide with topics that occupy normally developed girls. The music therapist could reflect in singing and playing a certain topic while the girls can respond by vocalization or by the use of AAC. Song writing is a successful technique for dealing with some of the topics. During these groups a combination of structured and familiar activities and more improvised are recommended. The variety in musical activities can help the group develop as a group but also in taking care of individual needs.

Inclusion through music therapy

Individuals with RS seek interaction and social attention with other children, this tendency results in children wanting to get closer to them. However, because they lack language, children are not always certain how to approach a child with RS. In a four year community music inclusion project [30] children with severe developmental disorders, including several girls with RS were integrated into a regular neighbouring elementary school during music activities. The project was initiated by this author, for the purpose of making social change in a community in a middle class city in Israel, where children with special needs were segregated from the community. Through the development of the music group the children learnt to know and to relate to each other through musical activities as mutual interest. The children without special needs asked many questions concerning the other children had, but as these were answered and the difficult barriers were lifted, the children gradually became closer to one another. The children with RS showed affection and compassion towards the other children.

The project had very positive results on the children, staff, parents and the community and lasted for many years. The music project was extended to other activities outside the music room and was moved into extensive integration activities in the community. The girls with RS who participated in the project became less dependent during the music group activities, they made new friends and were empowered by this experience. The following is an excerpt from the music integration project which can describe the relationships the children had built. It took place towards the end of the first year of the project and the elementary school children did not want to terminate the project. They decided to initiate a summer camp for all the children.

> Sharon, Nina, Amy, Abigail and Mira were sitting on the bench in the schoolyard when the cameraman and a reporter from the Israeli Public Television approached them. "We are here to ask you a few questions about your project. We heard that this group is planning a summer camp. How is it possible that out of all the summer camps there are in this town you chose to initiate one in the special education center? Sharon answered: "Most friends go together to summer camps, and now that we have Amy and Mira (and others) as our friends it is only natural that we would spend the summer together." Nina looked at Amy and said (while holding Amy's hand): "Do you have any idea how much I have learned from this girl?" "How is this possible, she doesn't even talk?" asked the reporter. "We can't even begin to explain this. You won't understand" replied Nina.

Through integration we can see that it isn't only individuals with RS who can benefit from the experience but also the other children. This type of music integration group was a group empowerment.

Music therapy to enhance functional skills

Individual with RS' emotional well being is strengthened by music therapy; however the music therapist can also assist to strengthen her functional skills.

Since music is so motivating for the person with RS the use of musical instruments could be used to achieve object holding for long durations. This could be achieved through playing the xylophone, drums and other percussion instruments. This could be transferred into object holding in other functional areas such as holding feeding utensils during meal times.

The use of switches during music therapy sessions could be widened into every day situation when the person with RS could be using a switch to operate a tape recorder/CD to hear favourite songs. Later this ability could be widened into operating other types of electronical equipment.

Songs in music therapy could be used to enhance the use of Assistive Augmentative Communication (AAC). Whereas the songs that are sung to the client by the therapist have a character of emotional expressivity, the use of communicative devices within music therapy sessions has a different character. The Big Mac and Step by Step devices could be used as communication interactive devices to hear a favourite song. Any song could be recorded into the device and the client could actively 'sing' the song with someone else; a turn taking interactive game. Most of the songs are structured in short phrases and easy to follow. Let's take for example the song 'Happy Birthday'. The first phrase 'happy birthday to you' could be sung by the person engaged with the girl, then she presses the device and hears the next phrase 'happy birthday to you', then the person sings the next phrase 'happy birthday dear Natalie' and the girl presses the device for the last phrase 'happy birthday to me'. This type of turn-taking experience gives the client a feeling that her voice is being heard. It gives her the ability to have a shared experience in the song and to control her singing parts even though she actually doesn't sing. It is not only emotional satisfying; it is also an important learning experience and a way of relating to others.

Co-therapy. Music therapy in collaboration with other therapies

Earlier in this chapter we saw that during assessment and evaluation music therapy can work in conjunction with other professionals. The music can motivate the client to bring forth resources that otherwise may be difficult to detect. Her communicative, cognitive, learning and motor abilities can be brought to higher levels through the accompaniment and the support of the music therapist. In different settings it could be advised to work in co-therapy for the same reason as mentioned earlier but in a more focused way. This means that the music therapist can work together with the physical therapist, occupational therapist or speech and language therapist. The purpose of these types of settings will typically be to promote work in other areas, in addition to emotional/expressive musical skills. In order to work in co-therapy it is recommended that both therapists are established therapists with ample clinical experience.

In a paper [31] the authors; a music therapist and a physical therapist, described work principles in a longitudinal case study with a girl with RS. Both therapists had worked separately with the girl previous to their joint work. The music therapist found it challenging to work alone with the girl due to her physical challenges. The physical therapist found the girl uncooperative, which resulted in gradual lowering the demands and the sessions became shortened. Both therapists had separate and mutual goals in which they attended to and adjusted according to the girl's physical and emotional needs every session. The result of this therapy was that the girl improved in all areas (communicative, emotionally and physically) while fully participating in long and intensive sessions.

This example shows the benefit of co-therapy for some individuals with RS. Working in co-therapy is not an easy task for the therapists who arrive to the session from different backgrounds. It is recommended that the therapists discuss before and after each session in order to improve their co-work so that the client can benefit from the merging of the therapists. A video recording of the mutual sessions is recommended as tutorial material for the therapists to observe and improve.

Conclusions

Music therapy is recommended for individuals with RS. They respond emotionally to musical interactions, share these emotions and expressivity with the therapist and as a result expand and open up new venues for communication and learning.

Individuals with RS can benefit from individual or group music therapy sessions, however these have different purposes. Group work can be in the form of integration with normally developed children or in groups with people with special needs as well as in groups with only individuals with RS.

When working with this population it is important to work within a frame of age appropriate music as well as music that they choose. This doesn't only mean to engage them only with songs and activities that are age appropriate, but also age appropriate messages which may occupy them.

The chapter attempted to convey possibilities in how to engage in music therapy with individuals with RS. Through a healthy mutual relationship between the client and the therapist while the music can serve as a bridge into new venues for emotional, communicative, social, functional, or educational development.

References

[1]   Amir RE, Van den Veyver IB, Wan M, Tran CQ, Francke U, Zoghbi HY. Rett syndrome is caused by mutations in X-linked MECP2, encoding methyl-CpG-binding protein 2. Nat Genet 1999;23(2): 185-8.

[2]   Amir RE, Van Den Veyve IB, Schultz R, Malicki DM, Tran CQ, Dahle EJ. Influence of mutation type and X chromosome inactivation on Rett syndrome phenotypes. Ann Neurol 2000;47: 670-9.

[3]   Hagberg B. Rett Syndrome: Clinical and biological aspects. London: Mac Keith Press, 1993.

[4]   Engerstrom IW, Kerr A. Workshop on autonomic function in Rett Syndrome, Swedish Rett center, Frösön, Sweden. Brain Dev 1998; 20:323-6.

[5]   Lotan M. Management for Rett syndrome. Tel Aviv, IL: Rotem Publ, 2006. [Hebrew]

[6]   Rett A. Grundlagen der Musiktherapie und Music-Psychologie 1982. Stuutgart: G Harrer, 1982. [German]

[7]   Elefant C. Speechless yet communicative: Revealing the person behind the disability of Rett syndrome through clinical research on songs in music therapy. In: Aldridge D, Di Franco G, Ruud E, Wigram T, eds. Music Therapy in Europe. Rome: ISMEZ, 2001.

[8]   Elefant C. Enhancing communication in girls with Rett syndrome through songs in music therapy. Dissertation. Aalborg: Aalborg Univ, 2002.

[9]   Elefant C, Wigram T. Learning ability in children with Rett syndrome. Brain Dev 2005;27: 97-101.

[10]   Hadsell NA, Coleman KA. Rett syndrome: A challenge for music therapists. Music Ther Perspect 1988;5:52- 6.

[11]   Montague J. Music therapy in the treatment of Rett syndrome. Glasgow: UK Rett Syndr Assoc, 1988.

[12]   Wesecky A. Music therapy for children with Rett syndrome. Am J Med Genetics 1986;24:253-7.

[13]   Wigram T. Music therapy for a girl with Rett's syndrome: Balancing structure and freedom. In: Bruscia K, ed. Case studies in music therapy. Gilsum, NH: Barcelona Publ, 1991:39-55

[14]   Hill SA. The relevance and value of music therapy for children with Rett syndrome. Br J Spec Educ 1997;24(3):124-8.

[15]   Lindberg B. Understanding Rett syndrome A practical guide for parents, teachers and therapists, 2nd. rev ed. Cambridge, MA: Hogrefe, 2006.

[16]   Wigram T. A model of assessment and differential diagnosis of handicap in children through the medium of music therapy. In: Wigram T, Saperston B, West R, eds. The art and science of music therapy: A handbook. Chur, Switzerland: Harwood Acad Publ, 1995:181-93.

[17]   Lotan M, Manor-Binyamini I, Elefant C, Wine J, Saraf E, Yoshei T The Israeli Rett Syndrome Center. Evaluation and transdisciplinary play-based assessment. ScientificWorldJournal 2006;6:1302-13.

[18]   Wigram T, Elefant C. Therapeutic dialogues in music: Nurturing musicality of communication in children with autistic spectrum disorder and Rett syndrome. In: Malloch S, Trevarthen C, eds. Communicative musicality: Exploring the basis of human companionship, Oxford: Oxford Univ Press, 2009.

[19]   Malloch SN. Mother and infants and communicative musicality. Musicae Scientiae Special Issue, 1999-2000:29-57.

[20]   Trevarthen C, Malloch S. Musicality and music before three: Human vitality and invention shared with pride. Zero to Three 2002;25(1):10-8.

[21]   Elefant C, Lotan M. Music and physical therapies in Rett syndrome: A transdisciplinary approach. Spec Educ Rehabil J 1998;13(2):89-97. [Hebrew]

[22]   WigramT, Cass H. Music therapy within the assessment process for a therapy clinic for people with Rett syndrome. Presentation, Rett Syndr World Conf, Sweden, 1996.

[23]   Burford B, Trevarthen C. Evoking communication in Rett syndrome: Comparisons with conversations and games in mother-infant interaction. Eur Child Adolesc Psychiatry 1997;6(Suppl.1):26-30.

[24]   Holdsworth J. Responsiveness to music in 21 girls and women with Rett syndrome. Unpublished paper. Hull, UK: Dept Psychol, Univ Hull, 1999.

[25]   Merker B, Bergstrom-Isacsson, M, Witt Engerstrom, I. Music and the Rett disorder: The Swedish Rett Center survey. Nord J Music Ther 2001;10(1):42-53.

[26]   Woodyatt G, Ozanne A. Communication abilities and Rett syndrome. J Autism Dev Disord 1992;22:155-73.

[27]   Woodyatt G, Ozanne A. Intentionality and communication in four children with Rett syndrome. Aust NZ J Dev Disabil 1994;19:173-83.

[28]   Mount RH, Hastings RP, Reilly S, Cass H, Charman T. Behavioral and emotional features in Rett syndrome. Disabil Rehabil 2001;23(3/4):129-38.

[29]   Elefant C. The use of single case designs in testing a specific hypothesis. In: Aldridge D, ed. Case study designs in music therapy. London: Jessica Kingsley, 2005:145-62.

[30]   StigeB, Ansdell G, Elefant C, Pavlicevic M. Where music helps. Community music therapy in action and reflection. London: Ashgate Publisher, 2010.

[31]   Elefant C, Lotan M. Rett syndrome: Dual intervention. Music and physical therapy. Nord J Music Ther 2004;13(2):172-82.

In: Rett Syndrome: Therapeutic Interventions
Editors: Meir Lotan and Joav Merrick

ISBN: 978-1-61728-080-1
©2011 Nova Science Publishers, Inc.

Chapter XII

Rett Syndrome: Hydrotherapy Across the Life Span with a Review of the Literature and Three Case Studies

Meir Lotan, BPT, MScPT, PhD[*,1,2,3]
and Caroline Barmatz, BPT, HT, MHA[4]

[1]Israel Rett Center, National Evaluation Team, Chaim Sheba Medical Center, Tel HaShomer, Ramat Gan; [2]Zvi Quittman Residential Centers, Israel Elwyn, Jerusalem, [3]Department of Physical Therapy, Ariel University Campus, Ariel, [4]Therapeutic Rehabilitation Pool, Chaim Sheba Medical Center, Tel Hashomer, Ramat-Gan, Israel

Rett Syndrome (RS) is a genetic disorder mainly affecting females, who are challenged by several difficulties in many areas of their daily lives. Their neurological and orthopedic disabilities require extensive physical care but their fear of movement, typical of many with this disorder, leaves them extremely anxious about external uncontrolled movements. Therefore, in order to ease them into physical treatment, some kind of mediation is warranted. One of the favored environments for individuals with RS is the hydrotherapeutic pool. The warm water helps reduce spasticity and softens rigid tissues while assisting in calming the client if she is anxious of movement. Water provides the individual with RS intense stimulation while enabling free and easy movement, without fear of falling and without the use of assistive devices. Spending time in a pool puts the individual with RS in a normative place. Water provides her with new and exciting experiences, enabling her to function in ways that she is unable to achieve outside the water. In some cases, the water enables the person with RS to express her lost and sometimes latent motor-skills. The aim of this chapter is to describe clinical characteristics of individuals with RS and to present their challenges. Its intention is to explain the importance of water as a mediating environment for managing clients with

* Correspondence: Meir Lotan, BPT, MScPT, PhD, Department of Physical Therapy, Ariel University Campus, IL-40700 Ariel, Israel. E-mail: ml_pt_rs@netvision.net.il

RS, to describe commonalities in the hydrotherapeutic intervention for this population and present case-studies that exemplify hydrotherapeutic intervention for three individuals with RS at different ages and in different functional levels.

Introduction

Rett Syndrome (RS) is a complex neurological disorder resulting from a genetic fault [1] that occurs mostly in females and affects them throughout their lives. The syndrome is named after an Austrian physician, Andreas Rett, who, in 1966, was first to identify the syndrome [2]. Since the discovery of the genetic cause for RS [3], diagnosis of RS is found positive in 90% of individuals showing the clinical characteristics of the disorder but in many cases it still relies on descriptive criteria first suggested by Hagberg and Witt Ingerstrom from Sweden [4,5]. The general goals of hydrotherapy are to encourage the person with RS to reach her highest level of independence, to keep her physically fit (as a tool for independence and maintaining general health) and to improve her quality of life. This chapter will describe the existing literature on hydrotherapy with the disabled population in general with a focus on individuals with RS. Since the literature is scarce, the chapter will rely mainly on the authors' clinical experience for the last 15 years with individuals with RS of all ages.

Stages in rett syndrome

Since this chapter describes aquatic intervention for individuals with RS at different ages, the next paragraph will characterize the development of RS in the four classic stages and the way they focus the hydrotherapeutic intervention.

Stage I (onset). The primary development of most individuals with RS is, in many cases, similar to the norm. At this stage, the symptoms of RS are just emerging and are mostly vague [6,7]. At this point, the child usually displays hypotonia and might even show improved finger-use. In most cases, the girl will not alarm even the specialist physician [8]. The second stage is where the difficulties begin to emerge and need to receive more attention.

Stage II (Destructive). This stage can have a rapid onset and is a very difficult period for the child with RS and her family. The child at that stage completely lacks orientation, her senses are severely disturbed and her body betrays her [9]. Although a relatively short period (weeks or a few months), this stage is the girl's most difficult experience. Getting into warm water at this stage may ease her discomfort. Although it is questionable if functional goals can be achieved during this stormy period, it is worth trying and achieving relaxation at that stage is a possible goal. Since co-operation with her therapist is highly dependent upon interpersonal relations, the therapist should try and bond with the child in preparation for future, more challenging meetings.

Stage III (plateau). This stage is relatively calm. The extreme physical/emotional situation typical of stage II now seems to balance. The duration of this stage is long (years) and this enables the person with RS to achieve progress and to actively prevent possible future problems. A vast variety of possible treatment goals might be found appropriate at stage III.

Stage IV (late motor-deterioration). It is emphasized here that RS is not considered to be a degenerative disease and therefore the fourth stage is not obligatory and, according to experts in the field of RS, it is possible that with intensive well-aimed intervention, this stage might be delayed or even eliminated in many individuals with RS [10,11]. At this stage, in some people with RS, late motor-deterioration that requires increased physiotherapy may be noticed. Several cases have been reported, where girls with RS lost their ability to walk, but were able to improve their functional mobility and regain the lost abilities [12,13]. In one case–study, the rehabilitation of lost walking-skills was achieved with a 43 year-old individual after two decades of immobility [12]. It is important to stress that the inability to walk increases the risk of secondary complications such as scoliosis, pelvic and limb deformities, pulmonary problems, reduced bowel movements and blood flow to internal organs and enhances muscle wasting [14-17]. Therefore, it is extremely important to keep the person with RS as active as possible.

Hydrotherapeutic advantages

Despite differences in phenotypic expression among individuals with RS and the need to individualize an intervention plan for each client, our experience suggests that in many cases it is possible to identify common characteristics for this group of clients and therefore some mutual therapeutic goals for many individuals diagnosed with RS. Moreover, the positive effects of the hydrotherapeutic environment on the swimmer with RS [18,19] has for a long time been described and these can be well-matched to the clinical picture presented by many with RS.

Relaxation

The relaxing effect, whilst in a supine position in the swimming pool, occurs as a result of a yet unclear process, which causes obvious calming effects on heart-rate, respiration and blood pressure [20]. Studies have shown that the parasympathetic system is relatively hypoactive in individuals with RS due to immaturity of the brain stem [21], apparently leaving the children in a constant state of stress. On top of that, most individuals with RS are in constant motion and often display repetitive movements (especially hand-movements) that, for the most part, persist throughout the persons waking-hours. Decreasing the sympathetic system's activity, while enhancing intense respiration, might boost the parasympathetic system, thus balancing the autonomic system's activity. The water delivers many elements that help the swimmer to relax, such as the support given to the body by the water's hydrostatic pressure [22], the sense of weightlessness due to buoyancy [23], the warmth of the water [23] and the slow, rhythmic, movements of the therapist's support and passive manipulation (such as the Watsu techniques). In water, the swimmer with RS feels her stressed muscles calm and released; there is a decrease in her stereotyped movements and a reduction in her fears of uncontrolled movement by external manipulators (the therapist). The water is like a peaceful island in the midst of the RS chaos [23]. It gently embraces the girl and takes away the pain, fear and uncertainty, at least for the duration of the treatment. The personal touch, the eye-contact and the therapist's well-trained, secure hands are all beneficial. Getting the child to relax is of the utmost importance at Stage II, for children with RS display a great deal of irritability at this stage. Yet the person with RS who lacks the ability to verbally communicate, might, at times, become extremely upset without being able to inform her care-giver the reason behind such behavior. At such moments, a quiet treatment can save many hours of pain, tears and discomfort.

The normality of swimming

The values of swimming for the general population have been defined as survival, fitness and joy, by Elkington [24]. These values are the same for those with RS. Swimming enables the integration of the person with limitations within a normal setting. The activity in water is perceived by the swimmer, her family and their surroundings as a "normal" activity. Taking part in such an activity enhances positive notions of the girl about her ability to integrate into society, thereby improving her self-esteem and self-confidence. With these advantages, swimming and experiencing the water environment is recommended for the child with RS and her family from a young age.

Enabling exploration of the environment

It is common knowledge that limitations in movement diminish the young child's experience and delays development in all areas. This has been corroborated by researchers studying the connection between motor skills and perceptual development [25,26], who found that limitations in physical activity limit perceptual development. Internalizing the outer world is usually achieved through one's active experience, and due to their physical limitations, individuals with RS who lack normal movement, experience the world around them in a narrow perspective. Therefore, it is not surprising that their development in all areas is extremely limited. Since movement is easier and freer in the water, it allows the person with RS to explore her surroundings. Moreover, movement through the water gives the swimmer more sensory feedback due to the thickness of the water (in comparison movement through air). She might also generalize or carry over such behavior to land activities and improve her movement out of water as well. This in turn might help change her negative attitude towards movement. When the person with RS learns to move freely in water and sometimes even swim, she can join a swimming group or other water-based activity groups and thus improve her social abilities. In addition, her ability to move and use her body more freely can give her satisfaction and joy thereby raising her self-esteem and improve her self-confidence [22].

Freeing the swimmer from her limitations

When ambulating, the individual with RS has to confront her unreliable sensory processes (apraxia), her fear of movement, her fluctuating muscle tone and the poor muscular control, attributed to ataxia. The accumulation of such challenges inflicts severe functional limitations upon the individual with RS [27]. In the water, the equipment used to assist the girl in her everyday life, such as wheelchairs, splints and walkers, is not required, thus freeing her from her physical limitations. Free movement in water is a way to build strong and healthy body awareness. Getting used to the water is also important and allows the person with RS to participate more freely in her family's activities, such as going to the beach and swimming-pool.

Psychological effects

Improvements in quality of life and emotional well-being due to physical activity on land have been repeatedly reported [28-30] and similar results have been found in relation to swimming activity [31]. The elements mentioned above are particularly helpful in cases of people with intensified muscle-tone and children who fear movement - two common characteristics of individuals with RS. In water, the swimmer with RS feels relaxed and the water relaxes her tense muscles, eases her movement and reduces her fear of motion. Most individuals with RS lack verbal ability and are, therefore, challenged in conveying even the simplest messages. The aquatic experience can provide a safe environment for the person with RS thereby reducing anxiety and frustration caused by daily difficulties and failures. Such changes might lead to improvement in morale and self-esteem [31], a state of mind that, in turn, improves her quality of life.

Improving hand-use

Most individuals with RS acquire some form of hand-function in their post-gestational period. Such hand-function could be grip, finger feeding, turning the page of a book, using a phone–dial, or keypad. From the age of eight months, up to four years of age, these children gradually lose hand-function. The assumption is that the poor functional abilities of individuals with RS are not derived from lack of ability but rather from the combination of Apraxia, Ataxia, lack of experience [12] and learned helplessness. Hence, despite the deterioration of functional hand–use, individuals with RS can and should be taught repeatedly to re-acquire new hand skills [32]. Survival in the pool necessitates prolonged firm, functional grips over different types of buoys and holding on to the edge of the pool, thereby encouraging hand-function that might be generalized to land-based activities.

Reducing pain

The person with RS might develop contractures [33,34], therefore necessitating different exercises to elongate shortened muscles and reduce limb deformities. Because of the water's warmth, rhythmic movement and viscosity, carrying out exercises that cause pain when performed on land should be considered a part of the hydro-therapeutic intervention. This is particularly true during the fourth stage of RS, when many people with RS might become more and more rigid.

Reducing spasticity

During childhood most individuals with RS present low muscle tone. In later years 40% of them have been found to increase muscle-tone and become rigid or spastic; 30% of them have dystonic muscle-tone [35]. Exercising in warm water decreases muscular spasticity, thereby allowing active healthy muscle fiber to strengthen and build up. This is especially true during adult years of individuals with RS, when many of them become more and more rigid and their muscles atrophied.

Preventing potential orthopedic problems (and treating existing ones)

People with RS might display the orthopedic problems of Scoliosis, Kyphosis, hip dislocation and deformation of the palms and/or feet.

Scoliosis can be found in 80%-85% of the total cases [5,36], especially among non-mobile individuals. Since a clear connection has been established between lack of mobility and severity of Scoliosis [36], it is very important to provide motivation for walking [37]. Since an intensive physical program has been found to halt and even regress the progression of scoliosis in an individual with RS [38], the implementation of such a program in the pool is highly recommended. Kyphosis is more common among people with RS who can walk but is usually not as severe and motor-disabling as Scoliosis [5].

In any case, the therapist can use water as a support system that warms and softens rigid tissues, thereby preparing the body for the needed handling while the therapist can skillfully manipulate the client's body. The deformation that often occurs in the palms and feet and dislocation of the hips usually occur in non-mobile individuals [33] and requires careful attention and specific treatments.

Preserving and improving joint range of motion

Those with RS are at high risk of developing deformities, especially in the spine and extremities [34] as a result of their sedentary life-style and, in some cases, their inability to move. Thanks to the viscosity of the water and lack of gravitational forces, the spine is better protected while working in an open kinematic chain, as is the case in hydrotherapy. Such exercises are extremely helpful in the case of existing articular pain. An intensive program aimed at increasing articular range of motion might set the foundation for general functional improvement.

Re-learning lost functions

Apraxia is a broad term referring to situations in which one is having difficulties in performing a motor-act on-demand or in learning a new function. It is derived from a deficit in sensory (tactile, proprioceptive, vestibular) information processing, causing a skewed body scheme, impairing the child's motor planning [39]. This difficulty affects the person with RS in all functional areas (feeding, ambulating, speech, hand function) and complicates the learning of new skills. Nevertheless, since the affected female with RS maintains the ability to learn new skills [8,40], it is recommended that new functional abilities be routinely exercised until she achieves an automated ability to perform a desired function. Due to the water's density and buoyancy, movements in water are slowed down, thus giving more sensory input and prolonging reaction time.

This characteristic enables secure and easier work in the process of learning different movements. It is important to recognize that people with limitations feel less clumsy in water, specifically because they are free of layers of clothing and limiting equipment, such as splints or crutches. The hydrostatic pressure provides the person with RS with good support and allows her to move freely in the pool. In this way, individuals with RS who have lost their ability to walk can exercise in the water with this activity and maybe even regain the lost ability. The major aim when practicing walking is to maintain the highest level of walking for the longest periods possible [41]. The water's support can be very helpful for the person with RS who lacks balance when out of the pool. Walking in water allows the individual with RS to exercise without injury or danger of falling. It is known that some individuals with RS who lost their walking ability, regained it after a period of immobility [12,21] and due to the above mentioned positive attributes of the water, it is possible that aquatic therapy may enable such progress.

Improving general physical activity and developing stamina

When individuals with Intellectual and Developmental Disability (IDD) have been compared to peers without IDD, they have been found continuously to be less active and, as a result, in a poorer physical condition [42-45]. Moreover, the sensory challenges (fear of movement) typical of individuals with RS are powerful setbacks in their being active. These factors drive the person with RS towards an inactive lifestyle, thereby leaving her muscular system deteriorated and weak, leading to further loss of her mobile abilities. When the physical ability of the individual with RS to move outside the water declines, it is helpful to increase her activity in the water and swimming could be considered as a good alternative to walking. Swimming encourages limb movement, prevents articular stiffness or contractures, strengthens muscles and improves cardio-pulmonary fitness [22-24]. These elements are highly important for overall health in any human being. Yet, the combined dangers of reduced mobility and enhanced spasticity, common in adults with RS, are a strong indicator of the benefits of implementing an aquatic program. Since the connection between better physical fitness and functional abilities of individuals with RS has been reported [46], improving physical condition, especially stamina, is extremely desirable for this population. Water resistance requires muscle activation whilst at the same time providing a motivating, enjoyable and safe environment in which to activate the individual with RS.

Improving limb circulation

It is well known that individuals with RS have poor circulation of the extremities, which is manifested by small, cold, swollen, ulcerated and blue-ish/red feet [19]. The warmth of the water, movement and pressure applied by active muscles, together with the hydrostatic pressure, can improve circulation and reduce edematic feet.

Socialization

Most individuals with RS are very friendly but their communication (especially of those who are not mobile) with their friends and class-mates might be technically difficult, due to their physical limitations. The mobility enabled by the water and the structure of the treatment in the pool enables the therapist to create conditions that encourage group-work. Since individuals with RS are very friendly and love to interact with adults and peers, working in pairs or in small groups is highly recommended for this population.

Maintaining ability to perform transitions [47]

One of the primary motor-losses of individuals with RS is experienced in transitions. Transitions include changes from a standing to a sitting position, from sitting to standing, from standing to walking and so forth. Therefore, during the treatment, one should include repetitive elements of movement and position-changes on a regular basis [41].

Enabling controlled breathing

Breathing control is important for all swimmers in all water activities [22], but it is specifically significant for individuals with RS who display various forms of breathing irregularities [48] such as hyperventilation, breath holding, air swallowing and abruptly blowing out large quantities of air and saliva [21]. Aquatic therapy treatment, especially submersion, enables the person with RS to exercise control over her body and lungs. It also allows her to maintain a regular breathing rhythm and might even teach her to control the rate and depth of her breathing outside the water. From our experience, most individuals with RS are able to learn how to control their breathing and eventually some might even enjoy their ability to dive during the aquatic treatment.

Re-assembling "mid-line" [49]

Body perception of many individuals with RS differs from the norm. It seems as if their proprioceptive system is skewed, giving them a sensation of their mid-line that is different from where it actually is. Sometimes they tilt so far to one side or backwards that one might easily rule out the possibility of independent seating [41], standing and walking. Aquatic therapy treatment enables the therapist to work with the person with RS on her distorted "mid-line" perception with or without the use of instruments. The therapist can use the water's surface as a solid line to which the swimmer can relate, by walking through it, moving below or above it. It is preferable that the swimmer is kept as active as possible, thereby stimulating the sensory\receptive system into establishing a more balanced body scheme.

Normalizing sensation

People with RS are often characterized by an unbalanced sensory system. This phenomenon cannot be seen but has been referred to in the past [9,50]. Individuals with RS display decreased pain sensation and hypersensitivity to touch on their faces, especially around the mouth. It was suggested by Lindberg that their fear of movement might be caused by dysfunctional vestibular perception [9], yet the authors believe that the main fault in RS perception rests within an irregular proprioceptive system causing a distracted body scheme; a vital component in accepting and relating to the world (apraxia). The water embraces the swimmer and provides her with sensory stability. Since the water has a more massive presence than air, the body's presence is solidified. In water, the swimmer with RS can move freely and peacefully, while experiencing maximum sensory feedback and allowing the warm water to relax her nervous system, thereby enhancing the occurrence of sensory integration [39].

Improving equilibrium and co-ordination

Among her other challenges, the individual with RS is diagnosed with ataxia. Ataxia is caused by damaged areas in the nervous system that control movement. The presence of ataxia causes the individual to experience a failure of muscle control over the limbs, resulting in a lack of balance and co-ordination and a disturbance of gait [51]. The ability to control the muscles is essential for supporting the body's posture in various positions and in movement. Lacking this ability can create severe motor limitations. The water supports the body and slows down limb and body movements, thereby allowing the swimmer with RS to react in her usually slow pace. Due to the enhanced sensation and the safety of the pool, the person with RS can practice and improve her difficulties in these areas.

Summary

From the numerous intervention possibilities suggested thus far, it appears that the person with RS might find it easier to address many of her challenges through aquatic intervention. Therefore, hydrotherapeutic intervention is highly recommended for this population. The next section of the chapter will discuss the course of an intervention program implemented at the Sheba hydrotherapeutic rehabilitation center with three individuals with RS at different ages and functional abilities.

Sheba hydrotherapeutic rehabilitation center

Sheba Medical Center is the largest and most comprehensive medical center in Israel, at which a unique approach combines acute care and rehabilitation within the same medical center. The hydrotherapeutic pool is part of the Department of Neurological Rehabilitation at Chaim Sheba Hospital, which provides treatment to patients from the time of injury to in-patient, out-patient, community integration and long-term follow-up periods. The hydrotherapeutic center treats patients with conditions of spinal cord injury, brain injury, stroke, multiple sclerosis, other neurological disorders and medically chronic spinal cord injured patients.

The criteria for patient admission to the pool are rehabilitation potential, medical stability and cognitive ability to participate in a rehabilitation program. The facility includes two modern and well-equipped therapeutic swimming pools that are used for hydrotherapeutic intervention. The staff at the center is specifically trained in hydrotherapy treatment techniques. The treatment includes exercises assisted by the buoyancy of the warm water.

Case study 1

RZ, a first-born in a family, with two other siblings (males), was born in 2000 and diagnosed with RS in 2004. RZ has been to several educational facilities and started receiving hydrotherapy intervention at the age of five.

State at admission to hydrotherapeutic intervention

RZ was diagnosed with severe spasticity, according to the Ashworth test [52], ranging from 4 in the lower extremities to 3 at the upper extremities. The spasticity is constantly accompanied with intense ataxic tremor of the limbs that escalates when RZ is exited or anxious. She is unable independently to change positions from lying, crawl, sit unsupported and is non-ambulant. RZ usually prefers to stay in one position and, when being moved, she shows signs of extreme distress (extensive tremor accompanied with apneas that later change to hyperventilation) especially when her limbs are being moved. She shows incidence of sudden apneas that might lead to bluish lips. The goals for hydrotherapeutic intervention were:

- Encouragement of movement towards independent movement in the water
- Improvement and maintenance of range of motion
- Enhancement of communication (choosing the order of activities),
- Improvement of breath control
- Movement in the water while in a supine position, supported at the shoulder's level

Therapeutic intervention

Table XII-1 is a summation of three years of hydrotherapy intervention. All sessions were conducted in a structured manner, each including a constant set of tasks, yet all were done while singing and maintaining the child's enthusiasm and eagerness to participate.

Table XII-1. Description of hydrotherapy sessions for RZ over a three year period

Activities	First year	Second year	Third year
Entering the pool	The child enters the pool from the side, supported at the pelvis, whilst encouraged with verbal and sensorial prompting	The child enters the pool from the side, supported at the pelvis, whilst encouraged with verbal and sensorial prompting	The child enters the pool from the side, supported at the pelvis, whilst encouraged with verbal and sensorial prompting
Position change	Changes from a vertical to a supine position with support at the pelvis	Changes from a vertical to a supine position with support at the pelvis	Changes from a vertical to a supine position with support at the shoulders*
Movement along pool-side	Movement while holding pool-side with pelvic support	Movement while holding pool-side with pelvic support	Movement while holding pool-side with pelvic support
Floating ability	Complete support	Floats on her back for five seconds with support at pelvic level*	Floats on her back for ten seconds with support at shoulder level*
Breath control	No breath control	When seated on the therapist's lap, puts mouth in the water on demand* She is as yet unable to control her breathing patterns	When seated on the therapist's lap, puts mouth in the water on demand* She is as yet unable to control her breathing patterns
Free movement	Minimal movement	When in supine position, turns her head to the side on demand*	When in supine position, turns her head to both sides on demand and gently splashes the water with her legs*
Communication	Inconsistent communication in relation to activities	Maintains eye contact throughout the activity, and communicates her wishes in relation to order of activities*	Maintains eye contact throughout the activity, and communicates her wishes in relation to order of activities
Climbing onto a large floatation device	Minimal movement	Minimal movement	Climbing onto a large floatation device support at pelvic level*
Walking in the water	Minimal movement	Minimal movement	Walking two-three steps, held at the pelvis when water is at shoulder level*

*Changes between years are marked and underlined

Summation of hydrotherapy intervention for RZ

The reports suggest that during this period RZ had learned to improve her communication abilities by communicating her wishes (through eye-pointing) to the therapist, thereby achieving a sense of control over the situation. Her ability to control her body gradually improved and she was able to move more freely in the water, thereby achieving functional abilities such as climbing onto a floatation device and moving her body in the water. Her ability to walk in the water was transferred to other areas and during that time and thereafter she has also shown the ability to take some steps (supported at shoulder level) on land and to go up and down a flight of stairs (fully supported). In comparison to other manual and motor-activities and therapy sessions (R.Z also receives conventional physical therapy, hippotherapy, in which she is usually tense and anxious), she enjoyed coming to the pool and receiving hydrotherapy.

Case study 2

OC was born in 1985. She has been receiving hydrotherapy intervention since childhood. She had never walked. She also had a severe scoliosis necessitating orthopedic surgery at the age of 15. She receives physical therapy intervention that focuses on sitting unsupported and standing supported as a means by which to maintain bone strength and maximize muscular activity and manual intervention to maintain and enhance limb range of movement. Her right hip joint is dislocated thereby reduction in right leg movements can be observed. OC has a very distinct character and can clearly display her desire to be left untouched and unmoved.

State at admission to hydrotherapeutic intervention

OC is a wheelchair user and has suffered a few pathological fractures due to osteoporosis. She presents only a limited amount of movement and a reduced range of movement in the trunk and extremities. The goals for hydrotherapeutic intervention for OC:

- Walking in the water
- Movement in the water to enhance range of movement
- Raising levels of activity
- Enhancing physical fitness

OC receives once-weekly, half-hour sessions in the swimming pool. In the pool, her resentment of movement is completely reduced and OC enjoys the smooth movement of her body in different positions. A considerable part of the session is focused on walking. Since OC has never walked on land, the steps that she can take when submerged gives her immense joy while enabling her (within one session) to exert a higher level of activity than she demonstrates during a week on land.

Summation of hydrotherapy intervention for OC

The goals for OC and the treatment have been kept stable for the past years. Yet, it seems that the few goals aimed at by the hydrotherapist are a valuable addition to the physical therapy intervention and that those intervention programs support one-another. Her resistance to being moved outside the pool is completely overturned once OC is in the water, thus enabling elevated levels of activity and making this type of intervention extremely valuable for her.

Case study 3

SR is an only child to her parents. She was born in 1965 and diagnosed with RS in 2005 at the age of 39. SR has been enrolled in several educational facilities and started receiving hydrotherapy intervention in the last few years. SR can walk with slight assistance and go up and down a few steps with assistance.

State at admission to hydrotherapeutic intervention

SR was diagnosed with severe Kyphoscoliosis that was treated in 1981 by the fixing of the spinal angel at 55^0 Cobb through a Harrington's rod procedure. Despite recent backaches (as reported by her parents) which renew a need for occasional assistance during ambulation, she has the ability to walk. She never had epilepsy. Her muscle-tone is characterized by spasticity associated with rigidity. The goals for hydrotherapeutic intervention for SR:

- Co-operation with hydrotherapist
- Movement in the water
- Interaction with therapist and peers
- Exposure to different stimuli.

SR receives twice-weekly, half-hour sessions in the swimming pool. Since people with RS are in need of a stable framework, her therapist is kept unchanged. As SR cannot change positions in the water and does not put her head in the water, most of the intervention focuses on standing and walking with erect posture.

Summation of hydrotherapy intervention for SR

The goals for SR and the treatment have been kept stable for the past years. From the goals and their stability, it seems that the pool team was not looking to initiate change but rather maintain and generalize existing abilities.

Discussion

When reviewing the literature and the above mentioned case-studies, one can learn that the hydrotherapeutic environment can assist individuals with RS in many of the challenging areas in need of improvement, as a result of the disorder.

When we examine the three case-studies, we see that, as the individual with RS is growing, the goals of the therapeutic team are gradually reduced (this is not specific to RS or to hydrotherapy but rather characterizes most therapeutic intervention for individuals with a disability). An intervention program that aims at achievable goals is one that is tailored for a client with RS, however limited she might be. A more subtle, less demanding path is taken when this child is a teenager or a grown woman. However, the authors as therapists believe that this trend should change and that habilitation should be the goal for the hydrotherapeutic intervention at all ages rather than maintenance. Nevertheless, all three cases indicate the advantages of hydrotherapy at all ages for individuals with RS.

The main advantages of hydrotherapy as we see them, lie in the fact that the water as well as the therapists, can mediate movement for the person with RS. Such a relaxed ambience, for a population that is usually so petrified of movement, enables the client with RS to gain control over her body, thereby improving her functional abilities. Moreover, the water provides a more intense sensory feedback (which is extremely important for a client with dispraxia). Such gains, when accompanied by improved communication skills, enhance the child's control over her body, thereby achieving a feeling of self-worth and empowerment. Therefore, the aquatic environment is highly recommended for all persons with RS.

References

[1]   Amir RE, Van Den Veyver IB, Wan M, Tran CQ, Franke U, Zoghbi H. Rett syndrome is caused by mutations in X-linked MECP2, encoding methyl CpG binding protein 2. Nat Genet 1999;23:185–8.

[2]   Rett A. Uber ein eigartiges hirnatrophisches Syndrom bei Hyperammoniamie in Kindesalter. Wien Med Wochenschr 1966;116:723–38. [German]

[3]   Amir RE, Van Den Veyver IB, Schultz R, Malicki DM, Tran CQ, et al. Influence of mutation type and X chromosome inactivation on phenotypes. Ann Neurol 2000;47:670-9.

[4]   International RS Association Web site:www.http://rettsyndrome.org/

[5]   Hagberg B. Rett syndrome clinical and biological aspects. London: Mac K Press, 1993.

[6]   Einspieler C. Signs of Rett disorder in the first six month of life. A lecture presented at the international course on Rett syndrome, Ostersund, Sweden, 2003 Jun 16-18.

[7]   Burford B. Identifying early signs of Rett disorder and their implications for development. A lecture presented at the international course on Rett syndrome, Ostersund, Sweden, 2003 Jun 16-18.

[8]   Leonard H, Fyfe S, Leonard S, Msall M. Functional status, medical impairments, and rehabilitation resources in 84 females with Rett syndrome: a snapshot across the world from the parental perspective. Disabil Rehabil 2001;23:107-17.

[9]   Lindberg B. Understanding Rett syndrome: A practice guide for parents, teachers and therapists. Toronto: Hognefe Huber, 2006.

[10]   Kerr AM. Reflections on the constraints and opportunities in therapy in Rett syndrome. ScientificWorldJournal 2006;6:992-7.

[11]   Ben Zeev B. Lessons from Rett syndrome and the MECP2 gene as a model for a neurodevelopemental disorder. Ann Conf Rare Dis, Sheba Hospital, Ramat-Gan, Israel, 2004 Dec 09.

[12]   Jacobsen K, Viken A, Von Tetchner S. Rett syndrome and aging: A case study. Disabil Rehabil 2001;23(3/4):160-6.

[13]   Larsson G, Engerström IW. Gross motor ability in Rett syndrome-the power of expectation, motivation and planning. Brain Dev 2001;23 Suppl 1:S77-81.

[14]   Creditor MC. Hazards of hospitalization of the elderly. Ann Intern Med 1993;118:219-23.

[15]   Hoenig HM, Rubenstein LZ. Hospital-associated deconditioning and dysfunction. J Am Geriatr Soc 1991;39:220-2.

[16]   Harper CM, Lyles YM. Physiology and complications of bed rest. J Am Geriatr Soc 1988;36:1047-54.

[17]   Mobily P, Skemp Kelley LS. Iatrogenesis in the elderly: factors of immobility. J Gerontol Nurs 1991;17:5-11.

[18]   Lotan M, Hadar-Frumer M. Aquatic Rehabilitation for Individuals with Rett syndrome. Aquatic Physical Therapy 2004;Dec:6-16.

[19]   Lotan M. Management for Rett syndrome. Tel Aviv: Tamar Publ, 2006. [Hebrew]

[20]   Nishimura M, Onodera S. Effects of supine floating on heart rate, blood pressure and cardiac autonomic nervous system activity. J Gravit Physiol 2000l;7(2):P171-2.

[21]   Engerstrom IW, Kerr A. Workshop on autonomic function in Rett syndrome. Swedish Rett Center, Frösön, Sweden. Brain Dev 1998;20:323-6.

[22]   Campion MR. Hydrotherapy in pediatrics, 2nd ed. Newton, MA: Butterworth Heinemann, 1991.

[23]   Lotan M, Hadar-Frumer M. Aquatic rehabilitation for individuals with Rett syndrome; 2002, E-book at: www.rettsyndrome.org/main/aquatic-rehab.htm

[24]   Elkington H. Swimming: A handbook for teachers. Cambridge: Cambridge Univ Press, 1978.

[25]   Rosenbloom I. The consequences of impaired movement: A hypothesis and review. In: Holt K, ed. Movement and child development. London: Heinemann, 1975:8-13.

[26]   Held R. Plasticity in sensory motor problems. Sci Am 1965;213 (84):1-16.

[27]   Lotan M, Ben-Zeev B. Rett syndrome. A review with emphasis on clinical characteristics and intervention ScientificWorldJournal 2006;6:1517-41.

[28]   Faulkner G, Biddle S. Exercise as an adjunct treatment for schizophrenia: a review of the literature. J Ment Health 1999;8:441-57.

[29]   Hutchinson DS, Skrinar GS, Cross C. The role of improved physical fitness in rehabilitation and recovery. Psychiatr Rehabil J 1999;22:355-9.

[30]   Skrinar GS, Unger KV, Hutchinson DS, Faignebaum, AD. Effects of exercise training in young adults with psychiatric disabilities. Can J Rehabil 1992;5:151-7.

[31]   Berger BG, Owen DR. Mood alteration with swimming - swimmers really do "feel better". Psychosom Med 1983;45(5):425-33.

[32]   Piazza CC, Nederson C, Fisher W. Teaching self-feeding skills to patients with Rett syndrome. Dev Med Child Neurol 1993;35:991-6.

[33]   Sponseller P. Orthopedic Update in Rett syndrome. Available at IRSA web site http://www.rettsyndrome.org/main/orthopaedic-update.htm

[34]   Sponseller P. Orthopaedic update in Rett syndrome. Rett Gazette 2001;1:4-5.

[35]   Kerr A. The future for girls with Rett Syndrome. Int Rett Syndr Assoc Newsletter 1992;Summer:1314.

[36]   Rossin L. Effectiveness of therapeutic and surgical intervention in the treatment of scoliosis in Rett syndrome. A seminar work, Pittsburgh, PA: Univ Duquesne, 1997:1-19.

[37]   Weekes L. RS. A lecture given to parents. Sydney, Australia. February, 1997

[38]   Lotan M, Merrick J, Carmeli E. Scoliosis management in Rett syndrome. A case Study. ScientificWorldJournal 2005;5:264-73.

[39]   Ayres JA. Sensory integration and the child, 5th ed. Los Angeles, CA: Western Psychol Serv, 1982.

[40]   Elefant C, Wigram T. Learning ability in children with Rett syndrome. Brain Dev 2005;27(Suppl 1):S97-S101.

[41]   Beuchel K. Physical therapy and gross motor skills in RS. A handout received at the IRSA annual conference: Washington, DC, May, 2001.

[42]   Pitteti KH, Jackson JA, Stubbs NB, Campbell KD, Battar SS. Fitness levels of adult special Olympics participants. Adapt Phys Activ Q 1989;6:254-70.

[43]   Pitetti KH Tan DM. Effects of a minimally supervised exercise program for mentally retarded adults. Med Sci Sport Exer 1991;23(5):594-601.

[44]   Pitetti KH, Boneh S. Cardiovascular fitness as related to leg strength in adults with mental retardation. Med Sci Sport Exer 1995;27(3):423-8.

[45]   King D, Mace E. Acquisition and maintenance of exercise skills under normalized conditions by adults with moderate and severe mental retardation. Ment Retard 1990;28(5):311-7.

[46]   Lotan M, Isakov E, Merrick J. Improving functional skills and physical fitness in children with Rett syndrome. J Intell Disabil Res 2004;48(8):730-5.

[47]   Hanks SB. Physical therapy strategies. Presentation, IRSA 12th Ann Conf, Boston, MA, 1996 May 24-27, Tape 622-08.

[48]   Kerr AM, Julu PO. Recent insights into hyperventilation from the study of Rett syndrome. Arch Dis Child 1999;80:384-7.

[49]   Hanks SB. Motor disabilities in RS and physical therapy strategies. Brain Dev 1990;12:157-61.

[50]   Hunter K. The Rett syndrome Handbook, Washington DC: Int Rett Syndr Assoc, 1999.

[51]   NINDS ataxias and cerebellar or spinocerebellar degeneration information page available at: http://www.ninds.nih.gov/disorders/ataxia/ataxia.htm

[52]   Ashworth B. Preliminary trial of carisoprodol in multiple sclerosis. Practitioner 1964;192:540-2.

In: Rett Syndrome: Therapeutic Interventions
Editors: Meir Lotan and Joav Merrick

ISBN: 978-1-61728-080-1
©2011 Nova Science Publishers, Inc.

Chapter XIII

Rett Syndrome: Hippotherapy Intervention

Maciques Rodríguez Elaime, Med
and Lotan Meir, BPT, MScPT, PhD[*]

Cuban National Riding Rehabilitation Center, Havana, Cuba, Israel Rett Center, National Evaluation Team, Chaim Sheba Medical Center, Tel HaShomer, Ramat Gan, Zvi Quittman Residential Centers, Israel Elwyn, Jerusalem and Department of Physical Therapy, Ariel University Center of Samaria, Ariel, Israel

Most individuals with Rett syndrome (RS) present an ongoing need for therapeutic intervention. One of the therapeutic approaches suggested for this population is therapeutic horseback riding. Experience shows that this type of intervention is extremely enjoyable for the individual with RS. The current chapter presents the possible benefits of applying hippotherapy for individuals with developmental disabilities, the characteristics of RS that are compatible with this type of intervention; and three case studies describing a unique application of hippotherapy specially designed for this population. It should be emphasized that the present chapter is mostly based on the authors' clinical experience in their field of expertise with minimal support from research findings, as these are scarce. The chapter presents some case studies to illustrate the implementation of the theoretical background and reviews the literature on RS and therapeutic horseback riding. Due to scarcity of scientific sources to support the claims presented by the authors, scientific generalization should be made cautiously.

* Correspondence: Meir Lotan, BPT, MScPT, PhD, Department of Physical Therapy, Ariel University Campus, IL-40700 Ariel, Israel. E-mail: ml_pt_rs@netvision.net.il

Introduction

Rett Syndrome (RS) is a complex neurological disorder resulting from a genetic fault in the X chromosome [1,2], which occurs mainly in females. It is considered to be the second most common cause, after Down's Syndrome, for multi-disabling disorder in females [3,4]. RS is characterized by reduced functional abilities in fine and gross motor skills, reduction of verbal communicative abilities, along with the development of stereotypic hand movements, these occurring after a period of apparently normal development. Individuals with RS often develop seizures and show disturbed breathing patterns with hyperventilation, along with periodic apnoea, scoliosis, growth retardation, apraxia and an atacxic gait pattern [5]. The disorder affects all fields of daily function throughout life. Due to the complex nature of RS, individuals showing this disorder are subjected to different intervention modes for long durations. In light of the vast array of intervention methods and approaches available today for the family affected by RS, a selection process based on knowledgeable decision-making should be performed when deciding on an appropriate therapeutic intervention. One of the available therapeutic approaches for this population is therapeutic horseback riding, which is enjoyed by 17.4% of individuals with RS in Australia [6].

This chapter presents therapeutic horseback riding (THR) as well as aspects of Rett syndrome, which may coincide with known benefits of THR.

Therapeutic horseback riding

Animal assisted therapy (AAT) is a goal-directed intervention, in which an animal that meets specific criteria becomes an integral part of the treatment, facilitating the healing process and rehabilitation of clients with acute or chronic disease [7]. The use of horses in the realm of AAT is referred to as therapeutic horseback riding (THR). Hippotherapy is a form of THR used by licensed health professionals to treat individuals who have impaired postural control and coordination [8].

Therapeutic horseback riding is an alternative therapy for individuals with a variety of physical, emotional, cognitive and social needs. Implementation of THR requires the following steps:

- analyzing the patient's response,
- proper positioning of the patient on the horse and
- directing the horse's movement in order to achieve specific treatment goals.

There is an array of different programs which utilize horses and horseback riding for therapeutic benefits. These interventional programs are also referred to as "equine assisted therapy (EAT)", "equine facilitation psychotherapy (EFP)" or "hippotherapy".

Definitions

Therapeutic riding refers specifically to horseback riding lessons for people with special needs, in which the therapeutic benefits of riding are a result of acquiring riding skills. Because riding is such an enjoyable activity for so many people, therapeutic riding is also used as a quality of life improving therapy for people with degenerative diseases, as well as a 'fun therapy' for individuals and adults alike. Therefore, riding, like many other alternative therapies, may also be considered a form of recreational therapy.

Other forms of equine assisted therapy include Hippotherapy, in which a certified therapist uses the horse as a therapeutic tool; and equine facilitated psychotherapy, in which a certified mental health professional utilizes the horse in various ways for therapeutic benefit. Hippotherapy is a therapeutic practice; which uses the multi-dimensional movement of a horse to improve the neuromuscular function and sensory processing of the rider [9]. Unlike other types of therapeutic riding [10], such as remedial educational vaulting, equine-assisted therapy or recreational riding, hippotherapy does not focus on improving riding skills but rather on the achievement of specific therapeutic goals.

Hippotherapy is a highly diverse, rapidly growing field. Although it is still termed as"alternative, therapeutic intervention", horseback riding in general and hippotherapy specifically, have been recognized by many professionals as a very effective therapy approach [11].

Benefits of intervention

According to the American Hippotherapy Association [12] conditions which can be modified or improved by hippotherapy include: psychological [13], mental (issues related to arousal, motivation and attention), physical (e.g. balance and posture, muscle tone and joints, spasticity reduction, movement coordination, mobility and motor planning), [14-18], social and cognitive skills [18-20], as well as sensorial (sensori-motor dysfunction) and communicational functioning [18].

Individuals with RS are each very different from one-another, displaying a versatility of phenotypic expression. Therefore, each and every one of them should be evaluated properly, along with each having a specific intervention program individually tailored for her. Nevertheless, these individuals do show some commonalities which are suitable for intervention through the use of hippotherapy. The achievement of such clinical aspects will be addressed theoretically, with proper case studies integrated into the text in the following section of the chapter.

It is the authors' belief that in order for the individual with RS to be properly addressed therapeutically and for the intervention program to be delivered skilfully, the management program should take into account a few aspects common to most individuals with RS. Therefore, the following section will present common aspects of individuals with RS and adjacent therapeutic possibilities by means of hippotherapy with the different characteristics of RS are set out in alphabetical order.

Attention span

Individuals with RS have short attention spans [21] which may harm their ability to participate in, as well as gain from educational interaction. In different populations, findings reveal that hippotherapy has contributed to the improvement of attention span and concentration [22-24]. Such findings, if applied to individuals with RS, suggest possibilities for improved participation and educational achievement.

Balance, posture, and coordination

When in motion, the individual with RS has to confront her unreliable sensory process, fear of movement and fluctuating muscle tone, on top of her poor muscular control, attributed to ataxia. The accumulation of such challenges inflicts severe functional limitations upon the individual with RS. Therefore, many of them will find it hard to handle tasks, such as ascending or descending staircases, walking on uneven terrains, running and more. Since hippotherapy has been found to be successful in improving the balance and posture in other populations [16,25-27], it might show similar results for individuals with RS.

As the horse moves, the rider is constantly thrown off-balance and the task of the rider is to stay on the horse by controlling and coordinating postural response, reacting to the motion of the horse [25]. This exercise activates deep muscles not usually operated through conventional physical therapy. Because hippotherapy requires balance and good posture from all riders, students lacking good balance and posture will work on their balance issues from the very moment they mount. The three-dimensional rhythmical motion of the horse is very similar to the motion created in the human pelvis [25]. When balance is set as a therapeutic goal, the instructor will often employ various exercises and riding styles which work on balance and posture in many different ways. Because hippotherapy can be adapted to each student's needs, exercises for balance are quite versatile. Exercises may begin simply by sitting on the horse; advance to walking and keeping balance while trotting. By selecting certain movements, speed, direction, gait and physical characteristics of the horse, the skilled therapist can elicit versatile favorable responses [28]. By placing the rider in different positions on the horse, different sets of muscles can be activated. Pausing and initiating movements of the horse, changing speed and direction increase these benefits. When engaged in promoting advanced balance skills, the client can work on balance and posture through the use of exercises, such as grabbing rings while riding, riding with arms stretched out, riding with the eyes closed, riding backwards, etc. Challenging the rider enables him/her to improve physical capabilities both on and off the horse. Improvement in balance and posture due to Hippotherapy intervention was found in two groups of individuals diagnosed with C.P. [16, 25]. Similar results were found by Biery and Kaufman with a group of adolescents with intellectual disability [26].

Body scheme and sensory input

Due to the sensory imbalance of individuals with RS, it is presumed that their body scheme has developed in an awkward way. This can be concluded from the apraxia shown by many people with RS and from their skewed body perception [29,30] as reported by Hanks. Their fear of movement is probably caused by this same problem. Experiencing such sensory uncertainties on a continuous basis can lead to a sense of fear and insecurity during movement. To reduce some of the anxiety accompanying the daily transfers of the individual with RS, it is recommended that intense proprioceptive input (deep pressure) is applied to help the individual build up her proprioceptive perception and sense of orientation [31,32]. In one session, the rider can be asked both to interpret sensory information she receives from the horse, instructor or her environment and use this information in an appropriate manner, in relation to to her human, as well as animal companions. Lessons may focus on sensory information, such as various sensory intakes (e.g. motion, touch, smell, sound and sight). The movement of the horse is the key element in producing change in the rider [28]. This type of movement is rhythmical, continuous and is performed while the rider is actively stabilizing herself on the horse. Such an intervention program enables the therapist to change the client's sensory perception causing her to change from activating "her entire upper body as one unit", into achieving more isolated movements[28]. Therefore, the sensory input received by the rider throughout the hippotherapy session can organize her body scheme and hopefully help it mature, overflowing to other activities associated with movement within the daily lives of the individual with RS.

Breathing abnormalities

Most individuals (84%) with RS present some form of breathing abnormality [33], such as apnea, hyperventilation, breath-holding and bloating. These incidents are apparent during waking hours alone [34]. The underlying assumption is that the immature regulatory system supervising the breathing mechanism can supply the individual's needs during sleep, while breathing irregularities are the outcome of the incapability of the system in coping with functional changes necessary during day-time activities [35]. In a case study of an individual with RS included in a hippotherapy program, the therapist observed that the individual "used the wrong muscles to breathe". Changing the breathing pattern of the individual was set as one of the intervention goals and during the sessions, the individual "was able to breathe normally while riding" [28:3].

Cognitive function

People with various cognitive and sensory disabilities can be treated with hippotherapy. Some such disorders include intellectual disability, autism, brain damage, Down syndrome [36], developmental disorders such as RS, ADD/ADHD, dyslexia, learning disabilities, etc. Due to the fact that riding, in general, along with Hippotherapy, requires attention, reasoning skills and memory, Hippotherapy enables the rider to build knowledge as time progresses. The instructor can gradually advance the rider from completing simple tasks to acquiring complex skills which provide her with intellectual stimulation. Riding is a complex task, incorporating a huge amount of information in a small amount of time. It is believed that by cognitively challenging the individual with RS, advancements can also be made in this context.

Communication skills

Individuals with RS show the emotional and social need to communicate but this need is coated by their disabilities [37], making their communicative acts difficult for the human environment to decipher. Nevertheless, when their motivation is high enough and the human surrounding attentive, the individual with RS is able to convey her needs and wants, thereby greatly improving her quality of life [38,39]. Hippotherapy has been found effective in improving the communication abilities [40,41] and increasing verbal sounds [42] of other groups of clients. These abilities later transferred to home environments [41]. Therefore, it is possible to assume that this type of intervention will also yield positive results for individuals with RS in the area of communication.

Coordination and motor planning

During THR, when involved in advanced riding, the control of the horse requires a lot of co-ordination in order to achieve the desired response. Since the horse provides instant feedback to every action by the rider, it is easy to know when the correct cue has been given. Repetition of patterned movements required in controlling a horse quickens reflexes and aids in motor-planning. Such a construct of repetitive actions with immediate response (feedback from the horse) is compatible with the disparxic aspect of RS [32].

Emotional, social and psychological aspects

Anyone with emotional, social and psychological disabilities may benefit from hippotherapy. This type of intervention is usually referred to as equine facilitated psychotherapy (EFP) and is considered beneficial for a variety of mental and developmental issues including behavioural issues, attention deficit disorder, eating disorders, abuse issues and depression [43].

Relationships - Building a relationship with an animal can be very rewarding in many aspects; for a person with an emotional, social or psychological disability, the trust and loyalty an animal shows, illustrates to the rider how important these attributes are in personal relationships.

Socialization - Horseback riding presents the rider with the opportunity to interact with others, as well as to form meaningful relationships with the horse and the instructor. Thus, through such interaction, socialization is stimulated [44].

Empowerment and self-esteem - Horses may assist the rider to feel in control of the situation because a direct correlation exists between the rider's action and the horse's reaction. Self-esteem can be increased through acquiring new-found abilities which positively influence another being [44]. In this way, the experience of riding a horse can empower the rider.

Self-monitoring - Treatment of anxiety in particular is well suited for Hippotherapy. Since individuals with RS are constantly in a state of an under-active para-sympathetic system [45], they are continuously in a highly strained state. The relaxed rhythmic movements of the horse, as well as the overall relaxed atmosphere of the ranch, may assist the individual with RS to relax and may even help in self-monitoring her internal autonomic system.

These aspects of the riding experience are similar to other forms of animal-assisted therapy and can generally improve the quality of life of the client [13].

Since the individual with RS is seemingly developing normally at a young age, the reaction she experiences from the surrounding human environment is normal, thereby contributing to the development of a relatively mature emotional baseline [46]. Therefore, one of the strongest attributes of these individuals is their emotional state. Due to the fluctuations typical of RS, the individual always experiences a state of instability (expressed in constantly changing ill-functioning of her body, such as: repeated constipation, reduced ambulation, epilepsy and abnormal sleep patterns). This unstable situation may contribute to agitation, as well as other emotional episodes, sometimes presented by individuals with RS. Since Hippotherapy has been found to positively contribute to the emotional state of the rider [13,27], it may also contribute to the improvement of the emotional state of the individual with RS.

Fear of movement

The fear of movement shown by individuals with RS has been described in the past [35], as caused by dysfunction of the vestibular system [47], but it is believed by the second author to be connected to irregular and immature proprioceptive system (more on this topic can be found in the chapter regarding occupational therapy). As a consequence of this constant fear of movement, the individual becomes cautious and the fluency of her everyday life is thereby interrupted. In her article, Graffman states that: "On her initial visit, Kara was completely unable to tolerate movement of the horse without being completely supported" [28:3]. This description clearly presents the fear of movement common to many individuals with RS and yet, this situation was improved later on, in the progression of the sessions.

In accordance with the above mentioned case study we might assume that the repeated, controlled and rhythmic movement of the horse, as well as the motivation of the individual with RS to continue and participate in Hippotherapy, will allow her to become accustomed to external facilitation and thereby reduce her fear of movement.

Functional improvement

McGibbon and his associates [48] evaluated the effects of an eight-week program of Hippotherapy on performance through the gross motor function measure (GMFM), energy expenditure during walking and gait parameters, in five individuals with spastic cerebral palsy. All participants demonstrated significant decrease in energy expenditure during walking and significant increase in the GMFM walk/run/jump sub-test after hippotherapy. Similar results were also revealed by other researchers [15,49-51]. These improvements were sustained seven weeks after the termination of the intervention program [14,49]. In a case study of an individual with RS treated with hippotherapy, the author states that there was an improvement in functional mobility of the client on the floor [28], thereby demonstrating that individuals with RS can gain functional improvements through Hippotherapy intervention.

Hand use

From about 8 months up to 4 years of age, individuals with RS gradually lose most of their hand functions [21]. The assumption is that poor functional skills of individuals with RS are not derived from lack of ability but rather from the combination of Apraxia, lack of experience [52] and probably learned helplessness. Hence, despite hand functional loss, individuals with RS can and should be taught to acquire new manual skills [53]. The use of adapted equipment, such as a saddle with hand grips, incorporated into the challenging mission of the rider to stay on the horse [25], may initiate long periods of hand gripping throughout the Hippotherapy session. Another means of encouraging hand function is through positioning the rider on the moving horse when she is on all fours. To enhance the difficulty of such an exercise, the use of reaching and purposefully grasping stuffed animals could be introduced [28]. It might be hoped that such training may carry over to other daily activities which require long periods of hand function, such as independent eating and drinking.

Muscle tension and joint range of motion

The movement of the horse also requires the rider to gain good muscle tone and flexibility. The most obvious muscle regions which benefit from such exercise are the torso and buttocks, as well the lower extremities. Muscles are strengthened by the increased usage of muscle action that is involved in riding. Even though riding is an exercise, it is perceived by the rider as enjoyable and therefore the rider has an increased tolerance of, and motivation for, long durations of exercise.

Riding also affects smaller muscles and joints throughout the body, since it is an activity which encourages the participation of the entire body. Riders with low muscle tone and hyper-flexible joints will work on strengthening and tightening the muscles. The therapeutic objective with riders showing high muscle tone is to relax the muscles through the rhythmic movements of the horse's gait. The diverse gait pattern of the horse can be utilized to make the rider aware of different muscle groups. The improvements in function can also be accomplished through the use of different positioning on the horse (for example, positioning a patient astride the horse facing sideways or backward helps improve balance and pelvis alignment, whereas a prone position extends the trunk and neck muscles, while lying supine stretches chest muscles and might elicit a need to pull up into a sitting position). It is believed that as the rider learns different riding skills, muscle tone and flexibility are increasingly improved. The flexibility of the Hippotherapist enables riders with very different needs to benefit from the same motion while learning similar skills.

Muscle shortening

Muscle shortening is common in individuals with RS who have high muscle tone [54]. Furthermore, individuals with RS who start with low muscle tone can gradually increase it, therefore necessitating a change in intervention goals. Muscle shortening can be addressed by applying hippotherapy. The warmth of the horse's body, accompanied by the animal's constant rhythmic movements, while maintaining an abducted position of the hips, can be suggested as a maintenance program to counter the shortening of the adductor muscles of the thigh.

Muscle tone

Spasticity is reduced by rhythmic motion [55], such as that of the horse. The warmth of the horse's body may further contribute to relaxation, especially of the legs. Sitting astride a horse helps break up extensor spasms of the lower limbs. Holding the reins helps break flexor spasm patterns of the upper limbs. Many of the developmental vaulting positions enable the breaking of pathological patterns or the reduction of spasticity. A small amount of fatigue also helps decrease spasticity by producing relaxation.

Individuals with RS present abnormal muscle tone. Most individuals with RS change from very low muscle tone or even sever hypotonia, to high muscle tone (about 60%), including spasticity and/or rigidity [56]. Such unbalanced muscle tone accompanying ataxia and apraxia will severely affect the individual's posture and stability, thus severely harming her ability to function or self-ambulate. These difficulties necessitate intensive therapeutic intervention. Since hippotherapy has been found in the past to reduce muscle tone in other populations [16,27], it is possible to speculate that similar beneficial results will be found for individuals with RS.

Osteoporosis/osteopnia

Osteoporosis occurs frequently in females with RS and has been reported in very young individuals. Patients with Rett syndrome have been found to have decreased bone mineral density, compared to controls [57]. The poor bony structure of theses individuals increases the risk of pathological fractures [58]. It is expected that ambulatory individuals with RS will present better bone mineral density than non-ambulatory ones [59]. These findings support the need for intensive locomotion programs for individuals with RS, initiating at infancy and childhood. Due to the connection found between people with osteoporosis and weak back musculature [60, 61], it is recommended that any activity program for osteoporosis prevention should include back muscle exercise to enhance back strength. Since hippotherapy mainly exercises the torso, buttocks and lower extremities, it presents a unique opportunity for all individuals with RS (although especially for non-ambulatory ones) to practice active motion of the trunk. Another aspect of proper intervention in cases of osteoporosis is the use of proprioceptive dynamic posture training (PDPT) [62]. Since the active motion of the horse is constantly producing dynamic postural changes, it is probable that Hippotherapy will yield positive results for the rider with RS in relation to bone mineral density as well as achieve postural gains (more information regarding osteoporosis intervention in RS could be found in another chapter in this book).

Postural benefits

The most obvious and immediately recognizable benefits of hippotherapy are postural. Because riding is a physical activity, children and adults with special physical needs and various physical impairments can benefit from riding. Hippotherapy uses movement as a primary means of habilitation and has been found to improve functional abilities of individuals with cerebral palsy [15]. Hippotherapy is assumed to benefit people with many different physical disabilities, such as muscular dystrophy, cerebral palsy, multiple sclerosis, amputation, paralysis and spina bifida. There are also anecdotal reports of similar outcomes for individuals with Rett syndrome [28,63].

Since the movement of the horse is the critical change-effecting factor in the rider [28] and since individuals with movement dysfunctions such as RS have limited experience in rhythmical movements and present postural abnormalities, such movements by the horse during hippotherapy constitute a driving force for change. The motion of the horse provides the client with an abundance of diverse practice conditions [25], which, it is hoped, will influence the postural condition of the individual with RS.

Skeletal deformities

Over the years and with the progression of RS, some of the following skeletal problems might occur:

- Scoliosis – appears in 85% of individuals with RS, while a deviation of the spine of at least 10 degrees may be detected in all diagnosed with RS [5]. An early diagnosis, followed by an intense physical regime, was found useful in regressing the spinal deformity in one person with RS [64] and such intervention may lead to the prevention of surgery [65]. Intense physical intervention is recommended by all experts in the field of RS in this situation [64-69]. A pre-post investigation with a control group has revealed that Hippotherapy brought on significant improvement in symmetry of muscle activity in muscle groups displaying asymmetry prior to Hippotherapy, in a group of children with developmental disabilities [70]. It has also been reported that Hippotherapy is beneficial for improving mid-line stability [40] and shows a positive effect on the quantity, as well as the quality, of weight-bearing [71]. It is hypothesized that the scoliosis presented by individuals with RS is caused in part by asymmetrical muscle activity [54], as well as by a skewed proprioceptive perception [29, 30]. Therefore, it is possible that riding a horse will enhance symmetrical muscle activity in the trunk muscles of individuals with RS and, moreover, that the use of asymmetrical positioning on the horse can cause opposite asymmetrical muscle activity of the trunk, thereby presenting a useful, yet enjoyable activity for the rider with RS who is diagnosed with asymmetrical postures and scoliosis.

- Hip instability - this orthopedic problem is not extremely common in ambulating individuals with RS, yet it tends to present itself more in those who are non-ambulatory [54]. Hip instability and dislocation may be avoided through the use of preventive measures, such as a daily standing program, manually keeping the joint in the full range of motion, serial casting and the use of hydrotherapy to strengthen the muscle around the joint [72]. The posture of the rider on the horse is, by itself, a preventive measure against hip dislocation and since the rider is actively contracting her muscles around the hips and buttocks during the hippotherapy session, such an exercise may prevent hip instability.

Stereotypical hand movements

Manual mannerisms are obvious in all individuals diagnosed with RS and in actuality, constitute the trademark of this population. These movements are involuntary, do not include the use of objects (beside Angelman-type RS) and are not used for protection or as a response to a sensorial need [73].

Voluntarily stopping the hand movement is usually very difficult for the individual with RS, although some can withdraw from those continuous movements on demand for a short period. It is speculated that the cause of stereotypical movements is due to neuro/chemical imbalance in the dopaminergic/monoaminergic/cholinergic systems [74,75]. Despite the fact that in late stages of RS, the stereotypical movements subside, they can nonetheless still be observed [47]. Reducing the stereotypical hand movements may be achieved through the use of adapted equipment, such as a saddle with hand grips, as well as through the use of challenging positioning (e.g. standing on all fours) More information regarding stereotypical movements in RS could be found in another chapter in this book.

Hippotherapy and rett syndrome

Due to the specific characteristics of RS, the present section will address issues which should be taken into consideration when the trained hippotherapist initially meets the individual with RS.

- The complex nature of RS necessitates that the experienced therapist at the ranch or stable coordinate his/her therapeutic efforts with other members of the therapeutic team managing the individual with RS.
- The intervention itself should be performed by a qualified instructor.
- A thorough primary evaluation should be performed by a licensed physical, occupational or speech therapist. Such a primary evaluation enables the therapeutic team to set appropriate goals and select the matching exercises, thereby meeting the specific needs of each client.
- The duration of the sessions should be adapted to the individual with RS, as it is possible that the individual will need a few shorter sessions to begin with [28], before getting used to being active for a whole 45-minute session. The specifically RS adapted program introduced later in this chapter, suggest that the time on the horse it self, within a 45 minute session, should not exceed 25 minutes.
- Safety equipment should always be included, incorporating equestrian helmets, Devonshire stirrups, which are closed in the front in order to properly position feet and prevent them from sliding through, as well as the use of quick-release "peacock" stirrups, which unhook if a rider falls.
- Due to the highly developed emotional state of individuals with RS [46], it is suggested that sessions be presented through creative exercises, keeping the interaction a fun experience.
- The complex nature of RS necessitates a multi-disciplinary approach [76,77]. Hippotherapy sessions may be provided by licensed therapists, physicians, clinical psychologists or students who volunteer at the ranch or stable. Nevertheless, they should all be supervised by a qualified therapist.
- The complexity of the RS condition (such as epilepsy [4,78], as well as the fluctuating muscle tone [56]) is an additional good reason for an experienced handler to guide each horse, ready to aid the rider who loses her balance, or to assist in exercises and games.
- Due to the lack of vocal communication by most individuals with RS, it is suggested that during the session the therapist/instructor constantly monitors the rider's responses and instructs the handler to change the horse's direction and tempo accordingly, if these are found necessary.
- The para-professional team should keep careful progress evaluation on a regular basis and report regularly to family members and the referring physician.
- Due to the complex expression of RS and the many facets of its phenotypic expression, it is recommended that the Hippotherapy sessions incorporate more flexible therapeutic principles, providing the individual with RS with versatile forms of intervention.
- Individuals with RS are famous for their functional and emotional fluctuations. During moments in an activity (yet sometimes even for hours or days) the individual with RS seems lost and disconnected "as if her mind is covered by a cloud" wrapped around her, separating her from the world [47:77]. In some past cases, such behavior was found to reduce the staff's (caregivers and therapist alike) confidence in the individual's abilities. This phenomenon is caused by numerous factors associated with this disorder (e.g. functional setbacks, irregular sleeping patterns, medication, etc.) and the therapist should have confidence in the fact that the individual will reconnect and return to her previous functional abilities.

Contraindication

The following list of conditions is suggeted as contraindications for therapeutic horseback riding by the American Hippotherapy Association [8]:

- People weighing over 300 pounds or more than 20 percent of the horse's weight or morbid obesity (usually not common in RS)
- Quadriplegics lacking control over trunk muscles
- Brittle-boned osteoporosis (according to the instruction of a physician– apply caution)
- Patients, mainly Down syndrome cases with atlantoaxial instability acute herniated disks (not common in RS)
- Degenerated hip joints
- Curvature of the spine greater than 30 degrees, (according to the instruction of a physician – might need the use of supportive bracing)
- Acute arthritis (not common in RS)
- Heart problems
- Poor head, neck, and/or trunk control (the use of neck support may be suggested)
- People requiring medical equipment, such as an oxygen tank, suction machine, or ventilator (therapeutic intervention according to the instruction of a physician - not common in RS)
- Severe allergies or asthma to animal dander, molds, trees, etc. (therapeutic intervention according to physician instruction. The use of respiratory system protection may be warranted - not common in RS)
- Uncontrolled seizures (according to the instruction of a physician. The use of supportive equipment may be suggested)
- Severe behavior problems (usually not common in RS)
- Painful joints such as in RA disease (usually not common in RS, although pain reaction might be hard to detect in individuals with RS; apply intervention with sensibility and caution)
- Uncontrolled movements as in athetoid CP (usually not common in RS)
- Active alcoholic/drug users (not common in RS)
- Severe and painful scoliosis (common in RS so therefore the therapeutic intervention should be applied according to the instruction of a physician; may need the use of supportive bracing)
- Some psychiatric patients who are not in touch with their surroundings (not common in RS)
- Very low functioning students who cannot learn or follow directions (the passivity common to many with RS can be overcome by proper adaptation of session structure and the introduction of motivational aspects)
- Osteogenesis Imperfecta which is active where movement may cause fractures (not common in RS, yet the osteoporotic condition of the person with RS should be evaluated prior to initiation of Hippotherapy and proper caution should be taken when positioning the individual with RS over the horse)
- Advanced muscular dystrophy (not common in RS).

The last part of this chapter presents three individuals with RS who have received hippotherapy intervention by the first author at the Cuban National Riding Rehabilitation Center. A short review of this Center and its working procedures is presented.

Cuban national riding rehabilitation center

The Cuban National Riding Rehabilitation Center has its facilities outside the city of Havana. It has four horses specially trained for therapeutic riding. It has six professional members; two psychopedagogists, one speech therapist, one physiotherapist and two riding trainers.

About 50 clients participate in each therapy cycle. These therapeutic cycles are determined by the proposed objectives for each patient, the therapeutic program and the due dates for those objectives. Therapy organization is settled in the following way: those with autism, Down's syndrome, and individuals with intellectual disability (ID) receive two sessions per week and individuals with neurological originated syndromes, psychomotor retardation and Rett syndrome receive therapy three times a week. The clients at the Center benefit from a comprehensive program compiled with an assortment of games and educational, sport and art-related activities. Each session is usually 45 minutes in duration.

In addition to the rehabilitation program suggested for individuals with RS at the Cuban National Riding Rehabilitation Center, a recommended comprehensive supplementary program is constructed for the treatment of the children by the primary caregivers (mostly parents). The parents receive instructions on how to perform additional work with their children, thus establishing a carry-over of the achievements of the intervention program received at the center. Therapeutic sessions at the Cuban National Riding Rehabilitation Center are divided into three sections:

First section: Waiting time/preparatory intervention

At this point, initial rapport with the individual is achieved, thereby enabling the therapist to evaluate the individual's mood and disposition within daily activities. This initial contact can be established through music, water games, finger painting, puppets and other psycho-educational procedures (see figures XIII-1 and XIII-2).

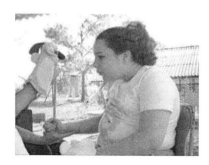

Figure XIII-1. waiting time prior to initiating intervention (The picture presents A.M. establishing rapport through the use of puppets to enhance eye contact).

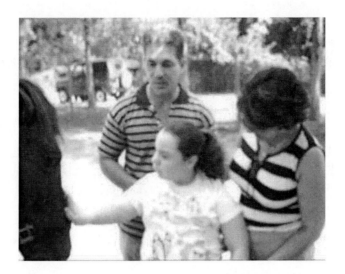

Figure XIII-2. Secure connection with the horse is achieved through the support of staff and parents during initial encounters.

In the case of individuals who present hypertonicity, tone reduction intervention is introduced with the objective of relaxing the muscles and enhancing joint range of motion (see figure XIII-3).

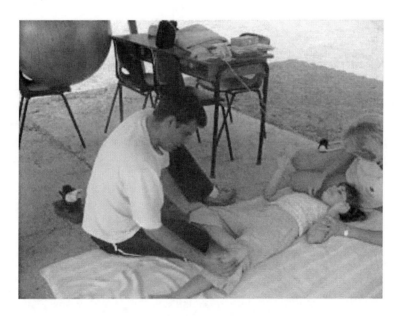

Figure XIII-3. Preparing the client with hypertonicity prior to intervention.

Second section: Riding time

During this section of the intervention program, Hippotherapy is implemented in accordance with the individual program designed for each client. It is important that riding time does not exceed 25 minutes, so as to avoid fatigue.

Third section: Assessment and Conclusion

This will permit consolidation of the achievements reached in the previous sections.

Evaluation process

The following schematic is a semi-subjective evaluation sheet that is being used by the National Riding Rehabilitation Center. The chart follows the child development across his program and enables the evaluation of motor development. This chart is adapted and re-edited from a hippotherapy evaluation scale created by Isabel Salama.

In all cases presented below, the same scale was used to evaluate the initial state of each participant as well as to assess accomplishments and final results (see figures XIII-1-3).

Table XIII-1. Hippotherapy evaluation scale

ÍTEMS	WEEK 1	WEEK 2	WEEK 3	WEEK 4	WEEK 5
Approaching the horse					
Mounting the horse					
Balance					
Muscular tone					
Postural adjustments					
Interactions with the therapists					
Latency Interval between stimulus and response					
Eye contact with the therapists					
Intentional use of hands					
Communication attempts					
Enjoyment shown during the activity					

Case story 1 (NV)

Antecedents: wanted pregnancy, Caesarean due to fetal position (rear) and non-expanding uterus neck. She was born without fetal suffering and weighed 8.5 pounds. The girl had a normal development, though she began to walk at the age of 18 months, mostly due to her being overweight. She does not present/display epilepsy. Age at diagnosis and first signs of Rett syndrome: 2 years and 6 months. Initial signs of RS: loss of attention-span and language ability, stereotypical movement of the hands (washing movements) along with the loss of their functional use.

Treatment prior to hippotherapy NV, did not receive any therapeutic intervention (including physiotherapy and special education). NV pharmacological therapeutic intervention included: carbamazepine (Tegretol or Tanfedin) as a preventive treatment.

On admission for intervention initiation she was 14 years of age, a young, affectionate and cheerful person who enjoys interaction with other people. She is highly attracted to musical sounds and enjoys it extremely, when she is spoken to. She also enjoys being touched and being paid attention to in search of physical contact with people with whom she is familiar. When someone indicates that he would like a hug from her, she will open up her arms and get closer to that person. NV recognizes her peers, family members and individuals, who are in daily contact with her. NV shows very good intentional communicative acts through her glance, body movements, and facial expressions. When NV feels uncomfortable, hungry or in pain, she will gesticulate by emitting deep sounds and cries.

She is able to convey her moods through eye glances or vocalizations and can maintain good eye contact. She obviously has the capacity to understand simple requests. She walks with an ataxic gait, can walk for long distances and is capable of going up and down stairs with minor help. When challenged by an obstacle, to succeed, she needs assistance in lifting her leg. When a new situation or environment is introduced to her, she displays great apprehension and fear, which leads to slowing down of her motor response. NV seldom falls. She displays general muscular hyper tonicity. She wears hand splints to prevent worsening of her finger deformities.

Reduced range of motion – NV is diagnosed with a right C scoliotic curvature of the spine of approximately 25 degrees. NV shows fear of positional changes and unknown people. This fear is expressed by anxious behavior and sweaty hands. After individual evaluation was performed with NV, the following therapeutic objectives were drawn up to address her needs and difficulties in psychomotor development. Therapeutic goals:

- Reduce hypertonicity
- Provide better equilibrium reactions
- Reduce scoliosis
- Improve independent gait

It is reiterated that, in addition to the rehabilitation program suggested for individuals with RS at our facility, NV's parents were involved in a comprehensive supplementary program. The parents received suggestions for possible exercises to be performed with NV at home. This program helped in achieving carry-over of the intervention program into other aspects of her life.

Intervention strategies were applied with the intent of increasing joint range of motion and reducing muscle tone through the relaxation of different muscular groups (see figuresXIII-4 and XIII-5). Applying various paces, cadences and ever- changing routes, while NV is mounted on the horse, in order to achieve postural adjustments. Enhancing controlled unbalance trunk activity to provoke her equilibrium reaction, in order for her to achieve correct posture on the horse. Applying changes in the pace of passage, along with abrupt stops to activate the protection answers and finally enhancing self-consciousness. Contraindications: Trotting should not be applied due to her hypertonicity

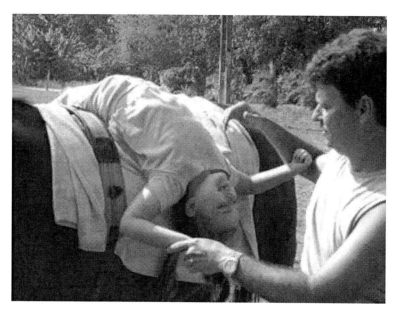

Figure XIII-4. Relaxing the back muscles and stretching abdominal ones at the beginning of the Hippotherapy session.

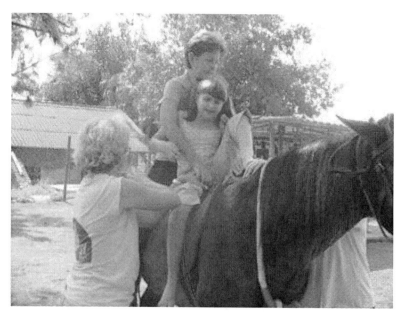

Figure XIII-5. Different positions to enhance joint range of motion and reduce spasticity.

The results with NV were very satisfactory and they became evident within three months of treatment initiation. The preparatory section of the intervention reduced her spasticity and enabled enhanced joint range of motion. This in-turn enabled better handling on the horse by the therapist, allowing work on the scoliosis and on balance. As a result NV was able to maintain a better balance on the horse. In fact, her trunk control was so improved that back riding (by the therapist) was discontinued and she commenced independent riding (with assistance/supervision). After only three months of intervention, NV was able to:

- Flex and extend her legs, arms and torso independently and without limitation
- Adopt a supine position on the horse (see figure XIII-4)
- Adopt a prone position transversally on the horse (see figure XIII-6)
- Lay back down on the floor and on the horse
- Improve her balance
- Minimize hand stereotypes and increase functional hand use during the exercise. She can also get hold of the horse's mane during medium walk and trot
- Lift her foot independently to overcome obstacles in her way, while walking
- Reduce her ataxic movement pattern, thereby normalizing her locomotion (see figure XIII-7)
- Regulate her response to sensorial stimuli
- Increase her ability to follow instructions
- Decrease her hyperventilation episodes
- Reduce self-injurious behavior
- Walk without help.

An important aspect of the intervention was the fact that after a year of therapeutic intervention, according to X-rays taken by her orthopedic surgeon, her scoliosis was reduced (from 25 degrees) to 10 degrees.

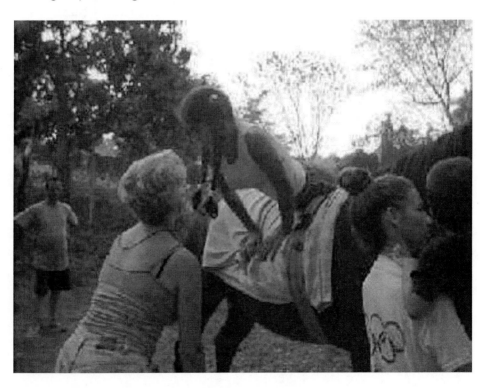

Figure XIII-6. Adopting a supine position transversally on the horse.

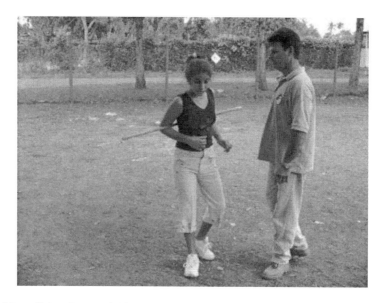

Figure XIII-7. Normalizing (less ataxic) locomotion.

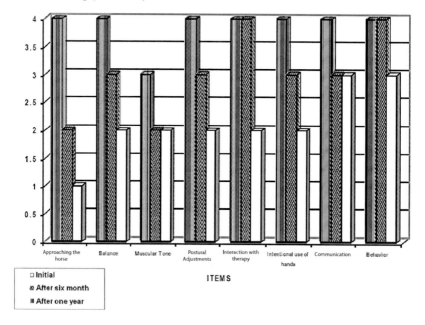

Figure XIII-8. NV Accomplishments during the first year of Hippotherapy.

Case story 2 (GC)

Antecedents: wanted pregnancy. GC was born weighing 7.5 pounds through a normal delivery. As an infant she had normal development for the duration of 15 months. She does not display epilepsy. Age at first signs: 15 month with initial signs of RS: Some autistic behaviors were manifested by GC. These conducts were refraining from eye contact, social withdrawal, lack of motivation for, or interest in, interactions with people or toys, loss of pre-acquired language and appearance of stereotypical hand movements. During manual mannerisms her hands are kept at body middle line and her stereotypical movements include hand mouthing followed by thigh banging.

Age at diagnosis of Rett syndrome was 2 years and 3 months with a genetic diagnosis (at the Genetic and Molecular Medicine Center, Pediatric Department of the University of Florence) of MECP2 mutation at T158M site. GC receives no medication, physiotherapy initiated at the age of 4 years and still performed at the present time.

On admission at age 6 years, GC enjoys contact with familiar people and differentiates between strangers and family. During her development, GC has never shown separation anxiety from her mother or relatives. She is usually of a good disposition, smiles when she feels fine and enjoys activities mostly when she is surrounded by her peers. She enjoys water games, playing on swings and walking around and when engaged in social happenings she shows socially accepted behavior. She has a special interest in music and dance and when she dislikes a certain type of music, she shows it by crying. She responds to simple requests. She is able to vocalize some sounds, mostly when she is upset, hungry or when the music stops. For example, she says "ya" when trying to express her dislike of something. GC is totally dependent with regard to ADL and hygiene. During meal times, GC chews with good lip closure. She has no diaper/nappy control.

CG showed hypotonic muscle tone in her upper extremities and trunk and maintains distonic muscle tone in the lower extremities with a slight tendency towards spasticity. GC can walk independently, though she usually appears as if wandering aimlessly. Her feet are inverted and supinated and, therefore, her weight-bearing is performed on the lateral side of the feet. She sometimes walks with her eyes closed or facing the floor. She is not capable of overcoming obstacles, so mostly she tries to avoid them and, therefore, often trips. Due to poor protective reactions, GC may hurt herself when falling and therefore, when ambulating, she is in need of constant monitoring.

When GC walks, she tends to recline her body backwards but, nevertheless, she maintains her balance. GC is able to ascend and descend stairs with moderate assistance. When seated she shows poor, floppy posture. GC is able to change from lying down to sitting (leaning through her left side without using her hands). From a sitting position on the floor, she needs assistance in order to achieve a standing position. At initiation of intervention, GC presented a minor left scoliosis of approximately 10 degrees. GC showed a short and fluctuating attention-span and our therapeutic goals were:

- Regulate muscular tone
- Improve equilibrium reactions
- Increase protective reactions

The intervention strategy for her were centered around the following:

- Looking for controlled "off-balance" postures to provoke her reaction, in order to achieve a correct position on the horse (see figure XIII-9)
- Changes in direction and speeds with abrupt stops to activate proper equilibrium reactions.

- Work in fetal position to strengthen and stretch the lower back muscles and work on the vestibular system, thereby enhancing balance and reducing spasticity.
- Work for 10 minutes with back-riding to achieve posture correction (see figure XIII-10).
- Change between prone and supine positions to fortify truncal muscular strength (see figure XIII-11).
- Activities around weight transference to enhance activity and postural reactions.
- Manipulative and corrective exercises to reduce the development of scoliosis (see figure XIII-12).

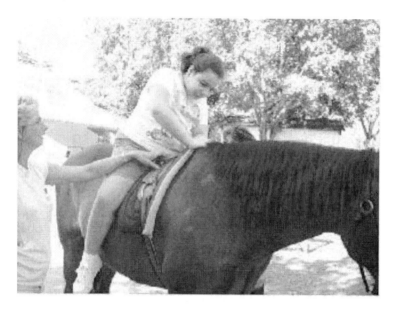

Figure XIII-9. Inducing balance shifts to provoke corrective postural reactions.

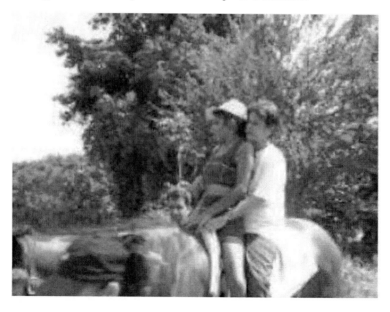

Figure XIII-10. Back riding to achieve posture correction.

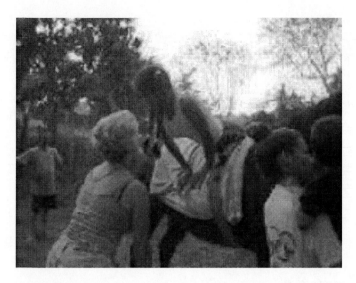

Figure XIII-11. Prone and supine positions.

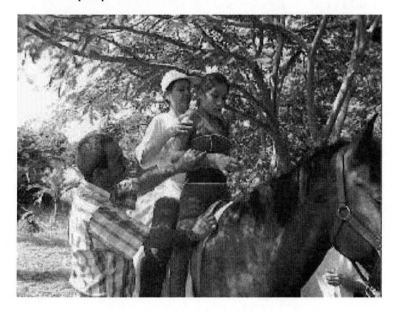

Figure XIII-12. Corrective exercises to reduce scoliosis.

The results with GC were slow to emerge and could only be observed in the long run. A substantial part of her achievement was due to the co-operation of her family in the training program. In six months of treatment, we have achieved: Better protective reactions, reduction in the number of falls, increased trunk muscular tone and better posture in sitting, reduced stereotypical mannerism on the horse, due to hand usage for holding the reins during trotting, increased functional hand use to grasp attractive objects while on the horse and reduced spasticity in lower limbs.

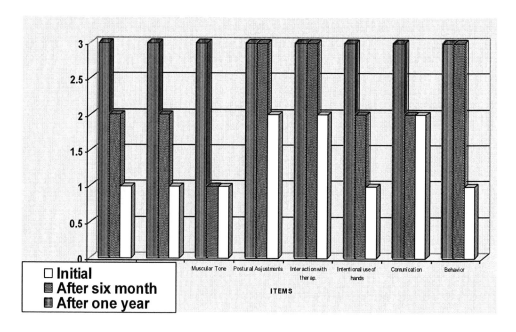

Figure XIII-13. GC Accomplishments during the first year of Hippotherapy.

Case story 3 (AM)

Antecedents: wanted pregnancy. AM was born weighing 8 pounds, through normal delivery. AM developed normally up to the age of two and a half years. On EEG epileptiform waves can be detected. However, she has never displayed an epileptic seizure. Age of first signs: Two years and six months with initial signs of RS: She began showing extreme autistic manifestations, such as severe behavioral disorders, irritability, arm fluttering, self-injurious behavior and became extremely withdrawn, as if she was locked within herself. A decline in functional abilities such as turning a page, ascending a staircase, and changing positions from and into a sitting position, was observed. A deterioration of gait was manifested by clumsiness expressed through widening of the base of support, and loss of interest in her physical surroundings. She showed General Psychomotor retardation. Stereotypical hand movements appeared at two and a half years of age, although her manual abilities gradually deteriorated throughout the following year. Manual Stereotypes are expressed by clapping.

Her diagnosis was difficult and passed through several stages and medical criteria. She was diagnosed as a "general development disorder of unknown cause", since, according to the neurologist, she did not fulfill all the diagnostic criteria of RS and only a few aspects were present; ataxic gait, epileptogenic brain waves, bruxism, and an affective dichotomy; laughing and crying for no reason. The genetic confirmation for RS was made only when AM was 8 years old in 2001 at the Pediatric Department of the Genetics and Molecular Medicine Center, University of Florence, which showed a mutation in axon 4 at MECP2 site R270X. neither parent was found to be carrying such a mutation.

AM received physical therapy intervention since her first regression period at the age of two and a half with the diagnosis of infantile autism and psychomotor retardation. The intervention was terminated, when AM had reached the age of five. She had been receiving anti-convulsive medication since she was five, as a preventive measure against challenging behaviors. The intervention was discontinued by her parents, when AM reached eight years of age.

On admission she was 9 years old and affectionate towards familiar people. She showed emotional dependency on both her parents. She has fluctuating mood swings, sadness being predominate. AM usually showed very little interest in her surroundings. In terms of communication, A.M. appears to signal slight non-verbal communicative acts. As surprising as it sounds, AM does not enjoy music, while on the other hand, enjoys poetry to be recited to her. She also enjoys water games and playing with puppets. When exposed to a new situation, AM experiences stress and pronounces the word "mother" out of distress.

AM avoids contact with anyone who is not a relative. Frequently, she shows aggressiveness and self-abuse behavior. She is easily irritated and is mostly in a bad disposition that manifests itself with frequent crying. During physical therapy, she helps a bit and all her movements are assisted, due to her low tone, passivity and the fact that she is over-weight.

AM is totally dependent on her human surrounding for accomplishing her ADL. During meal times, she presents good chewing abilities, as well as appropriate lip closure around a spoon. AM has a tendency towards living a sedentary lifestyle and can remain seated in front of the television set for hours on end, if not interrupted. She presents a kyphotic trunk and generalized hypotonicity, as well as obesity.

AM can transit from a lying down to a sitting position without the use of her hands, although she is in need of assistance when moving from a seated position on the floor to standing. When sitting on a chair, AM can rise independently to a standing position. AM maintains an independent wide-based gait with fluttering arms. She lacks the ability to ascend or descend a flight of stairs and reacts negatively when asked to participate in physical exercises, whereupon generally she cries throughout the activity. She is not able to avoid or overcome obstacles and when she is confronted by an obstacle, she usually tries to push it aside. Therapeutic goals:

- Regulate muscle tone
- Reduce challenging behaviors
- Improve balance

The intervention strategy for her were centered around the following:

- Positioning A.M in controlled unbalance postures to provoke her reaction, in order to try to get her to correct her position on the horse (see figure XIII-9)
- Working for 10 minutes in back-riding to correct her posture (see figure XIII-10)
- Activities related to weight shift
- Trotting.
- Working on proprioceptive activities (see figures XIII-14, XIII-15)
- Changing paths of the horse to enhance corrective reactions

The horse's pace was kept fast at all times and contraindications were changing positions to prone or lateral supine position due to her lordotic posture and obesity.

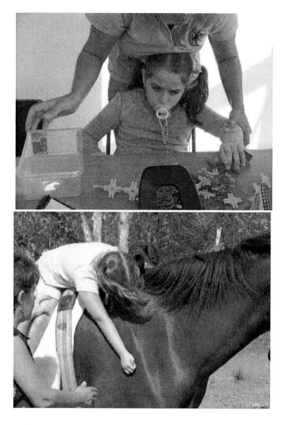

Figure XIII-14, XIII-15. Proprioceptive activities before and during intervention.

The results for AM are not very impressive. Some of the difficulties arose from the fact that the parents were having a hard time in supporting the therapeutic program at home, despite of our recommendation for a comprehensive program. AM still spends most of her time passively watching TV. Nevertheless some positive changes have been noted:

- She does not cry any more during physical therapy
- She holds better posture on the horse
- Her walking abilities have improved
- She is now able to accept trotting, (thereby regulating her muscle tone).
- Her attention span seems to increase, so therefore she is now able to spend more time following a game, especially when water and puppets are involved.
- A more balanced sensory system that can be observed by her reduced reactivity to touch, by accepting the touch of her therapist
- Her attunement to her surrounding has increased since she now reacts when her name is called.
- Reduction in self-provoked hyperventilation episodes.
- Reduction in challenging behaviors

The authors believe that the positive changes in her challenging behaviors were due to the combination of group intervention in which AM was participating before each session of hippotherapy. This included interations with other children and her parents (some painting, music, water games) and also due to the overall changes in her level of functioning that were the result of changes in her muscle tone, sensory system and posture, enabling her be in control when ambulating.

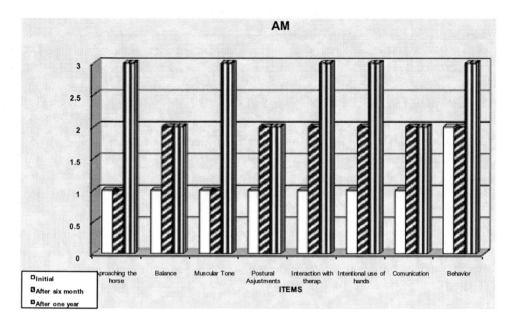

Figure XIII-16. AM Accomplishments during the first year of Hippotherapy.

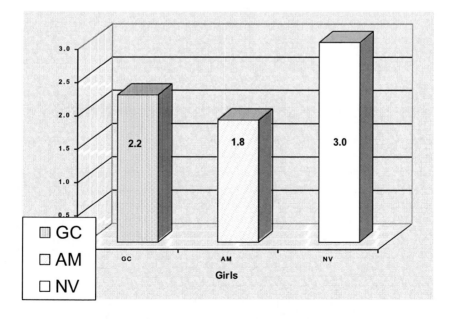

Figure XIII-17. A summary of accomplishments for all participants during the first year of Hippotherapy.

Conclusions

We were satisfied with the results achieved within one year of intervention of all the three cases. These achievements would not have been possible without the help of the families, who took part in the home program that improved the handling of the girls and supported the goals of the therapy team in performing the home program. The items evaluated reflected a significant improvement in the motor development of these girls, as well as posture and challenging behaviors, as is evident in figure 17.

The present chapter showed the use of THR in general, and more specifically, hippotherapy as means for therapeutic intervention for individuals with RS. The novelty of the chapter is due to the fact that the suggested approach was developed specifically for individuals with RS by the first author (MRE). Yet, it is reiterated that this is not a research report, but rather a review based on our experience in the realms of Rett syndrome and therapeutic horseback riding and therefore, scientific generalization is limited.

Nevertheless, accumulating evidence suggests that hippotherapy is gradually shifting from being of the "non-traditional" therapeutic approach to being a part of mainstream therapeutic intervention presented for individuals with developmental disabilities, such as those with RS. Scientific evidence, as well as experience, imply that hippotherapy is a beneficial intervention for individuals with RS and may suggest physical, sensorial, emotional and social improvements, when applied in an organized, goal-oriented intervention, thereby positively affecting the individual's and family's quality of life.

References

[1]   Amir RE, Van den Veyver IB, Wan M, Tran CQ, Francke U, Zoghbi HY. Rett syndrome is caused by mutations in X-linked MECP2, encoding methyl-CpG-binding protein 2. Nature Genetics 1999; 23(2):185-8.

[2]   Amir RE, Van Den Veyver IB, Schultz R, Malicki DM, Tran CQ, Dahle EJ, et al. Influence of mutation type and X chromosome inactivation on Rett syndrome phenotypes. Ann Neurology 2000;47:670-9.

[3]   Hagberg B. Rett syndrome: clinical peculiarities and biological mysteries. Acta Paediatr 1995;84:971–6.

[4]   Ellaway C, Christodoulou J. Rett syndrome: Clinical characteristics and recent genetic advances. Disabil Rehabil 2001;23:98-106.

[5]   Hagberg B. Rett syndrome: Clinical and biological aspects. London: Mac Keith, 1993.

[6]   Leonard S. The Australian Rett syndrome study inaugural report. Aust: Telethon Inst Child Health Res, 2002.

[7]   Rothe EQ, Vega BJ, Torres RM, Soler SMC, Pazos RMM. From kids and horses: Equine facilitated psychotherapy for children. Int J Clin Health Psychol 2005;5(2):373-83.

[8]   American Hippotherapy Association. Home page. Denver, CO: North American Riding for the Handicapped Association, 2000. Retrieved 2006 May 04, http://www.narha.org/.

[9]   MacPhail HEA, Edwards J, Golding J, Miller K, Mosier C, Zwiers T. Trunk postural reactions in children with and without cerebral palsy during therapeutic horseback riding. Pediatr Phys Ther 1998;10;143-7.

[10]   Copeland-Fitzpatrick J. Hippotherapy and therapeutic riding: An international review. In: North American Riding for the Handicapped Association, ed. Proceedings of the ninth international therapeutic riding congress. Denver, CO:1997:1-12.

[11]   Therapeutic Horseback Riding. Term definition at the wikipedia encyclopedia. Available on may 2006 From internet site: http://en.wikipedia.org/wiki/Therapeutic_Horseback_Riding

[12]   American hippotherapy association: A section of the North American riding for the handicap association. P.O.B 33150, Denver, CO 80233.

[13]   Bizub AL, Joy A, Davidson L. "It's like being in another world": demonstrating the benefits of therapeutic horseback riding for individuals with psychiatric disability. Psychiatr Rehabil J 2003;26(4):377-84.

[14]   Winchester P, Kendall K, Peters H, Sears N, Winkley T. The effect of therapeutic horseback riding on gross motor function and gait speed in children who are developmentally delayed. Phys Occup Ther Pediatr 2002;22(3-4):37-50.

[15]   Sterba JA, Rogers BT, France AP, Vokes DA. The effect of horseback riding on gross motor function measure (GMFM) in children with cerebral palsy. 54th Ann Meet Am Acad Cerebral Palsy Dev Med. Toronto, Canada, 2000.

[16]   Bertoti DB. Effect of therapeutic horseback riding on posture in children with cerebral palsy. Phys Ther 1988;68(10):1505-12.

[17]   Liptak GS. Complementary and alternative therapies for cerebral palsy. Ment Retard Dev Disabil Res Rev 2005;11(2):156-63.

[18]   Dismuke-Blakely, R. Hippotherapy as a treatment modality for speech/language therapy. In: North American Riding for the Handicapped Association, ed. Proceedings of the ninth international therapeutic riding congress. Denver, CO, 1997:195-9.

[19]   Cole KM, Gawlinski A. Animal-assisted therapy: the human-animal bond. AACN Clin Issues 2000;11(1):139-49.

[20]   Dossey L. The healing power of pets: a look at animal-assisted therapy. Altern Ther Health Med 1997;3(4):8-16.

[21]   Lindberg, B. Understanding Rett Syndrome: A practical guide for parents, teachers and therapists, 2nd ed. Toronto: Hognefe Huber, 2006.

[22]   MacKinnon JR, Noh S, Lariviere J, MacPhail A, Allan DE, Laliberte D. A study of therapeutic effects of horseback riding for children with cerebral palsy. Phys Occup Ther Pediatrics 1995;15(1):17-34.

[23]   Splinter-Watkins KL, Calhoun SC. Benefits of therapeutic horseback riding: An effective occupational therapy intervention for persons with developmental disabilities. Dev Disabil Spec Interest Section Quart 1999;22:1-3.

[24]   MacKinnon JR, Noh S, Lariviere J, MacPhail A, Allan DE, Laliberte D. A study of therapeutic effects of horseback riding for children with cerebral palsy. Phys Occup Ther Pediatr 1995;15(1):17-34.

[25]   Hachl V, Giuliani C, Lewis C. Influence of hippotherapy on the kinematics and functional performance of two children with cerebral palsy. Pediatric Phys Ther 1999;89:89-101.

[26]   Biery MJ, Kaufman N. The effect of therapeutic horseback riding on balance. Adapted Phys Act Quart 1989;6:221-9.

[27]   Hammer A, Nilsagård Y, Forsberg A, Pepa H, Skargren E, Öberg B. Evaluation of therapeutic riding (Sweden)/hippotherapy (United States). A single-subject experimental design study replicated in eleven patients with multiple sclerosis. Physiotherapy Theory and Practice 2005;21(1):51-77.

[28]   Graffman K. Hippotherapy: never heard of it. Rett Gazette 2003 Feb:3-4.

[29]   Hanks SB. Motor disabilities in the Rett Syndrome and physical therapy strategies. Brain Dev 1990;12:157-61.

[30]   Hanks SB. Physical therapy strategies. Paper presented at the IRSA 12th Ann Conf 1996 May 24-27 May, Boston, MA, tape 622-08.

[31]   Hanks SB. Why physical therapy? Rett Gazette, Spring 2001. Also available at IRSA web site: http://www.rettsyndrome.org/main/orthopaedic-update.htm

[32]   Lotan M. Silent angels: The management of individuals with Rett syndrome. Tel Aviv: Rotem Publ, Isr Rett Syndr Assoc, 2006. [Hebrew]

[33]   Mount RH, Hastings RP, Reilly S, Cass H, Charman T. Behavioral and emotional features in Rett syndrome. Disabil Rehabil 2001;23;129-38.

[34]   Elian M, Rudolf ND. EEG and respiration in Rett Syndrome. Acta Neurolgica Scand 1991;83:123-8.

[35]   Hunter K. The Rett syndrome handbook, Washington, DC: Int Rett Syndr Assoc, 1999.

[36]   Baker L. Medical considerations for therapeutic riding. NARHA Strides Magazine 1996:24-26.

[37]   Sigafoos J, Woodyatt G, Tucker M, Roberts-Pennell D, Pittendreigh N. Assessment of potential communication acts in three individuals with Rett syndrome. J Dev Phys Disabil 1999;12(3): 203-16.

[38]   Sigafoos J. Communication development and aberrant behavior in children with developmental disabilities. Educ Training Ment Retard Dev Dis 2000;35(2):168-76.

[39]   Sigafoos J, Woodyatt G, Keen D, Tait K, Tucker M, Roberts-Pennell D, Pittendreigh N. Identifying potential communicative acts in children with developmental and physical disabilities. Communication Disord Quart 2000;21(2):77-86.

[40]   Engel BT. The horse as a modality for occupational therapy. Occup Ther Health Care 1984;1:41-7.

[41]   Glazer HD, Clark MD, Stein DS. The impact of hippotherapy on grieving children. J Hospice Palliat Nurs 2004;6:171-5.

[42]   Lehrman J, Ross DB. Therapeutic riding for a student with multiple disabilities and visual impairment: A case study. J Visual Impair Blindness 2001;95:108.

[43]   Katcher AH, Wilkins GG. Animal-assisted therapy in the treatment of disruptive behavior disorder in children. In: Lundberg A, ed. The environment and mental health: A guide for clinicians. Mahwah, NJ: Laweence Erlbaum, pp.193-204, 1998.

[44]   Taylor SM. Equine facilitated psychotherapy: An emerging field. Dissertation. Winooski Park Colchester, VT: Saint Michael's College, 2001.

[45]   Engerstrom IW, Kerr A. Workshop on autonomic function in Rett Syndrome, Swedish Rett center, Fröson, Sweden. Brain Dev 1998;20:323-6.

[46]   Elefant C. Emotional/musical communication of children with RS. A lecture at an annual conference on RS. Ramat Gan, IL: Chaim Sheba Med Center, July 2005.

[47]   Lindberg B. Understanding Rett syndrome: A practical guide for parents, teachers and therapists. Toronto: Hognefe Huber, 1991.

[48]   McGibbon NH, Andrade CK, Widener G, Cintas HL. Effect of an equine-movement therapy program on gait, energy expenditure, and motor function in children with spastic cerebral palsy. Dev Med Child Neurol 1998;40(11):754-62.

[49]   Casady RL, Nichols-Larsen DS. The effect of hippotherapy on ten children with cerebral palsy. Pediatric Phys Ther 2004;16(3):165-72.

[50]   Would J. Improved gait in two children with cerebral palsy after hippotherapy: Two case reports. Sci Educ J Therapeut Riding 1998;51-8.

[51]   Would J. Improvements in walking and functional ability in children with cerebral palsy following hippotherapy: Research results. Int Symposium, Amiens, France: University Picardie, August 2002.

[52]   Jacobsen K, Viken A, Von Tetchner S. Rett syndrome and aging: A case study. Disabil Rehabil 2001;23(3/4):160-6.

[53]   Piazza CC, Nederson C, Fisher W. Teaching self-feeding skills to patients with Rett Syndrome. Dev Med Child Neurol 1993;35:991-6.

[54]   Sponseller P. Orthopedic update in Rett syndrome. Rett Gazette 2001, spring:1,4-5.

[55]   Schalow G. Non-drug induced spasticity reduction achieved by coordination dynamic therapy in CNS injury. Electromyogr Clin Neurophysiol 2002;42(5):281-93.

[56]   Kerr AM. The future for Rett Syndrome girls. Int Rett Syndr Assoc Newsletter1992:13-4.

[57]   Haas RH, Dixon SD, Sartoris DJ, Hennessy MJ. Osteopenia in Rett syndrome. J Pediatr 1997;131(5):771-4.

[58]   Budden SS, Gunness ME Bone histomorphometry in three females with Rett syndrome. Brain Dev 2001;23(Suppl 1):S133-7.

[59]   Cepollaro C, Gonnelli S, Bruni D, Pacini S, Martini S, Franci MB, Gennari L, Rossi S, Hayek G, Zappella M, Gennari C. Dual X-ray absorptiometry and bone ultrasonography in patients with Rett syndrome. Calcif Tissue Int 2001;69:259–62.

[60]   Sinaki M, Khosla S, Limburg PJ, Rogers JW, Murtaugh PA 1993 Muscle strength in osteoporotic versus normal women. Osteoporos Int 1993;3:8-12.

[61]   Sinaki M, Itoi E, Wahner HW, Wollan P, Gelzcer R, Mullan BP, Collins DA, Hodgson SF Stronger back muscles reduce the incidence of vertebral fractures: A prospective 10 year follow-up of postmenopausal women. Bone 2002;30:836-41.

[62]   Sinaki M, Lynn SG. Reducing the risk of falls through proprioceptive dynamic posture training in osteoporotic women with kyphotic posturing: A randomized pilot study. Am J Phys Med Rehabil 2002;81:241-6.

[63]   Maciques R. Hippotherapy: A rehabilitating therapy for the Rett syndrome. A case study. Newsletter UK Rett Assoc, 2004.

[64]   Lotan M, Merrick J, Carmeli E. Scoliosis management in Rett syndrome. A case study. ScientificWorld Journal 2005;5:264-73.

[65]   Budden SS. Management of Rett syndrome: A ten-year experience. Neuropediatrics 1995;26(2):75-7.

[66]   Lotan M, Elefant C. Physiotherapy and music therapy for a girl with Rett syndrome. A dual treatment approach. Fysioterapeuten 2006;2: 15-20. [Danish]

[67]   Weeks L. Rett Syndrome. A lecture given at Sydney Australia, February, 1997.

[68]   Rossin L. Effectiveness of therapeutic and surgical intervention in the treatment of scoliosis in Rett syndrome. A seminar work, University of Duquesne, 1997:1-19.

[69]   McClure MK, Battaglia C, McClure RJ. The relationship of cumulative motor asymmetries to scoliosis in Rett Syndrome. Am J Occup Ther 1998;52:196-204.

[70]   Benda W, McGibbon NH, Grant KL. Improvements in muscle symmetry in children with cerebral palsy after equine-assisted therapy (hippotherapy). J Altern Complement Med 2003;9(6):817-25.

[71]   Bertoti DB. Effect of therapeutic horseback riding on extremity weight bearing in a child with hemiplegic cerebral palsy: A case report as an example of clinical research. Pediatr Phys Ther 1991;3:219-24.

[72]   Lotan M, Hadar-Frumer M. Hydrotherapy for individuals with Rett syndrome. A guidebook for hydrotherapists. Raanana, IL: Beit Issie Shapiro Publ, 2002. [Hebrew]

[73]   Lotan M, Roth D. The effect of hand vibrators on the hand stereotypes and function in Rett syndrome. Two case studies. Isr Physiother Quart 1996;52:23-6. [Hebrew]

[74]   Nomura Y, Segawa M. Motor symptoms of the Rett syndrome: abnormal muscle tone, posture, locomotion and stereotyped movement. Brain Dev 1992;14(Suppl): S21-8.

[75]   Matsuishi T, Yamashita Y, Kusaga A. Neurobiology and neurochemistry of Rett syndrome. Brain Dev 2001;23(Suppl 1):S58-61.

[76]   Cass H, Reilly S, Owen L, Wisbeach A, Weekes L, Slonims V, Wigram T, Charman T. Findings from a multidisciplinary clinical case series of females with Rett syndrome. Dev Med Child Neurol 2003;45(5):325-37.

[77]   Lotan M, Manor-Binyamini I, Elefant C, Wine J, Saraf E, Yoshei T. The Israeli Rett Syndrome Center. Evaluation and transdisciplinary play-based assessment. ScientificWorldJournal 2006;6:1302–13.

[78]   Nieto MA, Candau RS, Prieto P. Contribution to studies of seizures in Rett Syndrome analysis of critical forms of four cases. Rev Neurol 1995;23:1185-9.

In: Rett Syndrome: Therapeutic Interventions
Editors: Meir Lotan and Joav Merrick

ISBN: 978-1-61728-080-1
©2011 Nova Science Publishers, Inc.

Chapter XIV

Rett syndrome: Therapeutic Options with Snoezelen

Meir Lotan, BPT, MScPT, PhD[*]

Israel Rett Center, National Evaluation Team, Chaim Sheba Medical Center, Tel HaShomer, Ramat Gan, Zvi Quittman Residential Centers, Israel Elwyn, Jerusalem and Department of Physical Therapy, Ariel University Campus, Ariel, Israel

Rett Syndrome (RS) is a neurological disorder resulting from an X-linked dominant mutation. It is characterized by a variety of physical and perceptual disabilities, resulting in a need for continuous intervention programs to be administered on a regular basis throughout life. Many people with Rett syndrome show fear of movement and therefore find it hard to accept external facilitation (so common in physical therapy intervention). In a search for novel intervention techniques, that might improve their ability to cope with difficulties in daily situations while reducing their difficulty in handling motion inflicted by an external physical facilitator, we examined the use of the Snoezelen room. The Snoezelen, also known as the controlled multi-sensory environment (CMSE), can provide a soothing environment that appeals to the individual with Rett syndrome while at the same time improve physical, sensorial and functional abilities. This chapter suggests various intervention goals which are appropriate for individuals with RS at different stages of the disorder. Since the management of young children with RS in the multi sensory environment has been discussed in length in the past, this article will mainly describe intervention with adults with RS focusing on three case studies. This chapter will review the available scientific materials on the topic of Snoezelen, incorporating clinical knowledge in the field of Rett syndrome and suggesting this approach as an appropriate intervention method for this population.

[*] Correspondence: Meir Lotan, BPT, MScPT, PhD, Department of Physical Therapy, Ariel University Campus, IL-40700 Ariel, Israel. E-mail: ml_pt_rs@netvision.net.il

Introduction

Rett Syndrome (RS) is a neurological disorder resulting from an X-linked dominant mutation [1], affecting mainly females and found in a variety of racial and ethnic groups worldwide [2]. RS is a frequent cause of neurological dysfunction in females, accounting for the second most common cause for multiple-disability among females, after Down's syndrome [3,4].

Individuals with this disorder show a variety of difficulties in motor planning and execution (apraxia), in function, in communication and have an array of orthopedic and neurological problems [5]. Since life expectancy in RS is evaluated as around 49 years [6] and due to the vast physical challenges experienced by children with this disorder, treatment (especially physical treatment) is essential, necessitating lifelong therapeutic intervention [7]. The secondary motor deterioration typical of adolescents with this disorder compels the increasing of such physical therapy (PT) intervention [8] and presents it as one of the most important treatments for individuals with RS. This notion is supported by the fact that PT is applied to almost 80% of girls with this disorder [7].

In spite of its importance, PT can be unpleasant and at times even invasive. Such elements of the treatment may induce unpleasant feelings, which the person is incapable of expressing. Individuals with RS function according to their highly developed emotional state [9] and when they dislike physical treatment they might react by resisting, to the point of falling asleep, long spells of hyperventilation episodes, or by evoking a seizure [10]. Due to sensorial difficulties, such as fear of movement, some individuals with RS take little pleasure in external facilitation and in many cases show resistance and fear of physical intervention [11]. Due to the above mentioned consideration, a novel intervention environment is hereby considered. One such approach, that could integrate the need for movement and sensorial needs of the individual with RS, while at the same time present a more calmer/emotional experience, is the Snoezelen, or the controlled multi-sensory environment (CMSE).

Controlled multi-sensory environment

The word Snoezelen is a combination of two Dutch words: Snoezel = to sniff like a dog and Doezelen = to doze. The word 'doze' indicates that a restful activity is involved and the word 'sniff' gives it the more dynamic sensorial aspect [12]. Ad Verheul, the Dutch originator of this technique, mentions that the name "Snoezelen" came up due to its nice ring and therefore clients caught onto the name very easily [12].

The CMSE is a partially-lit room that provides sensory stimulation to both the client and the therapist, where the senses are provided harmoniously, whether alone or combined. The sensory stimulus in Snoezelen is provided according to the client's choice, thus empowering the individual participating in such a program. The aim of the treatment is to find a balance between relaxation and activity within the framework of a safe, adapted environment by means of an enabling therapist [13].

We live our lives through our senses. It is by means of experiencing those senses that we develop an understanding about our environment [14]. Any form of sensorial disturbance that a person may exhibit, which will disturb his interaction with the environment, may influence his understanding and as a result, may disturb development. According to Longhorn [15], without sensation and arousal of the senses, people with disturbances will find it very difficult to comprehend the world around them and as a result, will have difficulty in learning.

The basic assumption is that the CMSE intrigues the client's interest and, therefore, she begins to explore and discover her surroundings. This exploration acts as a stepping- stone towards learning and development.

People with disabilities usually have minimal effect over their own lives and cannot create their own optimal environments. The Snoezelen gives them the opportunity to do so. By modeling the CMSE according to the client's preference, we create a safe and favored sensory experience for the individual with RS to explore [13].

Intervention in the Snoezelen among different populations with disabilities was found to be highly effective in addressing various problems [16]. Holtkamp and Kragt [17] undertook a study, where Snoezelen was applied with seventeen elderly people. Using a randomized cross-over design, they indicated a higher degree of well-being for the experimental group than for the control group. Shapiro et al [18] conducted an experimental cross-over design study with twenty children with intellectual disability (not including children with RS) exhibiting maladaptive behaviors. This research concluded that Snoezelen had a positive effect on these children as a therapeutic agent. The research included both behavioral and physiological measures. The results of their ambulatory heart rates suggested that the Snoezelen could balance heart rate, reducing it in children who were hyperactive and increasing it in children who were passive [18]. Snoezelen was also found to be effective in dealing with individuals with apraxia [19], yielding positive physical outcomes, such as improving gate and balance for those with physical disabilities [20]. It showed carry-over effects, generalizing into daily situations, for individuals presenting extreme agitation and challenging behaviors [21,22]. These indirect findings, as well as the author's experience [23,24], imply that this environment might be adjusted for individuals with RS at various ages and with a variety of difficulties.

Snoezelen and rett syndrome

It should be stressed that every child with RS is unique. Therefore, the individual clinical expression of this disorder necessitates a thorough evaluation for each child, prior to deciding on the type and content of intervention delivered for the child, preferably in a multi-disciplinary approach [25]. Despite such individual diversity, those with RS display some typical characteristics that might be appropriate to handle using treatments via the multi-sensory environment. Common challenges in dealing with this population should be screened according to the typical stages of the disorder.

When screening the literature, one might find hints as to intervention elements that experts in the field of RS have suggested as beneficial for this population:

- Close interpersonal contact [26] is recommended
- Quiet and reassuring environment may achieve reduction in anxiety and agitation in children with RS [27]
- Music is valuable as means of relaxation [28]
- The child (with RS) will respond best to tender, loving care which encourages activity in an interesting but quiet environment, during regression [28]

In a lecture by Kerr [29], the following suggestions for a desired intervention with this population were added to the above:

- Encourage and facilitate learning without pressurizing the child;
- Provide face-to-face contact, talking, singing, touching;
- Comfort the child and allow withdrawal during agitation;
- Encourage active supervised movement in soft play;
- Provide gentle movement of limbs and joints through their full range of motion.

When examining the CMSE and the concept of the enabling therapist, we find that it incorporates all the above elements and can serve as a potential intervention program for the individual with RS. A person with RS will respond positively to face-to-face contact, gentle caressing and communicative sounds, since those responses are programmed in every child from a young age [9]. Besides calming the agitated child, the interactions available in the multi-sensory environment might encourage the emergence of hidden skills, such as reaching out and initiation of hand manipulation, exploration behaviors and vocalization. General clinical guidelines when interacting with people with RS:

- The therapist should always be attuned to non-verbal language expressed by the eyes and face of the child [30], constantly talking to her and explaining what will happen next, while reinforcing her activities
- About 73% of children with RS present some form of epilepsy [30]. Thus, it is advisable to avoid different visual stimuli that might cause or induce a seizure (e.g. flickering lights)
- The role of the therapist in the multi-sensory environment is to create an interpersonal atmosphere in which the client feels unconditionally accepted [13].
- Music has constantly been found to be of enormous value for individuals with RS, at all levels of disability and ages [29,31-35]. The right kind of music can facilitate learning, relaxation or may, on the other hand, excite the child with RS. Advice regarding the recommended music for each individual should be pre-determined according to the therapeutic goals and might be obtained from parents, caregivers and the child's music therapist.
- The therapist should position him/herself according to the child's preferences and therapeutic needs. The therapist can be facing the child and communicating while massaging or moving her body and limbs[36] or can be behind the child, safely containing her with his arms, as described by Kerr and Burford [37].

Management

The importance of careful and specific evaluation is reiterated for each client before deciding her needs, difficulties and personal preferences. Nevertheless, most individuals with RS go through the stages listed below and some may present similar characteristic and disabilities. This next section will touch on such common features.

Stage I: Onset

The development of most RS females is close to normal; the symptoms of RS are just emerging at this stage and are somewhat vague. At this point, most children will display hypotonia and might even present improved finger usage. In most cases, the girl will usually not alarm even the most competent of physicians. The second stage is where the aberrant development emerges and the child's situation receives ample attention. The next stage can have a rapid onset and is a very difficult period for the girl and her family [36].

Stage II: Destructive stage/motor deterioration

Although relatively short (mostly spanning for weeks or up to few months), this stage is the girl's (as well as her family's) most difficult experience. Now she completely lacks orientation, her senses are severely disturbed and her body betrays her [10].

Getting into a quiet, dim-lit environment at this stage may ease the child's discomfort. A water-bed might serve as a peaceful "island in the midst of chaos" [36]; it warmly and gently embraces the girl and takes away the pain, fear and uncertainty for the duration of the treatment. The personal touch, the eye contact and the therapist's well-trained and secure hands are all beneficial. Although it is questionable if functional goals can be achieved at this stage, relaxation is a huge comfort. The therapist should try to bond with the child in preparation for future meetings.

The benefits of Snoezelen for young children with RS have already been discussed at length elsewhere [23] and will only be touched on at this point. At this stage of RS, abnormal neural activity can be detected in brain electrical measurements [38] and in bio-chemical components such as high levels of glutamate [39], causing the cortex and other brain area to go into an abnormally excitatory state [27,40]. The severity of such manifestations may be controlled by external intervention, which regulates incoming sensory input and balances the over-excited neural system. With increasing knowledge of RS within the medical community, the diagnosis of young children with RS is progressing, as can be seen in figure XIV-1 (published with permission) [41].

It is possible that in the near future, early diagnosis will enable early intervention for children with RS. If therapeutic measures are to be utilized at an earlier age there is a chance of minimizing damage to neural tissue. Such (calming) measures, if introduced to the small child with RS, are believed by experts in the field of neural development [40,42], to reduce the damage caused by this hyper-exited state of the brain tissue, enabling future development and advancement for the child as she enters calmer stages of the disorder (stage III). It is also hypothesized that such a relaxing intervention might have the capability to normalize the unbalanced sympathetic activity by elevating the basically low-vagal tone typical of RS [31]. The evidence regarding continued brain growth and the absence of major destructive processes [43,44] provide hope that appropriate calming techniques, implemented from a young age, will enable future brain development and possible future learning [45].

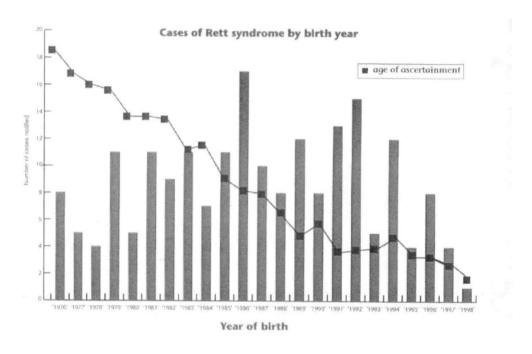

Figure XIV-1. Age of ascertainment of RS 1976- 1998.

Appropriate intervention goals for individual at stage II of RS would be relaxation. Individuals with RS tend to go through mood swings (although not all of them do and those who do are not always prone to them). At times we might see that the child is extremely upset, without our understanding of the cause of such behavior. Since communication in the majority of girls with RS is non-verbal and thus sometimes difficult to understand, it seems that a quiet treatment can save many hours of pain, tears, and discomfort (even if the cause remains enigmatic). It is important to mention that the emotional bonding between the girl and her therapist is extremely important. A loving and understanding therapist will win the girl's love and trust and, as a result, attain her cooperation, essential to effective treatment. With that notion in mind, the therapist should find the time to build an interpersonal relationship. The use of the water-bed with heated water, together with soft large pillows/bean begs can contain the child, enhancing a primal sense of a womb-like experience, which is very calming and is highly recommended. Auditory stimulation in accordance with child's preference will add in building up a sense of familiarity and safeness.

Case story 1 (relaxation)

DA is an adult woman (aged 63 years). DA showed the characteristics of the preserved speech variant of RS. She eats and walks independently but requires help in all other daily activities. DA lives in a residential setting in Jerusalem, Israel. Prior to intervention initiation, when DA was among her peers, she was frequently upset, expressing her unease by excessive body movements and long-lasting, loud shouts. Since no explanation could be determined to explain her tantrums, it was decided to start her on a Snoezelen intervention program, aimed at relaxing her, thus reducing her agitated behavior. DA received two half-hour individual sessions a week. The intervention in the Snoezelen room was performed with dim lights and calming soft music. The attention at the first part of the treatment (about 10 minutes) was focused on functional abilities and included a tour around the room (see figure XIV-2) walking (with assistance) on high mattresses exercising her equilibrium and walking abilities.

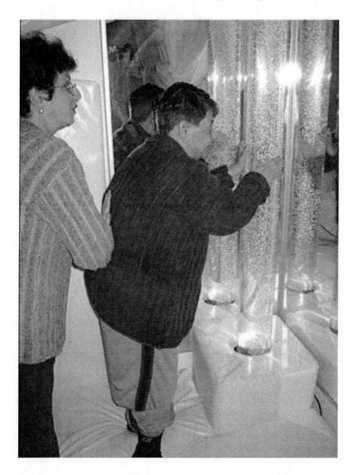

Figure XIV-2. Functional abilities in the multi-sensory environment.

This exercise was presented due to the author's impression that when stepping on the thick mattresses there was a change in her pattern of walking, from the regular wide-based large sway, straight–kneed gait typical of individuals with RS, to a more normal pattern of walking with bended knees. In the second part of the intervention DA lay on her back and received a slow and gentle massage to her extremities. This part of the treatment was aimed at reducing her tantrums. DA enjoyed herself during those treatments, came willingly to the Snoezelen room and was never upset during the interventions.

After three months of intervention, DA's agitation has diminished and she was much more relaxed throughout the day (see figure XIV-3). Due to the reduction and then complete cessation of tantrums, DA's intervention program was terminated in order to enable other clients of the residential setting to benefit from the advantages of the Snoezelen intervention.

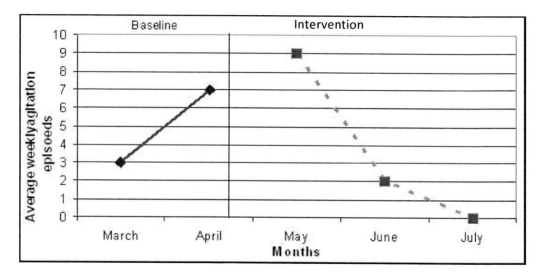

Figure XIV-3. Reduction in agitation due to Snoezelen intervention.

Stage III: Plateau

This stage is relatively long and calm. The radical physical/emotional situation now seems to have subsided and become more balanced. The duration of this stage is quite lengthy (spanning a period of years), which enables the girl to achieve some progress due to therapeutic intervention, while preventing possible future problems.

Appropriate intervention goals for individuals at stage III of RS would be **hand functions**. Stereotyped hand movements are present in 30%-72% of the waking hours of the child with RS [46]. These movements, together with apraxia and ataxia, reduce the likelihood of functional hand use. Thus, in order to activate the hands of the person with RS, it is important to try using various instruments and techniques. An environment that might favorably enhance manual use is the CMSE. Using different interesting visual stimuli like the 'optic fibers', 'infinity', 'fireworks' and 'electrical ball' might be found interesting enough for the client to try and use her hands. If the person with RS is able to crawl, performing such an activity on a thick mattress covering the floor of the room will facilitate intense proprioceptive stimulation to the hands and might pay off in terms of functional manual improvement. The 'bubbles pole' creates visual and vibrating stimulation simultaneously and might be used when treatment goals are aimed at enhancing hand function. Different visual stimulation (e.g. through the use of a projector) can be adjusted to illuminate the wall in front of the individual with RS, to enhance further manual function and exploration. The ability to select different slides to match individual client preference can further motivate her to use her hand.

Transitions are another issue at this stage. The primary functional loss of girls with RS is experienced in decreased ability to change her position [47,48]. Transitions include the changes from standing to a sitting position, from sitting to standing, from standing to walking and so forth. Therefore, during any functional treatment régime, one should include repetitive elements of active movement and position-changing, on a regular basis [8]. Walking is an extremely important function for individuals with RS, because it stimulates the work of internal organs and the digestive system, thus reducing constipation. Standing or walking in an upright position is of immense importance [49] and was found to be positively correlated in delaying the development of scoliosis [50] and reduction of osteoporosis in children with developmental disabilities [51]. Thick, unsteady mattresses create a rough terrain for the individual with RS to handle but at the same time allows her (as a person usually struggling with the control over her body) to experience walking without the risk of injuring herself, in case of a fall. Practicing transitions in the CMSE, with an adult without RS but with apraxia, has been found useful in enhancing functional independence and the ability to re-learn lost transitions [19].

Preventing potential orthopedic problems (and managing existing ones) should also be a focus at this stage. Girls with RS might display the following orthopedic problems: Scoliosis (a side-to-side/rotational curve of the spine), kyphosis (forward curve of the upper–thoracic–spine) and deformation of the palms and/or feet. Scoliosis can be found in 80-85% of individuals with RS [3,50], especially among non-mobile children [50,52]. Thus, it is very important to provide motivation for walking [49]. Kyphosis is more common among girls who can walk but is not as severe and movement-disabling as scoliosis [3]. In both cases, the therapist can apply gentle passive mobilization to the trunk, while using mattresses as a support system. If the therapist can manage to persuade the client with RS to lie on the waterbed on her stomach, this will be extremely beneficial in maintaining and increasing range of motion of the trunk, hips and shoulder towards extension. The deformation that often occurs in the palms and feet, as well as the dislocation of the hips, require careful attention and specific treatments. The water-bed might be useful in such cases, as well in assisting the therapist as a support system that warms and softens rigid tissues. At the same time, the tranquil and relaxed atmosphere in the multi-sensory room created by the dim lights, soothing music and gentle movements of the water-bed can calm the child. This effect will reduce the child's rigidity and can prevent disturbing and sometimes painful manual manipulations.

Re-assembling proprioceptive perception [53], as some girls with RS were described by Hanks as losing their sense of "mid-line". In such conditions the child senses her body differently positioned from where it actually is. Sometimes they tilt so far to one side or backwards that one might even rule out the possibility of independent sitting [8]. This condition prevents her from standing straight (since standing straight seems odd to her) and if the uneven posture is continuously maintained, it can cause damage such as scoliosis, kyphosis and even a loss of ability to sit, stand and walk. Due to the high frequency of scoliosis in this population [3,50], Hanks[47]suggested that every individual with RS should be routinely treated from childhood with deep symmetrical proprioceptive stimulation, as preventive intervention. Rolling on the mattresses is also an option for performing deep proprioceptive stimulation as part of the multi-sensory treatment and enables the therapist to work with the individual with RS on her "appropriate" proprioceptive perception with an electrical massager (if this appliance's sensation can be tolerated by the individual with RS) or without the use of instruments. Covering the child with a big bean-bag sack\pillow can also give intense proprioceptive input.

Equilibrium and coordination. Among her other challenges, the individual with RS is disabled by ataxia. Ataxia is characterized by reduced control over muscle activity in the usual, coordinated manner; that most of us perform automatically (mostly displayed by effected postural muscles). The ability to control these muscles is essential for supporting body posture in various positions and in movement. Lacking this ability can aggravate motor limitations. Knee-walking across the mattresses of the CMSE can improve equilibrium and trunk control, which is vital for most motor acts. It is postulated that the functional improvement observed after treadmill training in this population is due to enhanced trunk control [54]. Standing on all fours on the water-bed is a challenging exercise and will yield similar results. In addition, such an exercise gives proprioceptive input to the upper extremities and might also enhance hand usage.

Case story 2

BA, an adult woman aged 58, showing the characteristics of RS, living in a residential setting in Jerusalem, Israel. She is self-ambulant, but requires assistance in all other ADL functions. She is extremely kyphotic. In the recent months prior to intervention initiation, staff informed the therapeutic department that she had started to show signs of old age, manifested in increased kyphosis and falls. After discussing the situation, an intervention program was initiated both at BA's dormitory, and in the CMSE. The aims of the program were to reduce falls and to improve posture. The staff was advised to put BA on her stomach for 20 minutes every day, during nap times. In the Snoezelen, BA received two half-hour-long individual sessions a week. The lights were kept on and popular music was played in the background. During those sessions BA would walk around the room, stepping on the thick mattresses in order to improve her balance and she was assisted in obtaining motivating objects, which were placed on high shelves across the room (the objects were mainly made up of various small musical and illuminating gadgets, which BA particularly likes), in order to enhance active extension of the arms and upper thorax (see figure XIV-4).

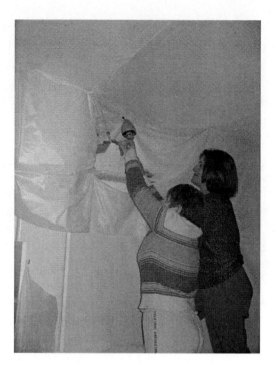

Figure XIV-4. Collecting motivating objects from high shelves.

The program has been going on for two years now and is still under way today. According to collected data over a period of 6 years, falls that dramatically increased during 2004, which resulted in the Snoezelen intervention, have completely ceased and are no longer a problem for BA (see figure XIV-5), although, visually, her posture does not seem to change.

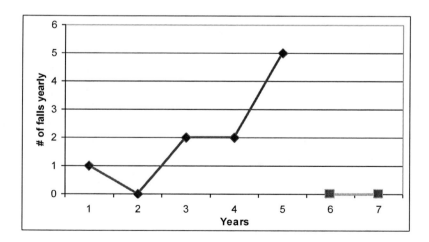

Figure XIV-5. Reduction in falls due to Snoezelen intervention.

Sensation. Individuals with RS are often characterized by an unbalanced sensory system. This phenomenon has never been thoroughly investigated but nevertheless, it has been well documented, mainly via parental reports. Many individuals with RS display decreased pain sensation and hypersensitivity to touch over their faces [55], especially around the mouth [10]. Their fear of movement was suggested by Lindberg as caused by a dysfunction of the vestibular system [10]. Yet it seems to the author (ML) that this limitation should mostly be attributed to deficiencies within the proprioceptive system. As a consequence of her fear of movement, the individual is cautious and the fluency of her everyday life is interrupted. The unclear/disorienting messages received at the cortex level causes the brain to create a distracted body scheme, a vital component in accepting and relating to the world. Without it, the individual is affected by apraxia [14]. The fear of movement can also be express by "proprioceptive distress" presented by a fear of external movement and facilitation of the body and limbs and ambulation over altered surfaces (more information regarding this topic could be found within the chapter dealing with occupational therapy in this book). Embracing the child should provide her with deep proprioceptive sensory stability and this secure sensation should be maintained as the basic 'sanctuary' until the child is acclimatized with the environment, the therapist and the intervention program. In extreme cases of fear of movement, this relaxed and familiar posture should be the point from which slow rhythmic movement starts and to which it returns. After a sense of security in this familiar situation is achieved, the girl who is generally afraid of movement might agree to more physically powerful, free-flowing movements. When the child is completely confident in this situation (in other words, most parts of her nervous system are relaxed and learning can become possible), the sensory feedback enables an integration and organization of her sensory system [14]. Routinely revisiting the CMAE and reestablishing confidence in movement might ensure positive results in her daily activities. From my experience, individuals with RS, who have shown an obvious and paralyzing rejection of movement by an external facilitator prior to the intervention, handled in the above-mentioned manner in the CMSE, have become gradually accustomed to movement and to the experience of motion.

Stage IV: Late motor deterioration

At this stage, which occurs in some girls and women, late motor deterioration that requires increased physiotherapy may be noticed. Several cases have been reported, where girls with RS lost their ability to walk but were able to improve their functional mobility and regain ambulation [48,56,57]. In one case study, the rehabilitation of lost walking skill was achieved with a 43 year old individual after two decades of immobility [58]. It is important to stress that the inability to walk increases the risk of secondary complications, such as scoliosis, pelvic deformities, pulmonary (lung) problems, reduced bowel movements and blood flow to internal organs and lower limbs. Thus, it is extremely important to keep individuals with RS ambulant.

The need for extensive intervention collides with her aversion to physical intervention, while the CMSE, with its relaxing effect, can help the child\young woman in liking or at least in enduring the obligatory physical manipulations. Despite new difficulties, new areas are open to improvement, such as a decrease in repetitive hand movements and the improvement of social and communicative skills. In Stage IV, therefore, one should address the problems reported in Stage III, if appropriate, and with increased intensity (if necessary), but without neglecting new areas of possible improvements, such as communication and social skills.

Communication [59]. Most girls with RS do not communicate verbally. However, they like to communicate with others, especially adults and it is easier for them to communicate in a one-on-one situation (individual treatment). During therapy in the multi-sensory environment, if communication enhancement is to be achieved, the therapist should be in front of the girl, facing her and maintaining direct eye-contact with her. The therapist should be attuned to non-verbal cues expressed by the eyes and face, constantly talking to her, explaining what will happen next and reinforcing her by commenting to her communicative acts. Moving across the CMSE can be performed according to the child's preference using a set of plastic cards (see figure XIV-6 - showing different areas of the room) pointed out by the child's eye-gaze or hand. Such activity might have a carry-over application in enhancing assisted communication within daily situations [60].

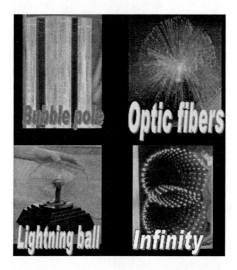

Figure XIV-6. Enhancing communication and choice-making through cards.

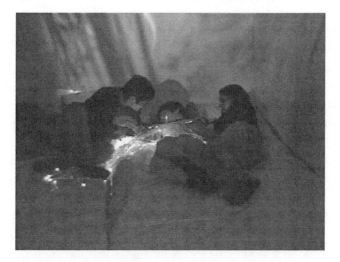

Figure XIV-7. Familial encounters in the Snoezelen.

Social skills. Girls with RS are very friendly but their communication (especially girls that are not mobile) with their friends, peers and classmates is technically difficult. Better communicative ability can be developed during treatment in the CMSE. Reinforcing relationships with others is important at all times and during every treatment but is highly significant at Stage IV of RS. Getting friends and/or family members to be present in the CMSE (see figure XIV-7) can enhance joy and happiness in the life of that person and the close human circles wherein she shares her life. Such closeness can take the mind off of daily hardships, thus recharging mental strengths for the ongoing struggle of living with RS [55].

Spasticity and range of motion (see case study 3). At an older age, individuals with RS tend to develop high muscle-tone. Reducing this spasticity/rigidity requires a relaxed and secure atmosphere, deep manual pressure and slow, continuous rhythmic movements, which can be achieved using the water-bed. The music-bed can be used for the same purpose, since the vibration of the loudspeakers can induce muscle-tone reduction. Muscle-tone reduction has been found useful especially when using vibro-acoustics [35].

Case story 3

MB, is a 24 year-old female diagnosed with RS and living in a residential facility. MB has never walked, has no functional abilities and shows severe musculo-skeletal contractures, both in the trunk and limbs. In recent years, her contractures had deteriorated to the point her caregivers started to complain that even dressing and undressing her had become a very tedious task, not to mention the pain these every day occurrences seemed to cause. The constant fear of adding to her daily encounters the suffering of a pathological fracture due to the fragility of RS bones [61-63] was unremittingly present.

In the light of this situation, a program for increasing her articular range of motion was initiated in the physical therapy room. Despite the fact that this intervention program took into account her long-lasting condition and her fragility and was delivered in the gentlest manner, it became apparent after the first few sessions that MB was not enjoying the intervention. On top of that, only minimal movements could be performed on her limbs and trunk, which made it clear that this form of intervention was not very efficient and that new intervention options should be considered.

The next option to consider was the Snoezelen environment. MB was introduced to the Snoezelen environment in a slowly adaptive manner and started receiving manual intervention aimed at increasing her range of motion in two half -hour sessions per week. The treatment took place on the heated water-bed and was performed with dim lights and soft music. At the beginning of each treatment (5-10 minutes), MB's body was covered with a large bean-bag in order to enhance a feeling of security and supply proprioceptive sensory input, thus reducing muscle-tone and relaxing her body. During the remaining part of the intervention, manual range of movement exercises were performed (in the same manner as it was done before in the physical therapy room), while the slow rhythmic movements, dim lights and soft music remained constant. Judging by the look in her eyes and the type of smiles she wore, it was obvious that MB was enjoying the experience.

Table XIV-1. Difference in range of motion after a four month intervention

Body part	side	Direction of movement	Pre intervention 15/6/2004	Post intervention 13/10/2004
Shoulder	left	Flexion	65	90
		Abduction	19	180
		Elevation	90	113
		Int. Rotation	---	45
		External rotation	---	45
	Right	Flexion	75	180
		Abduction	180	180
		Elevation	62	90
		Internal Rotation	---	180
		External rotation	---	180
Elbow	left	Flexion	180	180
		Extension	100	113
	Right	Flexion	180	180
		Extension	107	105
Palm	left	Palmar flexion	80	80
		Palmar extension	10	22
		Ulnar dev.	45	45
		Radial Dev.	-10	0
	Right	Palmar flexion	0	20
		Palmar extension	90	90
		Ulnar dev.	45	45
		Radial Dev.	-10	0
M.C.P	left	Flexion	110	110
		Extension	-10	---
	Right	Flexion	32	---
		Extension	0	---
Legs				
Hip	left	Flexion	95	180
		Extension	-15	0
		Abduction	0	0
		Adduction	0	0
		Int Rotation	90	90
		External rotation	0	37
	Right	Flexion	40	180
		Extension	0	0
		Abduction	10	30
		Adduction	10	12
		Int Rotation	0	30
		External rotation	60	64
Knee	left	Flexion	180	180
		Extension	103	153
	Right	Flexion	150	155
		Extension	60	118
Ankle	left	Dorsi Flexion	32	25
		Plantar flexion	10	50
	Right	Dorsi Flexion	5	10
		Plantar flexion	40	40

A one way paired student T-Test have found a significant difference **P< 0.0003** between the pre-post measurements.

An examination of her joint range of motion (JROM) after the course of four months (see table XIV-1) revealed that an increase in JROM was established throughout her body, enough to ease the daily suffering of MB and alleviate her caregivers' difficulties. Moreover, this small change has been found statistically significant.

Conclusions

It is reiterated that the present chapter is a review of the available scientific materials on the topic of Snoezelen, incorporating the clinical knowledge of the author in the field of Rett syndrome and, therefore, scientific generalization should be limited. This chapter and other available literature on this topic [23,24] illustrate the possibility of using the controlled multi-sensory environment (CMSE/Snoezelen) as an appropriate intervention approach towards achieving a variety of remedial goals for young girls as well as adult women with RS. The fact that the multi-sensory environment enables the use of the two major motivational factors of individuals with RS (love for music and close human contact) is, by itself, a good reason for suggesting such a program for clients with RS. Moreover, it appears that when screening some of the major difficulties of individuals with RS, most of them might be cared for using this approach. Nevertheless, it is restated that any management program should be adapted to the individual client after a careful evaluation of her specific needs.

When evaluating the child with RS, it is also important to realize the possible future achievements and plan ahead, while deciding on new ways of intervention with those individuals [64]. Individuals with RS tend to have an over-active sympathetic system [65] constantly placing them in a state of highly-strained being, therefore using a soothing environment such as the Snoezelen on regular basis might contribute to relaxation and, as a result, an enhanced quality of life. An additional important element to be reflected upon, when considering the Snoezelen room as a therapeutic approach for individuals with RS, is our ability to change the setting according to each client's preferences, thus empowering her. It should be emphasized here that the use of Snoezelen as described in the present chapter adds to the original concept of the Snoezelen by using this approach in a more therapeutic manner than intended by the original initiators of this approach [12]. This manner of operating intervention in the CMSE is coined by the author as Therapeutic Snoezelen Intervention (TSI), which gives an added value for this environment as long as the therapeutic endeavors do not contradict the basic concept of the enabling therapist.

Acknowledgments

The author would like to thank the management of Israel Elwyn and the Elwyn residential centers for their cooperation and support in this project.

References

[1]   Amir RE, Van Den Veyver IB, Schultz R, Malicki DM, Tran CQ, Dahle EJ, et al. Influence of mutation type and X chromosome inactivation on Rett syndrome phenotypes. Ann Neurology 2000;47:670-9.

[2]   Hagberg B, Aicardi J, Dias K, Ramos O. A progressive syndrome of autism, dementia, ataxia, and loss of purposeful hand use in girls: Rett syndrome: report of 35 cases. Ann Neurology 1983;14: 471-9.

[3]   Hagberg B. Rett syndrome. Clinical and biological aspects. London: Mac Keith Press, 1993.

[4]   Ellaway C, Christodoulou J. Rett syndrome: Clinical characteristics and recent genetic advances. Disabil Rehabil 2001;23:98-106.

[5]   Budden SS. Management of Rett syndrome: A ten-year experience. Neuropediatrics 1995;26(2):75-7.

[6]   Percy AK. International research review. Presentation, IRSA 12th Ann Conf, 1996 May 24-27, Boston, MA, tape 622-15.

[7]   Leonard H, Fyfe S, Leonard S, Msall M. Functional status, medical impairments, and rehabilitation resources in 84 females with Rett syndrome: a snapshot across the world from the parental perspective. Disabil Rehabil 2001;23:107-17.

[8]   Beuchel K. Physical therapy and gross motor skills in Rett syndrome. Handout, IRDA Ann Conf, Washington, DC, 2001.

[9]   Elefant C. Emotional/musical communication of children with RS. Presentation, Ann Conf Rett Syndr, Sheba hospital, Ramat-Gan, Israel, July 2005.

[10]   Lindberg B. Understanding Rett syndrome: A practice guide for parents, teachers and therapists. Toronto: Hognefe Huber, 1991.

[11]   Lotan M, Elefant, C. Physiotherapy and music therapy for a girl with Rett syndrome – a dual treatment approach. Fysioterapeuten 2006;2:5-20. [Danish]

[12]   Verheul A, Hulsegge J. Snoezelen another world. Chsterfield: Rompa, 1987.

[13]   Shapiro M, Bacher S. The Snoezelen philosophy of Beit Issie Shapiro. The controlled multi-sensory environment. A guide book. Raanana, IL: Beit Issie Shapiro, 2004. [Hebrew]

[14]   Ayres JA. Sensory integration and the child, 5th ed. Los Angeles, CA: Western Psychol Serv, 1982.

[15]   Longhorn F. Planning a multi-sensory massage programme for very special people London: Catalyst Educ Resources, 1993.

[16]   Lotan M, Yelon-Haimovich S, Gold C. Meta analysis on the efficiency of Snoezelen intervention for individual with intellectual disabilities. Unpublished data.

[17]   Burns I, Cox H, Plant H. Leisure or therapeutics? Snoezelen and the care of older persons with dementia. Int J Nurs Pract 2000;6(3):118-26.

[18]   Shapiro M, Parush S, Green M, Roth D. The efficacy of the "Snoezelen" in inhibiting maladaptive behaviours and facilitating adaptive behaviors in children who are mentally retarded. Br J Dev Disabil 1997;43(2):140-53.

[19]   Lotan M, Burshtein S. Snoezelen as physical therapy intervention for senior citizens with cognitive impairment. Presentation, AAMR Ann Conf, Chicago, IL, 2003 May 21-23.

[20]   Lotan M, Burshtein S, Cahana C. The multi-sensory environment (Snoezelen) as means to improve motor/functional abilities in individuals with cognitive impairment. Two case studies. Isr J Phys Ther 2003;5(2):24-30. [Hebrew]

[21]   21.   Lotan M, Burshtein S.Happiness is merely the base, not the limit of the multi-sensory environment. Presentation, Third Natl Conf Intellect Disabil, Jerusalem, 2003 Jun 9-10.

[22]   Lotan M, Burshtein S, Cahana C, Shapiro M. The multi-sensory environment as means to reduce mal-adaptive behaviors in individuals with cognitive impairment. Two case studies. Isr J Occupat Ther 2004;13(1):H43-H56. [Hebrew]

[23]   Lotan M, Shapiro M. Management of young children with Rett disorder in the controlled multi-sensory (Snoezelen) environment. Brain Dev 2005;27(Suppl 1):S88-S94.

[24]   Lotan M, Merrick J. Rett syndrome Management with Snoezelen or controlled multi-sensory environment: A review. Int J Adolesc Med Health 2004;16(1):5-12.

[25]   Lotan M, Wein J, Elefant C, Sharf A, Yoshei Y. The Rett syndrome evaluation center in Israel. A play based assessment model. Presentation, Ann Isr Phys Ther Assoc Conf, Dead Sea, IL, 2005.

[26]   Kerr AM, Belichenko P, Woodcock T, Woodcock M. Mind and brain in Rett disorder. Brain Dev 2001;23:s44-9.

[27]   Kerr AM. Annotation: Rett syndrome: recent progress and implications for research and clinical practice. J Child Psychol Child Psychiat 2002;43(3):277-87.

[28]   Kerr AM. How can we help the youngest ones with Rett disorder? Presentation, Ann RDAUK Fam Weekend, Northampton, UK, Oct 2002.

[29]   Elefant C. Music, choice making and communication in Rett syndrome. Presentation, Int Course Rett Syndr, Ostersund, Sweden, 2003 Jun 16-18.

[30]   Kerr AM. Infant development in Rett syndrome. Presentation, Int Course Rett Syndr, Ostersund, Sweden, 2003 Jun 16-18.

[31]   Bergstrom-Isacsson M. Ways to resolve agitation. Presentation, Int Course Rett Syndr, Ostersund, Sweden, 2003 Jun 16-18.

[32]   Merker B, Bergstrom-Isacsson M, Witt Engerstrom I. Music and the Rett disorder: the Swedish Rett Center survey. Nord J Music Ther 2001;10(1):42-53.

[33]   Wigram T. Assessment and treatment of a girl with Rett syndrome. In: Bruscia K, ed. Case studies in music therapy. Gilsum, NH: Barcelona Publ, 1991.

[34]   Wigram T. A model of assessment and differential diagnosis of handicap in children through the medium of music therapy. In: Wigram T, Saperston B, West R, eds. The art and science of music therapy: A handbook. Chur, Switzerland: Harwood Acad Publ, 1995.

[35]   Wigram T. Vibro-acoustics. Presentation, Int Conf Dev Disabil, Raanana, IL: Beit Issie Shapiro, 2002.

[36]   Lotan M, Hadar-Frumer M. Aquatic rehabilitation for individuals with Rett syndrome, 2002. An E-book at: www.rettsyndrome.org/main/aquatic-rehab.htm

[37]   Kerr AM, Burford B. Towards a full life with Rett disorder. Pediatr Rehabil 2001;4(4):157-68.

[38]   Cooper RA, Kerr AM, Amos PM. Rett syndrome: Critical examination of clinical features, serial E.E.G. and video-monitoring in understanding and management. Eur J Paediatr Neurol 1998;2:127-35.

[39]   Blue ME, Naidu S, Johnston MV. Development of amino acid receptors in frontal cortex from girls with Rett syndrome. Ann Neurology 1999;45:541-45.

[40]   Johnston M. Neurobiology of Rett syndrome, a disorder of synaptic development. Presentation, Int Course Rett Syndr, Ostersund, Sweden, 2003 Jun 16-18.

[41]   Leonard S. The Australian Rett syndrome study inaugural report. Aust: Telethon Inst Child Health Res, 2002.

[42]   Kaufmann WE, Johnston MV, Blue ME. MeCP2 expression and function during brain development: implications for Rett syndrome's pathogenesis and clinical evolution. Brain Dev 2005;27(Suppl 1):S77-S87.

[43]   Armstrong DD. The neuropathology of Rett syndrome. Overview 1994. Neuoropediatrics 1995;26:100-4.

[44]   Kaufmann WE, Taylor CV, Hohmann CF, Sanwal IB Naidu S. Abnormalities in neuronal maturation in Rett syndrome neocortex: preliminary molecular correlates. Eur Child Adolesc Psychiatry 1997;6:75-7.

[45]   Belichenco PV. The morphological substrate for communication. In: Kerr AM, Witt-Engerstrom I, eds. Rett disorder and the developing brain, Oxford: Oxford Univ Press, 2001:277-302.

[46]   Lotan M. Roth, D. The effect of hand vibrators on the hand stereotypes and function in Rett syndrome; Two case studies. Isr Physiother Quart 1996;52:23-6. [Hebrew]

[47]   Hanks SB. Why physical therapy? Rett Gazette, Spring 2001. Also available at IRSA web site: http://www.rettsyndrome.org/main/orthopaedic-update.htm

[48]   Hanks SB. Physical therapy strategies. Presentation, IRSA 12th Ann Conf, Boston, MA, 1996 May 24-27, Tape 622-08.

[49]   Weekes L. Rett syndrome. Presentation, Sydney, Aust, Feb 1997.

[50]   Rossin LK. Effectiveness of therapeutic and surgical intervention in the treatment of scoliosis in Rett syndrome. A seminar work, University of Duquesne; 1997:1-19.

[51]   Caulton JM, Ward KA, Alsop CW, Dunn G, Adams JE, Mughal MZ.A randomised controlled trial of standing programme on bone mineral density in non-ambulant children with cerebral palsy. Arch Dis Child 2004;89(2):131-5.

[52]   McClure MK, Battaglia C, McClure RS The relationship of cumulative motor asymmetries to scoliosis in Rett syndrome. J Occup Ther 1998;52(3):196-204.

[53]   Hanks SB. Motor disabilities in the Rett syndrome and physical therapy strategies. Brain Dev 1990;12:157-61.

[54]   Lotan M, Isakov E, Merrick J. Improving functional skills and physical fitness in children with Rett syndrome. J Intell Disabil Res 2004;48(8):730-5.

[55]   Hunter, K. The Rett syndrome handbook. Washington, DC: Int Rett Syndr Assoc, 1999.

[56]   Larsson G, Engerstrom IW. Gross motor ability in Rett syndrome- the power of expectation, motivation and planning. Brain Dev Dec 2001;23 (Suppl1):S77-S81.

[57]   Budden SS. Rett syndrome: habilitation and management reviewed. Eur Child Adolesc Psychiatry 1997;6(Suppl 1):103-7.

[58]   Jacobsen K, Viken A, Von Tetzchner S. Rett syndrome and aging: a case study. Disabil Rehabil 2001;23:160-6.

[59]   Elefant C. Speechless yet communicative: Revealing the person behind the disability of Rett syndrome through clinical research on songs in music therapy. In: Aldridge D, DiFranco G, Ruud E, Wigram T. eds. Music therapy in Europe. Rome: ISMEZ, 2001.

[60]   Gaines C. Making use of augmentative and alternative communication. Int Rett Syndr Assoc Newsletter Winter 1998:1,8.

[61]   Haas RH, Dixon SD, Sartoris DJ, Hennessy MJ. Osteopenia in Rett syndrome. J Pediatr 1997;131(5):771-4.

[62]   Leonard H, Thomson M, Glasson E, Fyfe S, Leonard S, Ellaway C, Christodouloon J, Bower C. Metacarpophalangeal pattern profile and bone age in Rett syndrome: Further radiological clues to the diagnosis. Am J Med Gen 1999;12(83):88-95.

[63]   Budden SS, Gunness ME. Bone histomorphometry in three females with Rett syndrome. Brain Dev 2001;23:S133-7.

[64]   Kerr, A. The future for girls with Rett syndrome. Int Rett Syndr Assoc Newsletter 1992;Summer:1314.

[65]   Engerstrom IW, Kerr A. Workshop on autonomic function in Rett syndrome, Swedish Rett Center, Frösön, Sweden. Brain Dev 1998;20:323-6.

Chapter XV

Rett Syndrome: Assistive Technology and Supplementary Treatment

Meir Lotan, BPT, MScPT, PhD[*]

Israeli Rett Center, National Evaluation Team, Chaim Sheba Medical Center, Tel Hashomer, Ramat Gan and Department of Physical Therapy, Ariel University Center of Samaria, Ariel, Israel

Rett Syndrome (RS) is a neurological disorder, affecting mainly females, caused by MECP2 mutations usually resulting in severe physical disability. Due to the physical challenges faced by the individual with RS and her family, her rehabilitation program should support her throughout different daily activities, contexts and surroundings. Habilitative interventions to reverse physical impairments include exercise of various types and different physical modalities. Nevertheless, in the vast majority of cases, hands-on therapeutic intervention opportunities are available for the client through a minute part of her waking hours. Hence, a supplementary system is required in order to engulf the child with a comprehensive network of support. Supplementary intervention can support physical impairment by introducing adaptive techniques, environmental modifications and assistive technologies. The therapy program of an individual with RS should include the use of assistive technology when such devices improve the user's performance. The term "supplementary management" relates to the fact that this intervention may be performed by non-professionals with the supervision of a qualified therapist. Such an intervention can further support the therapeutic goals of the client, at a time when direct intervention is not supplied. The present chapter will review the available literature on the topic of assistive technology, incorporating the clinical knowledge of the author in the field of RS.

* Correspondence: Meir Lotan, BPT, MScPT, PhD, Department of Physical Therapy, Ariel University Center of Samaria, IL-40700 Ariel, Israel. E-mail: ml_pt_rs@netvision.net.il

Introduction

Intervention for people with Rett Syndrome (RS) is aimed at compensating for and reduction of physical abilities and includes therapeutic intervention, adaptive techniques, environmental modifications and assistive technologies [1]. The intervention of health related disciplines, such as physiotherapy, occupational therapy, music therapy or others, should not be limited to what is administered in the treatment room or during individually applied sessions (also known as direct therapy). In order to attain a continuous effect, therapists and caring staff should work as a team with the family of the individual with RS to construct a comprehensive intervention program that includes both the educational facility as well as the individual's residence. Kerr [2] has asserted that exercise taught to care-givers is highly recommended throughout the life of the individual with RS and she suggests that regular activity is essential for the long-lasting health of this population [2].

The aim of this chapter is to present the use of assistive technology in order to construct a support network around the individual with RS. ("assistive technology" refers specifically to devices used to compensate for physical limitations. The term may be used narrowly to refer to special tools used to accomplish an activity [e.g., a walker] or it may include orthotics [e.g., braces, splints], as well as some adaptive techniques, which refer to modifications in the way an activity is carried out [1]. Such day-by-day and hour-to-hour support is advised, suggesting that everyone who is in contact with the individual with RS will be aware of her needs and supportive to her supplementary management program.

The term "supplementary management program" implies continuous care for the individual by use of time, intensity of appropriate handling and suitable assistive devices. A supplementary management program will accompany and support the client's therapeutic régime throughout the day. Such a program can help the individual with RS during all the wearying battles she must constantly wage against the limitations that RS imposes on her. Since RS is always present and never relents, treatment management should continue through every available minute of every day. This chapter will present possibilities for interventions that might be used even during the resting hours of the individual with RS, as well as utilizing her play and recreation time for the introduction of therapeutic elements without harming the joy of the user and the quality of her life.

The scope of this chapter is broad, with the intention of accommodating professionals as well as care-givers of individuals with RS and therefore, on occasion, could be found to be written by the experienced therapist in too much detail. When assistive devices are warranted, it is important that equipment and aids are prepared and chosen with the help of a multi-professional team that centers on the client, the family and other primary caregivers. Also involved in this process are the staff of the educational facility, agencies responsible for funding and members of the community who are in contact with the family. All these people must each contribute their part to attain the best possible results. All these aspects constitute the full scope of the supplementary management program.

Despite widespread use of assistive technology [3] in recent years for various populations, research on assistive technology, for the general user population as well as for individuals with RS, is relatively sparse and therefore, the scope of this chapter is mainly clinical. While reviewing available literature on issues of assistive technology, this chapter will present ideas that have been found successful for individuals with RS and might be found useful for others bearing the same diagnosis and who are in need of assistive technology.

Due to individual expression of RS and due to the ever-changing abilities and challenges facing this population, the therapist should not limit him\herself to conventions that have already been tried. When there are no existing solutions, there is a need to use imagination, to explore some crazy notions and to experiment with new ideas. In the words of Yalom[4], taken from another professional context but with the same spirit in mind, "inspire yourself to create a new treatment for each client." Anything that might get the client with RS to improve her disposition or performance is worth investigating.

Basic aspects of assistive technology

It is common knowledge that there are many negative aspects associated with the acquisition and use of assistive technology [5-8]. The main reasons that clients (in our case, the individual with RS and her family) abandon assistive technology is that they feel that the equipment does not meet their needs [9], the equipment is in disrepair, does not fit properly [10] or because they have difficulty operating or using it [11]. Therefore, and due to the complex nature of assistive technology and the ample factors associated with its purchase, it is advised that experienced health related professionals, knowledgeable in the area of assistive technology and RS, be involved in the process of adapting the most appropriate equipment. Furthermore, when choosing the appropriate assistive technology, the following factors should be taken into consideration:

- The child's physical profile (deformities, motor ability and tendency towards pressure sores)
- Environmental circumstances (elevators, transportation vehicles, access paths)
- Behavioral needs (such as self-injurious behavior -SIB)
- Daily routine (numerous transitions vs. remaining in one location)
- Future needs (due to change of residence, available support, or changes in function)

Professional experts can help to ensure that the device fits the client and her unique needs, recommend how to use the device correctly and provide training for the proper and full use of the device. Depending on the type of equipment required, a qualified therapist should assess the individual and make a recommendation to the organization responsible for the provision of the equipment or to the person or agency that has requested the assessment.

The complexity of the procedure necessitates that details are clarified before purchasing and adapting any technological aids [12] (see figure XV-1). It is important to weigh the advantages of the device. If we know how to provide a client with a bed that will keep her from falling out, a lift to prevent a care-giver from suffering backaches or a standing frame that can help the person to avoid future surgery for lengthening of the Achilles tendon, then we have achieved our objective. Daily practice and use of suitable aids will enable the client to attain improvement and prevent deterioration.

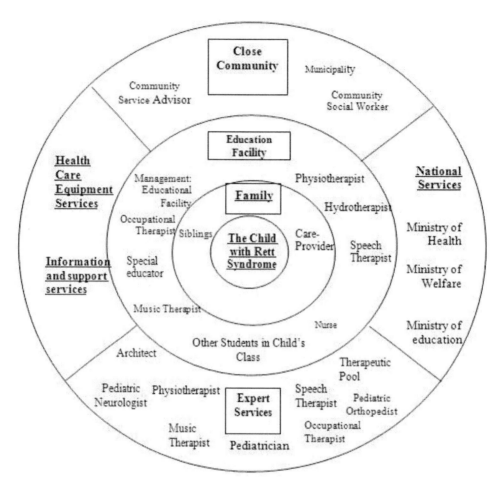

Figure XV-1. Schematic drawing of the different participants influencing supplementary treatment and assistive technology for individuals with RS, presenting the complexity of this issue and the many bodies involved in administering assistive technology for the individual with RS (adapted from Hedman[13]).

Assistive technology and rett syndrome

The Australian RS study [14] has gathered information regarding the use of assistive technology among individuals with RS. Their findings suggested that the majority of individuals with RS are using such appliances (see figure XV-2).

Despite the obvious need for such appliances to assist in the daily lives of individuals with RS, many have commented that "they had difficulty in obtaining the equipment…." The commonly mentioned obstacles in acquiring assistive technology were "the financial expenses and challenges associated with acquiring this equipment" [14]. Due to such difficulties, this chapter aims to introduce the elaborate process involved in the proper purchase, adaptation and use of such appliances, with special focus on individuals with RS. There are ten basic steps involved in choosing or adapting assistive technology:

- Identifying the problem
- Determining realistic objectives in a discussion with the client's human surroundings
- Performing a functional evaluation
- Planning the required intervention
- Choosing suitable technological aids
- Attaining funds
- Delivering the equipment and instructing the staff and/or family in its use
- Installing the equipment
- Practicing the use of the equipment
- Performing follow-up assessment

The stages that precede the purchase of assistive technology are critical and are therefore discussed here in detail.

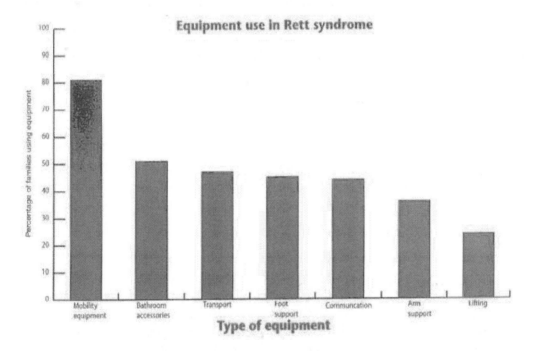

Figure XV-2. Equipment used by individuals with RS.

Identifying the problem

This stage is also connected to the second step of the above: defining the desired objective (the individual with RS will be able to walk independently in-house, using her hart walker; the individual with RS will be able to feed herself, throughout mealtime using an adapted spoon). This stage involves performing a preliminary evaluation that will enable identification of the existing strengths and difficulties in achieving the desired objective.

Performing a functional and environmental evaluation

This evaluation should identify functional difficulties and ways through which they might be alleviated. This evaluation should take into account the abilities and disabilities of the person with RS, her human support factors (such as care-givers, parents, siblings and the educational staff), her various living environments (home, school, community) and the frequency and mode of transportation between these environments[12,15].

Determining realistic objectives

After the preliminary evaluation, objectives that can be achieved without the use of aids can be determined. The basic concept is that assistive technology should be used as infrequently as possible, but according to client capability and demand. Only when the therapist has identified existing difficulties in attaining functional abilities through independent function and only after the thorough investigation into the use of adaptive techniques has been explored, then the use of assistive technology should be considered.

Planning the necessary intervention

The evaluation helps us to decide if it is preferable to begin an intensive rehabilitation program to increase the person's independent functional abilities or to conclude that the objective cannot be attained without technical aids. It is important to assess each person and to choose treatment strategies that are compatible to her personal needs and abilities [16].

Choosing suitable assistive technology

After the completion of the evaluation and the arrival at conclusions regarding the need for assistive technology, we must search the available selection and find the aids that are suitable to the needs of each person within her various life surroundings, modes of transport and other aspects of her need. If professionals or institutions who deal with assistive technology have not yet been consulted, this is the time to get them involved. Choosing assistive technology demands a wise, educated decision, based on consultation with a variety of experts [17], as can be viewed in figure XV-1. Attention should be paid to the following issues:

- Compatibility — with the patient's present needs, her age and her expected future development.
- Choice — Assess the numerous choices that are available and consult with a professional. Sometimes equipment can be borrowed in order to assess its suitability before purchasing it. Due to the unbalanced sensory system of the individual with RS and her difficulties adjusting to new situations [18], this option is strongly advised.
- Safety and quality — Ensure that the device is stable and has no dangerous, sharp corners or any small parts that might get lost or swallowed. Preference should be given to equipment that bears a stamp of approval by official agencies.

- Adjustments — Consider the number of times it will be necessary to re-adapt the equipment during the period of time it will be in use. Can this be done easily? Will these changes have any effect on its usability or safety?
- Comfort — Can the equipment be used comfortably? Can the client easily utilize it? Could the material from which it is made endanger the user? Is its structure comfortable? Can the care-giver operate and maintain it easily?
- Acceptance — It is important that the equipment be acceptable to the individual with RS who will be using it and by her caregivers and parents. Rejection of assistive technology by users for various reasons will quickly terminate its use even if the device itself is of assistance to the user. The opinion of the individual with RS regarding the designated instrumentation could be examined through the use of Assistive Augmentative Communication (AAC).
- Transport and storage — Equipment must be of a size and weight that can meet everyday needs, such as transport and/or storage. (A heavy wheelchair or a large rollator may be abandoned due the difficulty of transporting it on a daily basis.)
- Cleaning — Ensure that there are no small cracks or areas that will be difficult to keep clean, leading to abandonment of the equipment due to inappropriate appearance or smell.
- Repair and replacement parts — Check the cost of replacement parts before they are actually needed, in order to avoid unexpected expenses later on.
- The vendor (equipment supplier) — It is important to verify with other clients the trustworthiness of the vendor and get answers to important questions, such as: "Will maintenance personnel come to the client's home or must the equipment be brought to a repair shop or laboratory for repair?" "Are replacement parts readily available or should they be imported from abroad, thereby lengthening the duration of each breakdown?" It is important to clarify the previous track record that the supplier has in respect of this type of technology. Can they insure the equipment against damages? Do they offer training for the use of the device and, if so, what is the cost of such training? Is the device already in stock or will there be a wait of several weeks or months until it arrives?
- Instruction — Is there a need for instruction before using the device? How long does the instruction take? What are the cognitive demands of instruction and who will receive it (the individual's care-givers, parents or the user herself)?
- Attaining funds — Many assistive technology devices are extremely expensive. Funding for the equipment and the sources available should be assessed at the beginning of the process! A situation in which we have completed the assessment only to find that the necessary equipment is beyond the financial means should be avoided, since it will cause disappointment to all involved.
- Delivering the equipment and instructing the caregivers and/or family — As mentioned earlier, sources of information should be clarified before purchasing a piece of equipment. In many cases, renting a piece of equipment for several weeks can help to determine if it is suitable for the client. If an aid is purchased for an individual with RS, it must be ensured that everyone involved in her care receives clear instructions from the manufacturer and the therapist involved regarding its use, operation and maintenance. In some cases, there is no specific available device that can exactly provide the user's needs. When this is the case, it should be clarified in advance as to whether or not the manufacturer can provide for the equipment special alterations that are unavailable when buying it and how much these alterations will

cost. If the manufacturer cannot make the necessary alterations, help should be sought from organizations/experts that provide specially adapted equipment which can not be readily purchased.

- Installing the equipment — The device (powered wheelchair, elevator or adapted vehicle) should be installed by an experienced service-person and a warranty should be obtained for the installation.
- Practicing the use of the equipment — Any new piece of equipment demands a period of adaptation, particularly when dealing with individuals with RS who might show difficulties adapting to new situations. Often, users are unaware of the overall potential of the device and use it inappropriately due to insufficient initial practice, knowledge and\or training [19,20].
- Follow-up assessment — A trained health related professional should be invited for a follow-up examination about 2 weeks to 1 month after the assistive technology device has been put into use, even if it appears that the purchase and choice of equipment has been carried out successfully. This visit is intended to ensure that everyone involved is acquainted with the device and knows how to operate it in normal circumstances or in an emergency and that the device is providing suitable aid for the user with RS.

Supplementary management program using assistive technology

As previously stated, the person with RS should be constantly supported in her functional needs and the goals of health related personnel intervention should be carried out continuously in order for the client to gain maximal therapeutic results. Such intervention is referred to as a supplementary management program and is performed by her human milieu of support during times when health related interventions are not directly applied. This form of intervention can be introduced by using different assistive technology devices and the following part of the chapter will screen different aids in accordance with different postures of the individual with RS. Photos will be presented mostly when the assistive technology device in question or the method of use is unique to this population.

Lying down

Since 15–50% of individuals with RS are able to walk[21,22] it is hoped that they will spend only a small amount of time lying down. Nevertheless, if lying down is implemented, therapeutic thinking should turn the simple act of being on the mattress\bed to a situation involving therapeutic elements.

Prone lying

Prone lying can be utilized for improving and encouraging weight-bearing on the arms and strengthening trunk extensors. This position might inhibit stereotypical hand movements, as well as increase sensory information from the upper limbs, thereby enhancing body scheme. Prone lying should be encouraged before meals or before individual intervention sessions, during which the person with RS is expected to use her hands. For a person who is a constant wheelchair user, lying on the stomach can be employed as an alternative position, to cut down periods of prolonged sitting, thus avoiding the development of decubitus (pressure sores) and preventing flexion contractures of the hips. Using a wedge (see figure XV-3) can encourage safe, active play for children who suffer from extreme fear of movement and are afraid of transitioning from one position to another.

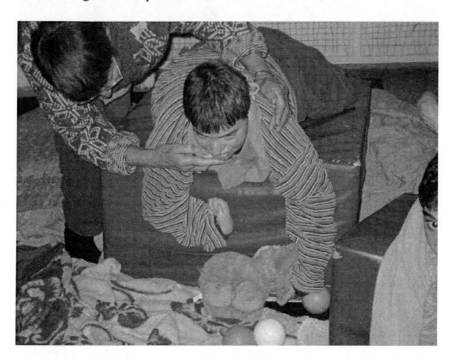

Figure XV-3. A child on a wedge.

Lying on the floor is a good position to encourage social contact with younger siblings; a point of strength and motivation for most individuals with RS. This position can also be utilized to encourage and motivate play. If the mat on which the person is lying is covered with interesting, colorful material, she will attempt to change the angle of her head and body and try touching it. Play can also be encouraged by placing several toys that she likes nearby, placing colored stickers on her hands, placing a bracelet with bells on her wrist or any other stimulation that will encourage intentional movement of the hands and fingers.

Lying on the stomach is a relatively safe position for an ataxic person who has difficulty controlling her movements. This position encourages the individual to use her hands while her body is fully supported. It will improve joint stability as well as contribute to normalizing muscle tone, while strengthening the upper back muscles. If we place a wedge under the person with RS, it will be easier for her to use her hands to push her body into maintaining an erect position. The person with RS can be encouraged to bear weight on her arms with relative ease by placing inflatable plastic swimming buoys or elbow supports on her forearms (see figure XV-4).

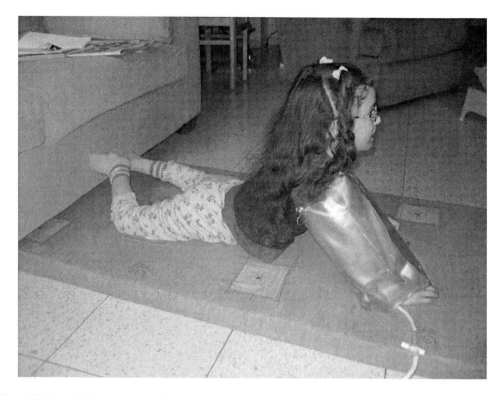

Figure XV-4. A child with plastic elbow supports.

It is important to place individuals with kyphosis or ones that constantly use a wheelchair (over 10 h/day) in this position on a daily basis. In the case of clients who have already developed flexion contractures of the hips/pelvis/lower back, the use of small pillows under the abdomen is recommended at initial trials in the new position, gradually decreasing the pillows in size. These could be placed under the pelvis until the individual with RS is able with minimal discomfort to assume a straighter position on the mat or surface.

The very hypotonic individual with RS might show considerable difficulty in maintaining an erect position while sitting. Exercising her upper trunk muscles might initially be possible only in prone position. In this posture, with the aid of an interesting motivational factor (a toy, TV, a family member), the person will strengthen her upper back musculature. Such a program, if performed on a daily basis and gradually increasing in duration, might later result in improved sitting ability.

Another possible position would be to place the person with RS on a massage bed with a hole for her head, with her hand on two sides of the head. In this posture, her whole body, including the shoulders and upper torso is erect. This position is recommended due to the tendency of individuals with RS to attain a kyphotic posture due to their constant hand mannerisms resulting also in shortened neck extensors muscles (see figure XV-5).

Caution: When assuming the position, it is important to prevent the neck from achieving a hyperextended position. This can be achieved if the individual's focus of interest (such as the TV screen) is properly situated. For instance, if the surface on which she is lying is a bit higher than the TV's level, she will also be using her upper trunk musculature in a straight posture, holding her head in an erect position. Another solution could be to place the TV under the bed.

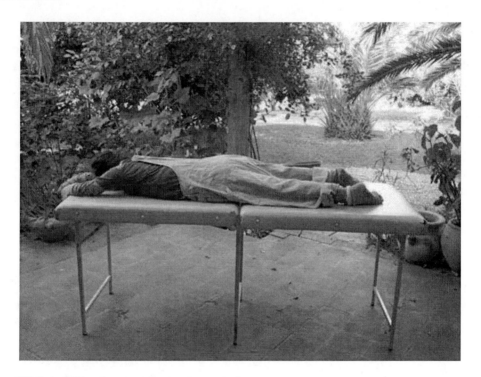

Figure XV-5. A child on her stomach on a therapy bed.

Supine lying

This position can be used to achieve numerous objectives such as socialization. In this position, the individual with RS can see playmates and young siblings can be encouraged to make close, intimate contact with their sister. Shiny toys that will draw visual attention or make noises, plush toy animals or other objects that will encourage her to reach out, can be placed above the person with RS when she is in supine lying.

Lying the client on her back is a good starting point for rolling her from side to side. This type of movement could be a part of a stimulation plan intended to reduce fear of movement and accustom the individual with RS to movement (many individuals with RS are afraid of movement and this fear is expressed by an anxiety towards external manipulation) [23]. Moving the person from side to side while she is on her back causes massive tactile stimulation that helps her to construct body schemas (particularly if she is active in performing part of the movement). Such exercise might make it easier for her to cope with manipulation by an external facilitator and for moving her body at other instances. The straightening of the thighs and knees and elongation of the anterior pelvis and stomach muscles are also attained in this position. Therefore, supine lying is an important position for individuals who spend an extended duration of time in a wheelchair. From this position, the person is able to change to side lying position.

Side lying

Lying on one side also achieves various treatment objectives. This position can be used for individuals who spend most of the day in a wheelchair. It is a good transitional position and can be used to prevent pressure sores in the buttocks area. It is also another position from which the individual with RS can view the world, experiencing a slightly different angle. Lying on one side encourages the raising of the head to the central axis, thereby strengthening the side muscles of the neck and trunk and improving head control (poor head control is typical of individuals with hypotonia). Maintaining this position while the care-giver/therapist/parent performs slow rhythmical movements will help in balancing muscle tone. Therefore, individuals who are extremely spastic or hypotonic can gain advantage from being placed in this position.

The static position of the lower extremities resting on the mattress enables a good, stable base for movement of the upper extremities and trunk against it. Therefore, this position can be introduced as part of a "range of motion" program for the individual with RS. Side lying stabilizes the body of the ataxic individual and might enable successful attempts of hand usage during play activities. Therefore, it is also important to place games, favorite toys, a mirror, family pictures, favorite foods or the family pet in front of her when she is lying in this position, in order to enhance functional hand movement.

Side lying is extremely important during instances when the shortening of soft tissues at the trunk is observed. If this condition is not dealt with, the client's back muscles on one side may become shortened, gradually leading to a loss of erect postures. Such a situation might terminate in loss of independent seating, standing and\or walking and the development of scoliosis. The person with RS should be placed in this position using special support, such as a small cylinder made out of a pillow, blanket, or rolled-up towel, with the affected side upward (i.e., an individual with a right-oriented scoliosis should be placed on her right side). This position mechanically elongates the tissues, thereby preventing or at least inhibiting the shortening of the trunk muscles.

A good, permanent side position can also be achieved at night by rolling a sheet around the client while she is lying on her side[24]. If the individual with RS does not mind, she might be placed in this position while resting or sleeping and by implementing such a program, the time-length invested in supplementary management program will be greatly extended. Another way to lengthen the treatment time for lying on one side is to use a U-shaped pillow to keep the person in the desired position. Using this type of pillow is an efficient method of treatment, when curvature of the spine develops (see figure XV-6).

This type of pillow can be made from stiff foam rubber, Styrofoam or soft plastic. The amount of firmness depends on the user's reaction and the amount of time she spends lying on that pillow. Lying on one side is a good starting point for getting up onto a side-sitting position. Side-sitting usually involves weight bearing on the arms, which is another important therapeutic element for individuals with RS.

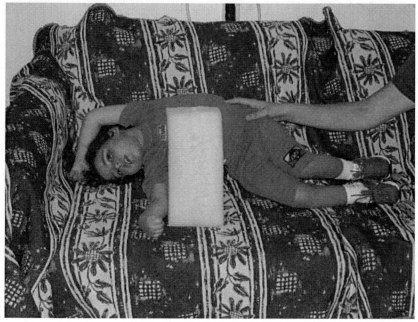

Figure XV-6. A child side lying with a U-shaped pillow.

Sitting

The objective of placing the person with RS in a sitting position is to provide external support and help her to function, despite her various limitations. Proper sitting solves existing problems, improves stability, and lessens the person's total disability. The objectives of correct sitting are [25]:

- To improve manual function
- To improve lung function
- To improve motor control of the mouth, thus improving eating and drinking
- To normalize muscle tone and improve balance of the trunk
- To improve proper movement, thus improving function
- To allow more time for leisure and socialization
- To improve the trunk and head control
- To improve quality and quantity of vocalization
- To enhance comfort and improve quality of life

A "seating system" is a general term describing any chair in which the person sits. Before adapting any type of chair, it is important to consider and analyze the user's everyday physical needs, as well as those of her caregivers and members of her family. Different sitting options are described for possible implementation in the next section (see the guidelines for integrating assistive technology described at the beginning of this chapter).

Puff chairs/bean-bags

Puff chairs are large bags fashioned out of cloth or leather, and filled with tiny Styrofoam balls. They can be molded into many shapes to support the person's entire body. When seated in a puff chair, the individual with RS feels secure, comfortable, and well contained. It is preferable to use this type of seating arrangement for short periods of time or for short dozing periods during the day, or in order to relax the back muscles after prolonged duration of functional activity (seating, standing, walking).

It is important to remember that this type of chair decreases the individual's mobility (which is already restricted due her objective physical limitations). When the individual with RS is placed in a partially prone position, her trunk is bent forward into a kyphotic position, which is prevalent among this population and therefore must be discouraged.

Individuals who are able to ambulate independently should not be encouraged to use puff chairs on a permanent basis. When a person is seated on such a bag, it is extremely difficult to get up from. Since the ability to perform transitional changes is one of the first mobility elements lost by individuals with RS [26,27], such passive placement for prolonged periods of time is not highly recommended

Side Seater

A side seat is a therapeutic device developed by the author for individuals with RS showing asymmetry of the trunk. Such intervention should be implemented as soon as an asymmetry of the trunk is noticeable [28].

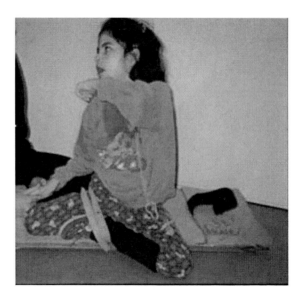

Figure XV-7. A side seater.

The device is designed to encourage asymmetric work of the trunk through balance reactions and is, therefore, an efficient tool for preventing, or at least reducing curvature of the spine among individuals with RS [28]. The position of the individual with RS in this device is stable, thus encouraging hand function and play. The straps that hold the person in place do not allow mobility. Therefore the seater is recommended for ambulant individuals only for short periods during the day. The height of the side support in this device should be adjusted against the height of the potential collapse point of the person's spine and should be designed to encourage active side flexion and extension (see figure XV-7).

Corner chair

This type of chair is usually made of wood. The corner chair offers strong support for the back and keeps it straight and perpendicular to the legs. This type of support to the trunk frees the hands to perform manual activities. A table (with a rim around it to prevent toys\communication devices, etc. from falling off) can be attached to the chair in order to encourage communication and play. The height of the back can be changed according to the height of the person sitting and the amount of support she needs. Therefore, this type of chair is also suitable for individuals with poor head control. The chair holds the person with RS in a full, seated position and thereby stretches the muscles of the lower back as well as the hamstrings. The chair keeps the person sitting in a stationary position and offers security but on the other hand, prevents movement. This type of chair may assist in giving the user with RS a symmetrical proprioceptive stimulus, establishing midline perception. Therefore, it could be used as a preventive measure for the development of skewed midline, leading to the development of scoliosis as suggested by Hanks [27].

The downside of this chair is that the user is unable to get herself out of it. It is not recommended that this type of chair be used for a person with self-ambulation abilities for long periods of time. When using this chair, the user must be strapped in so that her pelvis is at the back of the chair and her knees are only slightly bent. The care-giver/therapist/parent should be advised that if a waist-belt is not used to hold the person sitting in a proper seating position, she will slip forward, thereby encouraging the progression of a kyphotic curvature of the lower section of the spine.

Knee chair

This type of chair (see figure XV-8) is built so that it creates lumbar lordosis by tilting the pelvis forward (producing an anterior pelvic tilt). It offers support for the knees and pelvis but leaves the back free for activity while being supported due to the pelvic posture. Using such a chair should be considered as a means for preventing curvature of the spine and kyphosis [24]. These chairs can be used with rocker bottoms, intertwining stability and security with motion, and can be controlled by the user (the amount of movements caused by the users trunk sway will influence her rocking). This type of chair could be considered for use as a possible intervention management device for the person showing fear of movement (initially placing it over a thick carpet, gradually moving the chair to a firmer floor).

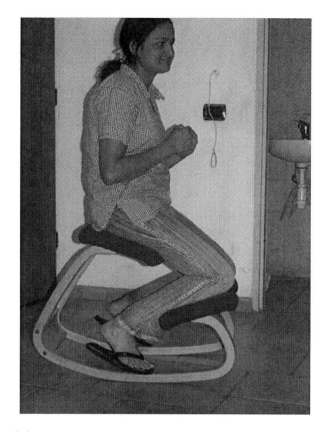

Figure XV-8. A knee chair.

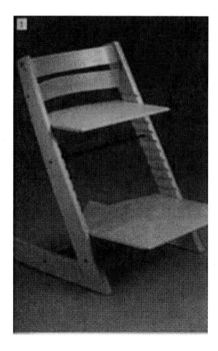

Figure XV-9. A trip trap chair.

Trip trap chair

This type of chair is recommended by many parents. It is aesthetic, it enables movement while the person is seated and its dimensions can be changed easily as the child grows, or in order to adjust it to the height of a family table (see figure XV-9).

This type of chair is suitable only for those with full trunk control, since no trunk support is present. The disadvantage of this chair is that its foot-rest is usually higher than the floor, creating a sort of a step, from which most individuals with RS find it difficult to descend. This step impairs the user's independence and movement. In the case of mobile individuals, it is preferable to consider a chair without a foot-rest so that the user is free to get up independently and walk away from the chair. Another possibility is to add a small staircase to this type of chair, thereby producing an opportunity to practice stair-climbing and descending before and after every use of the chair.

Stools

Individuals with RS have a tendency to lean against the nearest stable object around them, including, when seated, the backs of chairs. The author's experience has shown that in some individuals with RS, this phenomenon is exaggerated and leads to a permanent tendency at all situations to lean back, resulting in extension of the trunk when standing and walking, up to a point where independent walking and even sitting is lost. The ability to make transitions and change positions is one of the first motor functions lost by the individual with RS [26,27] and strong measures should be taken to keep the client as active as possible [2]. Seating the individual with RS on a stool is helpful in achieving such goals. Sitting on a stool obligates the individual to actively preserve balance of the trunk and prevents her from reverting to a permanently reclining position.

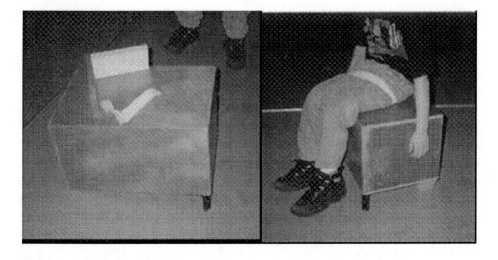

Figure XV-10. A child sitting on an active uneven stool.

If such level of trunk control can be achieved by individuals showing severe scoliosis, an uneven active seating surface can be introduced as a corrective measure against the development of scoliosis (see figure XV-10).

If the individual with RS possesses higher degrees of stability, it might be possible to consider the use of a T-chair as a regular practice.

Normal chairs

Any chair must be adapted to the specific needs of each user. For this reason and due to the fact that each individual with RS is different, there is no standard chair for them as a group. The basic guidelines when considering a chair for your child/client should be:

- Individuals with RS tend to lean towards available support. Therefore, any support, including chest vests, should be avoided as much as possible and active seating, even for parts of the day, should be constantly encouraged and implemented. If prolonged seating is difficult, start with short seating durations, which increase gradually as the child trunk control and muscle strength are improved.
- A belt should always be added as a means for appropriate pelvis positioning and if the seated person with RS is prone to epileptic seizures, a heavy-duty knuckle should be added to the belt as a safety measure.
- The client's feet must fully touch the floor in order to avoid shortening of the Achilles tendon, to provide constant sensory input and supply stability for function.
- The height of the foot-rests should allow for independent climbing and descending for individuals capable of such performance.
- Side supports might be added, if necessary, according to the person's trunk control and spinal deformities (although even in severe cases of scoliosis, it is highly recommended to try to achieve, as a daily intervention program, unsupported erect seating).
- The table at which the individual with RS is seated should not be too high as to limit hand function or too low as to encourage bending forward of the trunk, which can promote a kyphotic posture of the upper back. The rule of thumb is that the working surface (table) should be 5 cm (2 in.) lower than the elbows when the arms are held against the user's body. This height will enable her to control objects that are on the table and to engage in activities such as finger feeding, reaching for a cup (suited with a straw) and operating a communication board or a computer switch.

A heavy, stable chair should be considered for heavy individuals who are prone to epileptic seizures or are engaged in intense rocking and swaying movements. In order to add stability in such cases (epilepsy) without considerable addition to the chair's own weight, additional side supports can be added to the base of the chair to keep it from toppling over.

When a person with RS displays the first signs of curvature of the spine, intervention should be suggested immediately [28]. Asymmetrical corrections can be made to the side of the chair by raising the affected side (if the individual is showing right scoliosis, then the right side of the chair should be elevated to tilt the individuals weight to the left) and adding a side support at the level of the tip of her scoliosis (see figures XV-11, XV-12).

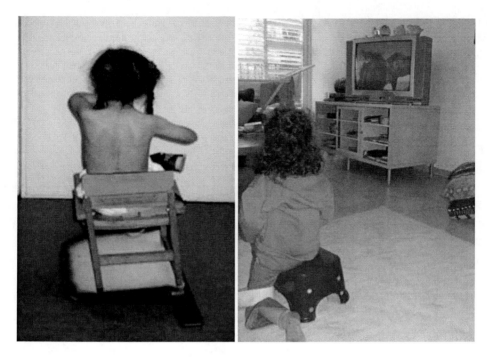

Figures XV-11, XV-12. Children with RS sitting on specially adapted chairs.

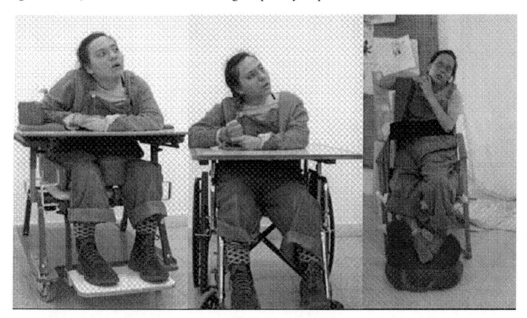

Figures XV-13-XV-15. A child with three different seating arrangements.

The point of this exercise is to encourage asymmetric muscle work against the direction of the curvature [29]. If the cause of the scoliosis is sensorial in origin, other measures should also be taken [30,31]. Usually, we would hope for the individual with RS to be as active as possible at all times or at least involved at a part-time activity program (such as an active seating arrangement). At the same time, we want her to keep her concentration focused on educational intervention and enjoy her meals as well as her recreation time (mostly spent in a comfortable chair). Furthermore, we do not want her to miss out on outdoor activities involving family and friends that might require walking beyond her capabilities (in such cases a wheelchair can be implemented). Therefore, in specific situations, the person with RS may need an array of seating arrangements to meet her different daily requirements (see figures XV-13-XV-15).

Wheelchairs

The initial decision to use a wheelchair is an extremely difficult one at most times and must be assessed after consulting with the parents as well as with the management staff. It is often easier to accept the first wheelchair if it is similar to a child's stroller, is non-disability oriented and appears as unthreatening as possible. A wheelchair, when appropriately administered, provides a good sitting position and mobility for the user who presents with limited ability to walk. It also provides support for individuals with postural problems or deformity while improving comfort, independence and safety during seated activities [32].

The author would like to emphasize here that moving from a stroller to a wheelchair should not mean giving up on walking altogether. One of the children with RS for whom I personally cared received her first wheelchair at the age of 8 due to her large physical stature and her extreme body sway making it difficult to control her movement through assisted ambulation. She is now 18 years old and still performs most of her daily ambulation by means of (assisted) walking due to the fact that her family kept her on a daily walking program.

Guidance from a therapist knowledgeable in wheelchairs and seating systems is advised whenever a client is prescribed a wheelchair but it is particularly important for individuals who are at risk of pressure sores, who show postural problems and/or difficulty with sitting balance and will use the wheelchair most or all of the time [1], as is the case with many individuals with RS. As stated before, each individual with RS is different from others with the same condition and, on top of that, the symptoms and phenotypic expression of the syndrome might change with age. Younger girls are mostly hypotonic and walking may be difficult for them; 15–50% of the girls with RS do not develop ambulation and are therefore in need of a proper seating arrangement appropriate for lengthy seated durations and transportation [22]. At an older age, some of them develop high muscle tone while others will show fluctuating/distonic muscle tone [33]. The first seating arrangement is usually an adapted baby stroller. Some young individuals with RS who are able to walk may also need a stroller for outdoor activities with their family; 25–85% of individuals with RS are expected to lose their ability to walk at a later age (when they reach stage IV of RS), therefore possibly needing a wheelchair [22,33]. The type of chair and any personal adaptations are determined by the user's physical condition and needs. There are three main types of manual wheelchairs:

- The basic wheelchair includes a folding sling seat and has removable footrests and armrests, yet sling seats may create discomfort, in the long run and can make it difficult to change position, increasing the risk of pressure sores [1]. Due to the slim stature of most individuals with RS and the potentially long durations in seated positions, a linear insert over the basic chair is recommended. Such an insert presents a stiff backrest and seat, supplying stability and support. When a linear insert is not suggested, a seat cushion should be used with the wheelchair. Special air and gel cushions are available to reduce risk of pressure sores in patients who have limited ability to shift their weight while seated [32]. This type of chair is suitable for individuals with minimal deformities and for those who present good trunk control.

- Wheelchairs with an adapted setup that is usually added with a modular insert. Other supports, such as a headrest, arm supports or a pommel (knee separator) can be added. This type of chair provides external support and stability, which (in some cases according to individual needs) may be asymmetrical, in order to adapt to the user's body curvatures. In this manner, pressure is distributed throughout the body, reducing the risk for developing pressure sores. This type of chair is padded with various combinations of foam.

- Custom-molded wheelchairs provide a seating arrangement totally adapted to the curvatures of the seated person's body and offer the most stable form of support. When this type of seating is well adapted, it enables the greatest distribution of pressure support and containment for the body. A great deal of time, knowledge and experience is required to produce and manufacture this type of chair. Custom-molded wheelchairs are made by using various methods of construction, such as vacuum pressure or through the use of a mixture of chemical materials. They are seldom prepared on site, and usually a mold of the user's body is sent to the factory for the assembly of such a seating arrangement.

In all types of chairs, proper positioning is important, but with this type of chair (custom molded), it is crucial that the person is always seated correctly since any change of position is liable to cause discomfort or pressure sores due to lack of compatibility between the chair and the user's body position. Due to the inability of most individuals with RS to convey their distress verbally, this type of seating arrangement should be accompanied by intense staff guidance. Evaluation should be performed by a physiotherapist using his/her knowledge of anatomy, kinesiology, biomechanics and principles of neuromuscular control and of stability and function [12,15,25].

The author is confident about the proficiency skills of physical/occupational therapists who are involved in the assembly of the appropriate seating system. Therefore, only specific elements regarding special issues typical of the client with RS that might effect the construction of such a seating arrangement will be mentioned in the section below.

- The final decision regarding the purchase and adaptability of the seating system for the individual with RS and to accommodate her daily activities should be made after a comprehensive examination as well as after consultation with parents, care-givers, teachers and managerial staff.

- If severe, uncontrolled seizures are present, proper measures should be taken (such as a chest vest or an upper trunk belt) to ensure the user's safety.

- A table is of extreme importance, in order to allow the user with RS to bear weight on her hands, for placing a communication board, for play-related activities and during meal times. Due to involuntary hand movements of the individual with RS, it is recommended that the table should have a high rim around its edge to prevent items from being accidentally pushed over.

- Some individuals with RS start as hypotonic; gradually some of them (about 40%) will develop spasticity and/or rigidity, mostly initiating from the shin muscles. About 30% will remain hypotonic, while the rest will show fluctuating/distonic muscle tone [33]. Due to such changes over different age periods, the seating system should be constructed taking the client's basic muscle tone into consideration and should be adapted according to the changes observed in muscle tone (regarding the amount of support, type of wheels, etc.).

- Due to the above-mentioned changes in muscle tone [33], and with relation to sensory abnormalities [34] and to functional fluctuations typical of the individual with RS, the aptness of the seating system should be assessed at delivery and reassessed periodically over a period of 6 months of use. This additional checkpoint is intended to ensure that the supplied system is fully innate with the flexible nature of RS.

- When the client is showing a tendency towards passivity and on the assumption she is intended to stay seated for long durations during each day, the chair should be fully adapted to pressure sore prevention (regarding appropriate cushioning and the ability for tilt-in-space of the seating system). Such adaptation is necessary due to sedentary behavior and to slim body composition typical of 85–90% of all individuals with RS [14]. The fact that this situation deteriorates with age [34,35,36] augments the issue of the management of individuals with RS as a population at risk of developing pressure sores.

- When the individual with RS is to use her seating system for many hours a day, the caregiver should be responsible for changing weight-bearing areas and alternate between different functional seating and resting positions, according to a preset program designed by the physical or occupational therapist.

- It has been occasionally reported that tilting the chair forward about 5 degrees improves head control, decreases deviation from the center line of the body and increases function [24]. Therefore, this option should be considered for the individual with RS.

- Some individuals with RS, mainly those who lack mobility and are extremely hypotonic, have a tendency towards external hip rotation [37]. This sometimes causes hip anterior displacement and is liable to result in instability of the hips, which may become painful and prevent ambulation. When such a condition is present or is expected, hip side supports should be used.

Motorized wheelchairs

Given the amount of involuntary movement presented by individuals with RS, as well as the difficulty in hand use, one might think that a powered chair is out of the question for this population, yet problems with upper extremity coordination could be accommodated through specialized controls [1]. Using head controls is one possible solution for granting an individual with RS the ability to propel a powered wheelchair independently. There are two reports regarding the use of motorized mobility by individuals with RS. One of them used a set of head controls; the other four jellybean switches [38]:

Joanne and her family started thinking about getting a powered wheelchair, when she was around four years of age as suggested by her physical therapist. Learning how to use the motorized wheel chair was done through "simulation training" under the supervision of a physical therapist for several months. After a period of time and a lot of convincing, Joanne got her own power chair, with three jellybean switches for driving, and an over-ride switch for the adult. Joanne has had her powered chair for two full years and she loves having her power chair even if it is something she does not use every day – it is something that is fun for her and that can give her a feeling of independence, yet it requires her attention and focus. Joanne is never left completely alone, but driving a powered wheelchair gives her the chance to make some choices without having to pass them through someone else. Her friends are envious of Joanne, because she can drive [38] (see figure XV-16).

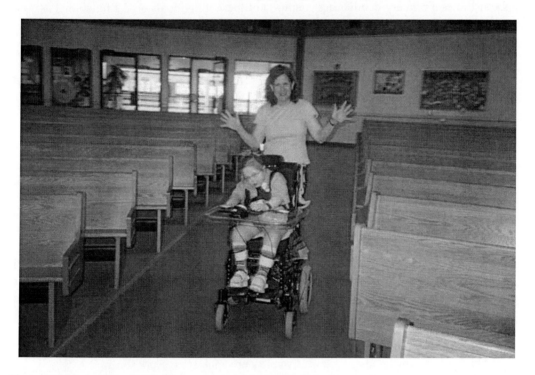

Figure XV-16. A child with RS driving a motorized wheelchair.

In the light of such a report, the possibility of an individual with RS using a motorized wheelchair should not be ruled out beforehand. Motorized wheelchairs and scooters are becoming increasingly common. Such devices are most helpful for individuals challenged by community mobility rather than in-home mobility and present sufficient control to enable independent, safe usage. In addition, if availability of a motorized wheelchair/scooter may increase participation of the individual with RS in activities that would be otherwise unavailable, its use should be considered. Secondary possible outcomes such as an increase in overall activity levels and a decrease in depression have been observed in other populations due to the use of powered mobility and should also be taken into account [31].

A wheelchair with sitting-to-standing position change enables the integration of two assistive technology devices into one and can be relevant when storage room is limited and the needs of the individual with RS necessitate both a transportation option and an enrolment in a daily standing program. Both manual and motorized wheelchairs are presently available with the ability to change the position of the user from a seated position to standing. The utility of the sitting-to-standing option for the average wheelchair user is unknown and these instruments cost considerably more than a standard wheelchair [1].

Standing

Standing is an important starting position for daily life and function. Some individuals with RS may present difficulties in standing and walking or cannot perform these functions at all. This constitutes a primary debilitating condition of these individuals on the functional as well as the social level, necessitating therapeutic intervention. Standing presents numerous advantages [39]:

- Standing encourages weight bearing, thus reducing the serious effects of osteoporosis [40,41]. Individuals with RS are known from a young age to have low bone mineral density [42,43]. Therefore, it is especially important to suggest a daily standing program for non-ambulant individuals, as a preventive measure.
- A regularly executed standing program may help to prevent contractures at the knees and hips for a wheelchair-bound individual. An individual with RS that uses a wheelchair for long durations daily should be walked on a regular basis [24] or, if not applicable, should at least be incorporated in a daily standing program.
- Standing is a muscle-tone-normalizing action [39]. Since individuals with RS present a diversity of tone changes [33], a person incorporated in a standing program will have the advantage of reduced tonal fluctuations.
- Standing improves the flow of blood to internal organs [39], thereby improving their functions [44,45]. Individuals with RS suffer from an array of intestinal problems [46] and those could favorably be affected when a standing program is implemented regularly.
- Standing involves a transition [47] (as opposed to sitting or lying down).
- For an individual who spends long daily durations in a seated position, standing is highly recommended as a preventive measure against pressure sores [48].
- Standing encourages equilibrium reactions and stability, thereby enhancing balance. Such improvements might constitute the first step towards walking for individuals with RS who are only capable of sitting and is, therefore, highly encouraged.
- Standing creates pressure directed towards the hip joints [49], thereby changing the angle of the femur from coxa valga to coxa vara, as well as building the acetabulum and preserving its healthy development [41]. Since asymmetry of the pelvis and hip displacement are orthopedic pathologies found among individuals with RS, particularly those who are not mobile [37], an habitual standing program is recommended for this population.
- Standing enables a change in one's perspective, enabling the client to experience her human environment at eye-level. Such a change might bear positive results regarding self-image, self-esteem and social skills [50].

- Individuals confined to wheelchairs belong to a risk group for diminished lung function. Since standing improves respiratory function [51], wheelchair-bound individuals with RS should be introduced to a routine standing program.
- Many individuals with RS display a shortening of the Achilles' tendon due to increased spasticity. Assuming a daily standing program while using a wedge under the client's feet (see figure XV-17) might prevent shortening of the gastrocnemius muscle, as well as reduce the need for daily unpleasant stretching exercises. If administered intensively and consistently, such an intervention might serve the individual with RS by avoiding the need for a Botox injection or surgery for Achilles tendon lengthening.

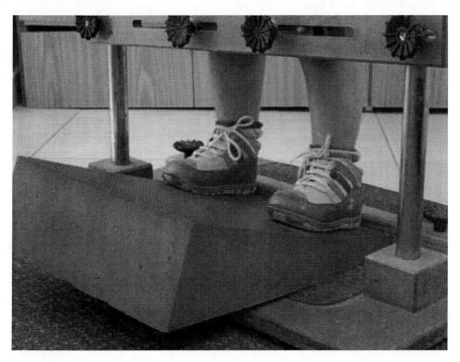

Figure XV-17. A child standing on a wedge.

- Numerous advantages of standing were reported for individuals with spinal cord injury [39], such as improved well-being, circulation, skin integrity, reflex activity, bowel and bladder function, digestion, sleep and reduced pain and fatigue. Other benefits reported for this population are in metabolic functions and psychological aspects [52]. It is possible that a standing program will yield similar benefits for individuals with RS.

Most orthopedic surgeons recommend that non-ambulant individuals will accumulate a daily standing duration of at least two hours in order for such exercise to bare results. Nevertheless, a recent study indicated that even shorter periods of standing, averaging at five hours weekly, are useful in achieving significant improvement in bone density [41].

An appropriate standing frame should be selected in accordance with the general criteria for choosing assistive technology, mentioned at the opening part of this chapter. The basic rule of thumb is to choose a standing frame that will offer the individual with RS the minimum amount of support possible and will obligate her to be as active as possible within the framework of her limitations. Using a table while the individual with RS is standing, for toys or a communication device, is recommended as long as the user does not lean on the table, preventing her from actively using her trunk muscles.

Caution: When instigating a standing program, one should acclimatize the individual with RS with the new unfamiliar situation (taking into account the difficulties individuals with RS present in such cases) as well as apply the program for minimal durations, gradually enhancing the effort demanded from the client. The duration of the standing activity is determined by the person with RS her self. When she is showing signs of weakness and slouches over the table, standing should be paused.

Standing frames

Tilt board

This kind of standing frame is designed for individuals who are very heavy or hypotonic and for those who show extremely poor trunk and head control. The tilt board is an electric or mechanical bed that can be tilted from a horizontal position to a vertical one. The client using this apparatus is placed on the board in a laying position. She is then elevated into a standing position, after being strapped by her knees and chest (and possibly with an extra safety belt at the pelvis level). A table can also be added so that the user can operate a switch or play while standing. This type of standing frame is usually used when the individual with RS is in need of massive support.

Supine/prone board

This type of standing frame can be leaned towards a table, wall or sofa with the individual with RS half lying on her stomach. The amount of support this type of standing frame offers can be changed according the client's head and trunk control and the angle of tilt. Such adaptations allow the person using the appliance to attain an optimal position. This type of standing frame also enables the individual with RS to be socially active; it can be leaned against the dining table, enabling her to eat and communicate with other members of the family during family gatherings. Most supine boards are equipped with wheels and can be moved from place to place. The prone board is preferable over a supine board for encouraging the activation of trunk extensors and thus is of great use for the kyphotic user.

Oswestry and adjustable oswestry

These are two types of rigid, stable, standing frames. The simpler form is extremely rigid, made of wood and supports the knees and pelvis. Additions can be made in order to allow for chest support. The height of the table can be changed in accordance with the user's needs.

The second type of standing frame (adjustable oswestry) is an improvement to the basic model and is made of stainless steel. This type of standing frame is foldable and is, therefore, easier to store. These two frames offer strong front and back support (however, they provide less support from the sides), while still enabling safe manual function. The table should be equipped with a high rim to prevent toys or other accessories from falling as a result of the client's unintentional hand movements. There are many kinds of standing frames (Richter, Bayreuth), including electric or mechanical frames that can raise the user from a seated position in her wheelchair to a standing position. All these standing frames' height can be adjusted according to the user's own height, with a range of 110–170 cm (44–68 in.). These standing frames are extremely heavy and difficult to move (even the ones that have wheels) and occupy a lot of space.

Pelvis-height standing frames/active standing frames

These standing frames support the user's knees and pelvis, with the back usually remaining free and active; an additional supportive belt at chest level or a table can be added. The simplest forms of active standing frames are mechanical and consist of a board and two vertical stainless steel rods with pelvis straps that can be adjusted to the individual's height. Knee supports can also be adjusted to the appropriate height and width of each user.

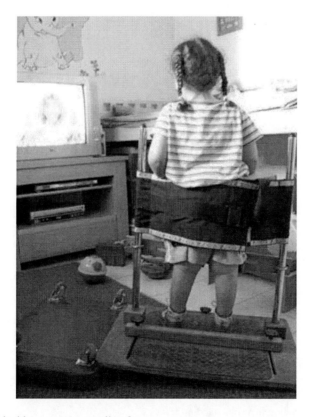

Figure XV-18. A child with an uneven standing frame.

More sophisticated models, such as the "flexistand major", are equipped with electronic lifts for lifting the user from the chair to a standing position. This type of frame can also be adjusted electronically to provide front, back, or side support, as well as for adjusting the height. If the person with RS begins to develop curvature of the spine, an asymmetric standing frame should be employed in order to encourage the use of muscles to counter the direction of the curvature (see figure XV-18). This method has been found useful in reducing scoliotic curvature [29].

Shin-standing frame

This type of standing frame was initiated by the author (see figure XV-19). It is suitable for a user who basically has moderate trunk control but requires minimal assistance or supervision in maintaining an erect posture. This type of standing frame can be made from a large old pair of AFO (ankle foot orthosis) splints attached to a wooden board. This standing frame supports the legs (the height of the splints, above or below the knees, is adjusted in accordance to the user's ability) and is designed to serve as a device for practicing standing and improving static balance abilities. It is difficult to control but offers good support for the hypotonic individual who possesses enough trunk control for maintaining this posture. After the person with RS has become accustomed to this type of standing frame, adjustments can be made, such as reducing the base of support (by narrowing the space between the splints or placing them in a variety of tandem positions on the wooden base); such changes enhance the users activity level.

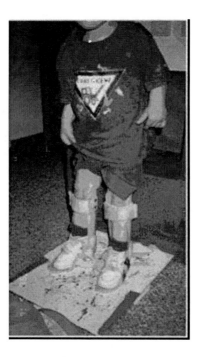

Figure XV-19. A child standing in a shin-standing frame.

The shin-standing frame can then be adapted to achieve higher levels of dynamic balance by inserting a screw underneath the center of board. This causes the base to move in different directions and standing on it becomes an active, challenging exercise. Slow, controlled movements in any direction are made possible by adding foam on the bottom of the base. The user can then feel relatively secure while moving slowly and gently, exercising and strengthening her trunk muscles and learning how to actively keep her balance, all at the same time.

Stationary standing area

A standing area is a device developed by the author. It is a safe and enclosed padded area that provides the user with RS with the opportunity to stand independently and even perform a few steps while safely and independently staying erect. Such a device can be made with a large barrel (individually adapted to the dimensions of each user and her standing abilities). It allows the user to remain in a standing position without requiring constant supervision or tight movement restrictions (As given by most standing frames). A motivational factor, such as a TV, game, audio recorder or communication device, can be placed within reach; so that the person standing in the device can stand or move while involved in a recreational activity (see figure XV-20).

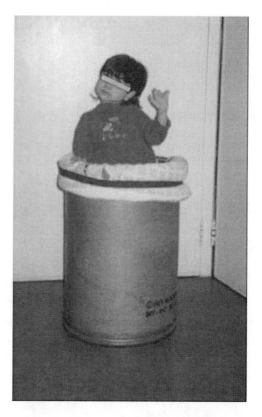

Figure XV-20. A child in a standing space.

A manual standing frame

This device was developed by the author especially for individuals with RS. It is made out of two poles, which the individual with RS holds with her hands. This type of standing frame is suitable for a user that has full control over her legs but is in need of assistance for standing or walking. The person with RS can hold the standing frame by herself or, as a safety measure, be strapped to the bars (in cases where hand usage is not fully reliable) (see figure XV-21). Side-to-side balance reactions can be achieved if the person with RS holds on to only one bar (see figure XV-22).

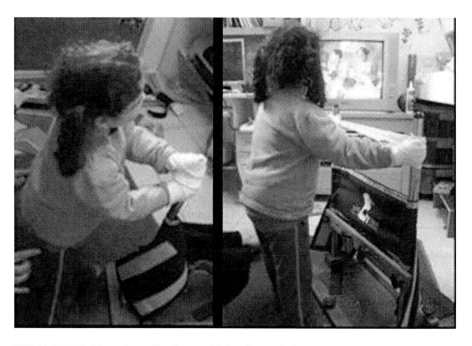

Figures XV-21, XV-22. Manual standing frame with hands attached.

Walking

One of the most immediate questions asked by parents of children with disabilities in general, as well as by parents of individuals with RS, is: "will she be able to walk?" Such a question stems from that fact that walking symbolizes independence and allows the individual to be embraced by society as a person with a problem as opposed to a non-mobile individual who is perceived as someone with a severe handicap [25]. Walking is crucial for any individual with developmental disability but is extremely important for the person with RS and it is highly recommended by experts in the field of RS[2]. If walking as an independent capability cannot be achieved, then short-distance therapeutic walking should be incorporated constantly into the supplementary management program. Walking, even therapeutic walking, has many benefits. Walking offers all the benefits of standing (see the previous section on standing), as well as the following advantages:

- Improving function and physical fitness — A daily, treadmill walking program was implemented for four children with RS for the duration of two months. Sessions lengthened for half an hour each, and provided the participants with comfortable walking speeds. The program was found to improve the physical fitness and functional abilities of all participants [53]. Training on a treadmill has been found to encourage independent walking in other populations [54,55] (more information on this topic could be found in the chapter regarding physical therapy).

- Preserving joint range of motion (ROM) — Walking improves ROM of the back, pelvis, hips, knees and ankles, and exercises many different joints [56]. Mobility is essential for individuals with RS who are in danger of joint contractures and should therefore be set as a primary therapeutic objective.

- Strengthening massive muscles of the lower limbs — The strengthening of muscular mass [57] reduces the secondary dangers of immobility, such as muscular atrophy. Bauer claims that the assembly of accumulating factors reducing the individual's level of activity, such as sedentary lifestyle, reduced functional abilities and physical fitness, medication and other factors presents an imminent danger for individuals with disabilities [58].

- Enhancing pulmonary activity — Using the muscles of the lower extremities, which are the largest muscles in the body, forces the lungs to work at higher capacities, resulting in improvement in lung capacity and function [57,59], thereby enhancing, in general, a more apt condition for the individual with RS.

- Improving heart function — Walking as an exercise of the large muscles of the lower extremities forces the heart to circulate blood to the extremities at higher rates, thereby enhancing aerobic capacity [60] and improving heart function [61,62]. It should be taken into account that 50%–100% of individuals with RS at stages III and IV present slight cardiac irregularities [63,64], such as elongated QT intervals. Therefore, after consulting with a physician, any controlled physical activities that stimulate and strengthen the heart muscle, are desirable.

- Positive prognosis for scoliosis — Scoliosis has been identified in 80%–85% of individuals with RS [22,65]. A negative connection was described between the person's ambulation abilities (especially her abilities to ascend or descend stairs) and the severity of scoliosis [22,65]. Therefore, intervention aimed at improving and maintaining ambulation abilities of the person with RS will have a positive effect on the severity of her scoliosis.

- Organization of body schemas — The action of ambulating enhances sensory stimulation of limbs and torso positioning. These proprioceptive messages are transferred to the neural system mostly when the individual is active. Therefore, walking is a continuous exercise that constantly reorganizes the neural system of the walker through different mechanisms [66,67]. It has been suggested [26,27] that due to sensory abnormalities leading to scoliosis in the majority of individuals with RS [22,65], sensory stimulations that enhance symmetrical sensations should be used from a young age as preventive measures for all individuals with RS. If executed properly, walking can enhance and preserve mid-line sensation.

- Improving blood circulation to the lower extremities — Individuals with RS present a dysfunctional autonomic system [68,69]. As a result, they show circulation problems of the lower and upper limbs. Walking improves circulation, helps muscle oxygenation and increases metabolism of the lower extremities, thus reducing ill-effects of the pathologic autonomic system of the feet (i.e., cold, edematous, bluish/red skin).

- Enhancing self-initiation and independence — One of the most common limitations of individuals with RS is their lack of initiative, with its accompanying dependency on others. Acquiring the ability to walk enables them to become less-dependent individuals, with an opportunity to explore/investigate their surroundings as they wish, reaching out and discovering the world. This is an ideal situation for any person and even more so for individuals with RS. For this reason, individuals with RS should be continuously trained to walk, preferably with the goal of achieving unassisted ambulation.
- Social acceptance — The manner in which a person gets about, by walking or in a wheelchair, influences the manner in which society views him/her. An individual who can walk and interact with others will have an advantage over a person confined to a wheelchair. If walking is not achieved, the individual with RS is dependent on others for initiating, approaching or creating positive social situations, thereby reducing her chances for social acceptance.
- Walking can be achieved at any age — According to parental reports on the RettNet, there are individuals with RS who have started walking at ages 3, 7 and even 18 years [70-72]. There are also reports of individuals with RS re-acquiring walking ability after years of using a wheelchair [26,46,73,74]. One case-study recounted a woman with RS who lost her ability to walk at age 20 years, but regained her ability at age 43 years, more than 20 years later [74].

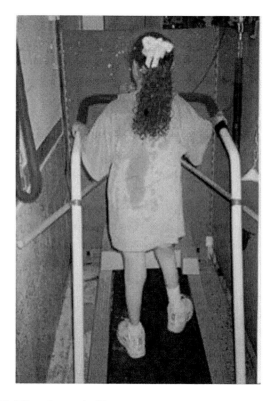

Figure XV-23. A child with RS on the treadmill.

The optimal type of walking is, of course, independent walking, free from the help of others or any mobility aids. Since some individuals with RS are in need of support at some stage, this part of the chapter will describe various types of walkers. If the person with RS is able to walk using this type of support, she should be allowed the freedom to walk independently, using a walker. Another tool that the author has used successfully for training individuals with RS to walk, is a treadmill (see figure XV-23), with extremely positive results in relation to function and aerobic conditions [53]. When properly placed, walking on a treadmill demands a minimum amount of supervision. The treadmill can be placed opposite the TV, in order to increase motivation of the user and elongate exercise duration.

Walking equipment

It should be emphasized that this chapter does not support the use of waking equipment but if taking the social, functional and physiological aspects into consideration, any type of mobility is preferable to sitting around leading a sedentary lifestyle. Therefore, if this is the only way to achieve mobility for the individual with RS, then adapting an appropriate walker should be considered.

It is common knowledge that walking frames are sometimes found less practical for use on all terrains and for dealing with daily situations, since they are difficult to maneuver in small spaces and cannot be used on a flight of stairs, thereby reducing the user's independence. Canes and crutches on the other hand are most useful when the gait problem is unilateral and/or mild but people who need bilateral canes may find that a walker works just as well and may even be easier to use [1]. There are several gait patterns that can be used with canes and crutches (e.g., swing through, opposition), some of which may be difficult to learn, especially for those with apraxia and ataxia (such as individuals with RS). If an incorrect gait pattern is used, the patient is at increased risk of falling and the crutches may not provide the correct support [1]. Therefore, due to the manual abilities and complex motor control associated with the use of these devices, they have been left outside the scope of the present chapter and the use of walkers as potential aids for the gait of the person with RS will be discussed.

Walkers can be used for two purposes:

- As part of a rehabilitation program wherein the user is recovering from an injury or operation.
- As a long-term aid for mobility when the user has a permanent difficulty with walking. This chapter will address mostly the latter, with special consideration for users with RS.

When rehabilitation is the aim of using a walking aid, then we anticipate that the process will assist gradual progress towards independent and unassisted walking. Such a process may commence with the use of a walking-frame in order to enhance the user's confidence and to enable her to gain experience. About 60% of individuals with RS achieve independent ambulation [2] but some may be in need of walking aids, while some may require such accessories at later ages, in case of deterioration in ambulation abilities. Due to the effect that

RS-attributed disabilities have on the individual's balance and co-ordination [22], mobility equipment may be required for long-term use.

A walker with no wheels at all (a four-point or pick-up walker) requires more energy and arm strength to use than the front-wheeled walker and is more complicated to use correctly[1], yet it offers little additional stability over a two-wheeled walker [76]. Most individual with RS show poor manual abilities and are dysparxic. Therefore the use of walkers (with no wheels) which requires the performance of sequential tasks (i.e., holding, lifting, and moving the walker forward, then advancing the legs, but not too much), might be too difficult for this population to master. Therefore, these appliances will be left outside the scope of the present chapter. Walking equipment may perform one or more functions, including:

- Providing greater stability and balance by extending a wider base of support
- Facilitating the walking pattern of the user, in terms of speed and evenness of stride
- Improving the user's upright body posture
- Increasing the confidence of the user in his/her walking ability

Safe use of walking equipment

Walking equipment should improve mobility. However, if an inappropriate walking device is used, if incorrect techniques are adopted or if the device is not suitable for a particular environment, the independence and safety of the user will be jeopardized. Factors that should be looked at to minimize the risk of falling while using a walking device include: arranging the home environment (loose rugs, irregular terrain and a cluttered floor area are all potential hazards), avoiding wet floors (walking equipment should not be used in wet floor areas) and wearing appropriate and supportive footwear.

General consideration regarding the use of rollators (wheeled walkers)

The following factors should be considered when choosing a walker:

- Research that examined several different types of walkers [77] has shown that the most important factors for adapting a walker to a person's needs are the user's clinical condition and home environment, rather than the conditions of the institution or educational facility.
- If a walker must be carried up and down a flight of stairs, it will soon be abandoned. If the daily activities and physical environment of the person with RS necessitates the use of stairs at home or in the institution or educational facility, then two rollators should be provided to use on different floors.
- Rollators usually occupy a lot of space and building larger rooms is not always financially or spatially possible. Therefore, handles should be attached to walls to support the user in small spaces, such as bathrooms, where the use of the rollator is excluded.

- A folding rollator should be chosen if the person travels daily by car or if her home is small and there is no place to store the rollator. (The rollators that take up the least amount of space are V-shaped walkers. These are also the easiest to maneuver but are less stable).
- Folding rollators must be checked when opened to ensure that they are locked so that they will not suddenly fold up when being used.
- In general cases of ataxia (other than RS), a reciprocal walker with a center axis (each side is moved alternately with the other) is sometimes recommended. It is difficult to control this type of walker and, for this reason it does not suit the needs of individuals with RS.
- When considering the physical environment of the potential user and whether or not the rollator is to be used in the bathroom, it is suggested that a rollator without a high anterior bar, in order to enable access to the toilet, be selected.
- The individual with poor trunk control should be given a rollator that provides enough stability. On the other hand, since initiative of many with RS is reduced, the best rollator to consider would be the one enabling maximum maneuverability. Therefore a delicate decision-making process should be performed to evaluate the suitable type of walker for each user with RS, in accordance with her functional abilities and attitude.
- The height of a walker should be carefully taken into consideration. If the frame is too high, the person will find it difficult to straighten her elbows sufficiently and will not receive enough body weight through the arms. On the other hand, if the frame is too low, it will encourage the person to bend over, resulting in poor posture. It is usually appropriate that the user's elbows are flexed at about 15 degrees when her hands are placed on the handles. In the case of a forearm-walking frame, the height of support should bring the elbows to a 90-degree angle [75].
- The height of the frame is an important element that can be altered for therapeutic needs. The physiotherapist may deliberately set up a frame at a "wrong" height. If the user with RS is kyphotic, she can be brought to a slightly more erect position by using elbow splints or by raising the height of the walker. For individuals with RS who tend to fall backwards, on the other hand, lowering the height of the walker will force them to keep their back slanting forward, thus improving their stability. If a person with RS tends to fall backwards, walking with the back slanting forward also helps to attain a corrective sensual feeling that will enable her to remain erect in the long run.
- The user should always be measured for the height of her walking frame when wearing appropriate and supportive footwear.
- Due to dyspraxia, the ability of those with RS to adjust properly to difficulties within their walking path may be limited. Therefore, it must be ensured that the walking area is flat and free of gaps, steps or other obstacles, at least during initial trials with the equipment. Regardless of all the above-mentioned safety precautions, if there is the slightest chance that the person might fall, close supervision should be administered.
- Light-weight walkers are easier to maneuver but, at the same time, are also less stable and are more liable to topple forward.
- Tipping an anterior walker forward might sometimes occur due to the user walking forward within the walking frame. If this danger becomes evident when the person with RS begins to walk, it is recommended that a mechanical limitation be placed to

prevent her from tipping forwards with the walking device. Examples for proper adjustments for such a problem are the use of elbow splints and the placing of a horizontal bar at pelvis level or the non-conventional use of a posterior walker (see figure XV-24)

- Since the manual abilities of the individual with RS are usually lacking, a basket can be attached to the rollator, enabling the user to carry things when she ambulates. Care should be taken not to overload the basket; as otherwise, the rollator could become unstable and overturn.

In many cases, the rollator needs to be altered in order to meet the needs of the individual with RS. These alterations include the following:

- Adding elbow splints — These splints can be either flexible or stiff and will help the user to keep her elbows straight or almost straight, thus bringing her hands to the proper position on the handles of the walker.
- Adding adapted handles — Grasping objects and holding them for long periods of time is difficult for most individuals with RS. For this reason, grasping is an important therapeutic element. Hand-rests and Velcro straps can be added to the handles of the walker to help the user grasp it for the prolonged durations.
- Adding a bar in front — As mentioned earlier, adding a bar at pelvis height can help in preventing the user from advancing too far forward and overturning the rollator as a result.
- Adding weights — If the person with RS uses the rollator throughout the day, it should be light-weight and foldable. If it is very heavy or large, it will impose difficulties for care-givers and will probably be abandoned. If the person with RS needs a heavy and stable walker to keep her balance, homemade or commercially purchased weights can be attached to the walker. The weights can be kept both at home and at the educational facility, attached at the base of the rollator when the user arrives and removed before she commutes, thereby creating a situation in which a light-weight walker is transported and heavy steady one is used for walking.
- Broadening the base — A rollator can be made more stable while still remaining light-weight by adding side-wheels similar to training wheels on a bicycle. This will broaden the base of the walker and add stability, without adding a lot of extra weight. If side-wheels are added to the rear bar of the rollator, they should be double hinged in a fashion that will allow passage in narrow doorways (no picture is available).
- Adapting the wheels — The wheels of the rollator should be made of material suitable for the type of surface/terrain on which the user walks. Small rubber wheels are sufficient for even floors. Larger wheels/castors are needed for traveling over rougher surfaces, such as gravel or brick-surfaced walks. Inflatable wheels should be used on extremely uneven surfaces but chances are that an individual who can successfully maneuver herself over surfaces of this type does not need a rollator at all.

The following section presents a list of rollators, ranging from simple, light-weight rollators to sophisticated ones. As explained before, this list will not include normal walkers (without wheels), since using these types of walkers demands a combination of abilities that are too difficult for most individuals with RS. All walkers described here have two or four wheels, and are rigid and stable.

Types of rollators

Basic rollators (two-wheeled walkers)

Standard aluminum rollators are square and have two front wheels, which move on one plane of movement and cannot swivel. Because of this, they cannot be used on un-paved surfaces or carpeting. The aluminum construction is lightweight and suitable for individuals who move around a lot. On the other hand, this type of rollator is not particularly strong or stable and should only be recommended for users with RS with minimal balance difficulties. Stainless steel rollators are more stable and durable and can be folded for easy transport and storage. However, these rollators are as difficult to steer as those made of aluminum when used on uneven surfaces.

Three-wheeled rollators

Three-wheeled walkers have greater maneuverability than four-wheeled walkers [78], but they do not offer the seating advantages of a four-wheeled walker and lack the stability of a two-wheeled walker. Three-wheeled walkers are particularly helpful for people who need more support than is provided by a cane and have to maneuver through narrow spaces, such as classrooms [1]. These rollators have the advantage of being compact and foldable for easy storage and have maximum mobility. On the other hand, their base is quite narrow and for that reason, they provide particularly poor stability, especially while turning. Some models are manufactured with brakes that lock as soon as weight is placed on the walker. Such an option offers a certain safety advantage.

Four-wheeled rollators

There are several types of four-wheeled rollators:

- Posterior rollators have four wheels; two front swiveling wheels and two non-swiveling rear wheels (ferrules). These wheels have brakes that are designed to prevent the user from stepping/falling backwards. These brakes are mostly not very efficient. The advantage of this type of rollator is that it provides stability and each step forward brings the rear bar into contact with the buttocks. This walker is usually made of aluminum and can be easily folded for storage. The open front-end enables the user to take broad, "normal" steps. A helmet should be considered for protection against falling injury. It is possible to use this walker in a non-conventional way (as an anterior rollator, for example) so as to achieve better stability. A forward inclination of the user can be applied as cautionary action against falling (backwards) and as a horizontal perimeter to prevent the user from stepping out of restraint (see figure XV-24).

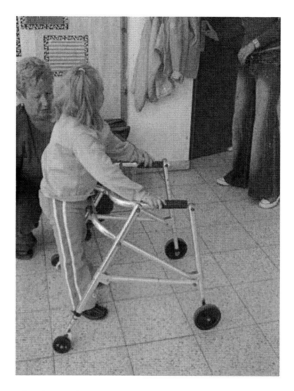

Figure XV-24. Non-conventional use of a posterior walker.

- Anterior (normal) rollators are extremely mobile and somewhat more stable than three-wheeled rollators. They can be fitted with a seat or basket and are therefore suitable for daily walks around the house or for taking short walks to a nearby playground/friend. Some have weight-operated brakes. The size and type of wheels should be chosen according to the dimensions of the user and the type of surface on which she usually walks. The more uneven the walking surface, the larger the wheels should be.

- Rollators with arm supports (platform armrest) are suitable for use by individuals with RS who have difficulty grasping objects. They are higher than normal rollators and are somewhat less stable and present an increase in the overall weight and bulk of the walker [1]. Due to a risk off over-turn, care must be taken when moving them over door-steps, carpets or other small obstacles. The armrest can be divided into two halves or can be used as one large area on which the individual can lean her entire weight. From my experience, this type of anterior leaning area tends to encourage the user to be more passive, while at the same time, hinders vision. A horizontal bar at pelvis height can also be added to this type of walker in order to prevent the user from moving too far forward. This offers the slight advantage of distributing weight equally on the front and rear edges of the rollators, adding greater stability.

- Rollators with trunk supports are usually made of steel and are extremely heavy, even though new plastic models are now available (see figure XV-25) which are much easier to maneuver. They have four wheels, two or four of which swivel (it is best to start with all four wheels locked to increase stability and gradually, when the user gains control, to enable pivoting to all wheels). Most are designed for indoor use and are intended for individuals with poor trunk control and poor balance. Due to the support they give to the user's trunk, these types of rollators seem unfit for passive individuals such as those with RS. Yet it is possible that a few months of daily training are needed to get the person with RS to "get the hang of it" as was the case with the child presented in figure XV-25.

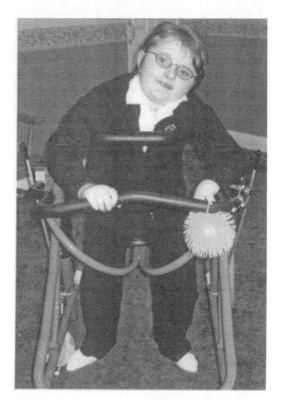

Figure XV-25. Use of rollator with trunk support by a child with RS.

There are three major types of rollators with trunk supports:

- Square steel frames — These rollators are equipped with removable and adjustable parts and accessories, such as front handles, a knee separator and hip supports. The height of the rollator and of the trunk support can be adjusted. Most of these rollators have leg-straps to prevent tight adduction during walking for individuals showing extreme adductor spasticity. Passive individuals are liable to sit and rest in the rollator rather than exercise; for those, alternate solutions should be considered. If the user is showing extreme flexor muscle tone, a rubber band tied to the rear poles while crossing her knees or having them tied at e ankle- level can immediately bring the user to perform leg movements. These movements, in turn, cause the rollator to move forward, causing the rubber bands to stretch.....and so on and so forth (see figure XV-26).

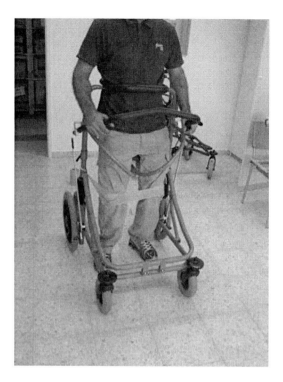

Figure XV-26. The use of elastic bands to enhance walking.

- Hart walker — The Hart walker is different from other types of rollators because it is especially designed to produce the user's walking ability from scratch. The user is held in place inside the rollator's frame by a corset for the trunk, as well as leg-support straps. The rollator has four wheels with a central bar that holds the support straps. When the user turns within the rollator, the front wheels turn with her. This type of rollator has brakes that lock automatically when the user bears weight on the walker, but unlock when she is supporting her own weight (the amount of weight that locks the brakes can be adjusted). One of the disadvantages of the Hart walker is that it takes some time to place the user in the walker and to remove her as well. This type of walker is suitable for individuals with poor trunk control, yet with motivation to walk.

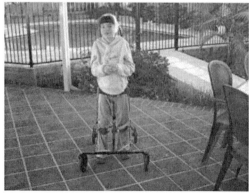
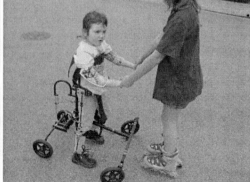

Figures XV-27 and XV-28. Children with RS using a Hart walker.

The Hart walker has the positive advantage of forcing the user to remain active. On the other hand, a person with RS who leans on the back straps will cause the brakes to lock and the walker will not move. Due to limitations in initiative displayed by many individuals with RS, it is questionable if this type of walker is suited for the majority of this population. Nevertheless, there are some who use it [79, 80] (see figures XV-27 and XV-28).

- Triangular walker — This type of walker is designed for users who cannot carry their own body-weight. The base is V-shaped and usually has small wheels. There is usually a central vertical support bar for the chest as well as a seat. The user sits on the seat with her body strapped in and pushes forward using small movements of her feet. This walker offers a maximum amount of support and passive individuals will not move this type of rollator unless they are encouraged with strong motivational incentives.

Cycles

Riding a cycle is an exciting experience that provides the rider with feelings of elation, familiarity with speed, independence and mobility [81]. Such feelings and experiences are particularly meaningful for people lacking the ability to self-ambulate. In addition to the above, using a cycle effectively constitutes an excellent form of physical training. Riding a cycle offers a form of outdoor enjoyment, an experience seldom shared by individuals with RS that are usually handicapped due to mobility problems. This form of recreation can be combined with a family/social activity, such as a picnic or get-together with other children at the playground. Riding a cycle can also improve hand function. Due to all of the above-mentioned advantages, it is highly recommended to consider the use of cycles for individuals with RS.

There are many different tricycles and bicycles on the market, so the "right" cycles are those that meet the needs of the specific person with RS (fitting her size, as well as providing the required trunk support, adjustability and appropriate foot rests), care-givers, and parents (price, size, weight).

Individuals with RS who experience fear of movement (Termed "proprioceptive defensiveness" by the author – see chapter regarding occupational therapy for more details) resulting from sensory problems should assume a sitting position providing extensive trunk support. Gradual cycle-riding experience wherein the user is well supported might actually help to reduce the person with RS's fear of movement. Consulting with an occupational therapist regarding this matter is recommended.

People with RS can learn to ride a cycle, acquiring a skill that can vary their daily experiences while improving their physical fitness in the meantime. When deciding to take on this task, it is recommended to begin gradually by first letting the person with RS experience the joy of other children using a cycle, by showing her cycles of different types, parked and ridden alike. Initial riding should be practiced in a quiet place, free of excessive stimulation. The person with RS may then be helped to mount the cycle (at her own pace!), remaining seated when it is stationary (a tricycle is preferable for maximal stability, thereby establishing a sense of security) and then gradually begin moving.

On many types of cycles, the pedals can be rotated both forward and as backward. During the first stages of learning, it is best if the pedals can only rotate uni-directionally (some cycles have this feature built in). Another possibility is to have the axle of the rear wheel fixed with this trait at a cycle repair shop.

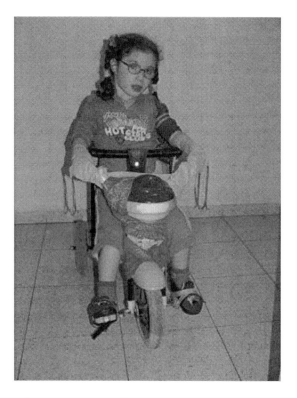

Figure XV-29. Using the cycle as a sensory experience.

It is recommended to begin riding with a tricycle equipped with good trunk support, a seat belt and pedals that can be strapped around the user's feet. At first, for the sake of building a sense of confidence by the user in the new activity, it is wise to set the handlebar in such a way that allows the cycle to move only in a straight line (some tricycles have this option built in). Gloves with Velcro strips can be used to help the user hold onto the handlebars. Another possibility that is not highly recommended is to eliminate use of the handlebars and to attach a rod to the hand-bar for pulling and external steering of the bike (some beginner bikes are manufactured with this option, see figure 29). Using this approach provides the user with the joy of movement, yet it carries the risk that the individual with RS will soon learn that she can allow herself to be passive, exerting little effort. A positive aspect of such an activity is the fact that pushing the cycle with the user's legs attached to the pedals causes alternating movements which might, in turn, enhance reciprocal gait. Therefore, such an exercise can be considered as a preliminary activity preceding gait training, for this population (see figure XV-29).

During the first stages, it is important to see that the person's trunk is well supported in order to enhance the individual's sense of security. If she enjoyed riding and would like to go again, these supports can gradually be reduced. As she becomes more and more secure, active seating should be tested in order to improve equilibrium reactions.

Songs about riding a cycle can add motivation and provide rhythm, as well as relax the individual with RS, in case the motion of the cycle makes her anxious. It is best to begin riding in a place with a slight incline, while going downhill the lightest touch on the pedals will move the cycle and she will gain immediate satisfaction and reward for her efforts.

Individuals who are especially sociable, such as most people with RS, can begin learning in a group or with a friend, since the company of another person riding with her or around her, can add motivation. It goes without saying that the user should always wear a safety helmet when riding.

There are several types of cycles that provide a solution for individuals with severe limitations who find it hard to ambulate or lack the sufficient control over their body and limbs to ride a cycle. This type of cycle enables the individual with RS to enjoy the exhilarating feeling of riding outdoors as well as participating in family outings and leisure activities.

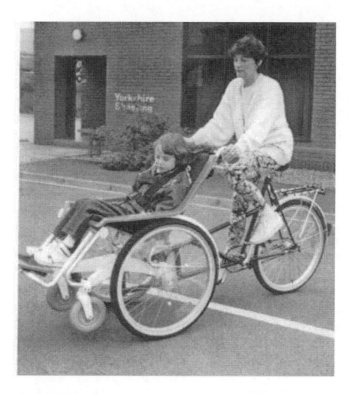

Figure XV-30. Duet wheelchair tricycles.

- Duet wheelchair tricycles have two wheels in front and one in back, a rear seat for the adult who operates and steers the cycle and a seat for the individual with RS situated in front (also referred to as Victorian tandems). The individual with RS can experience the speed, the wind on her face, enjoy the view and participate in activities with family or friends (see figure XV-30). This type of tricycle is more stable than tandem cycles and can be ridden more slowly. The person with RS can be left sitting on the tricycle even when it is not in motion, and the tricycle can be ridden at slow speeds suitable for all. The main advantage when using this type of cycle, is that person in the back can speak to the front rider with RS and address her while they are riding together

- Side-by-side tricycles have a wide seat with a backrest on which two people can sit side-by-side. Seat belts can be added for safety. In this sort of cycle, trunk support by the user is required (see figure XV-31).

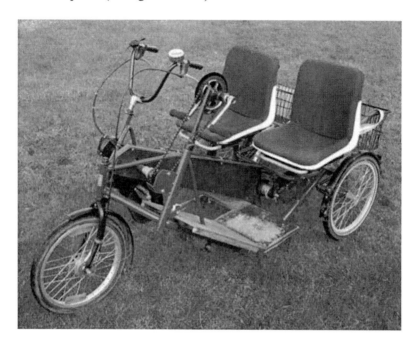

Figure XV-31. Side-by-side tricycles.

- Cycles with wheelchair attachments have a mechanism for easy attachment of the wheelchair to the side of the cycle's rear wheel or to a platform and enable individuals who lack the ability of actively riding a cycle to enjoy the outdoors (no picture is available).

Tandems and add-on trailer cycles

- Tandems are long cycles with two or more seats behind one another. These cycles allow people with multiple disabilities to enjoy the sensation of free riding. Leg motion can be achieved by strapping the user's feet to the pedals. Tandems can also be used in preparation for riding independently or for individuals who have difficulty using their hands and keeping balance. A trunk rest and seatbelts can be added for users who have difficulty keeping their balance and the user's hands can be strapped to the handlebars with Velcro straps to help her hold on. This type of cycle can be purchased in a more conventional; two- wheeled model, or an adjusted three-wheel version (see figure XV-32).

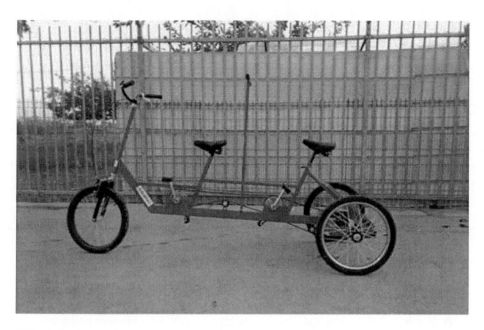

Figure XV-32. Tandem cycles.

- An add-on trailer is another option that enables the individual with RS to participate in family activities and enjoy the open doors and the feeling of movement even if she does not partake in the actual action of riding. This setup can be used for familiarizing a person with RS with riding\movement in general, and as an initial step towards commencement of riding (see figure XV-33).

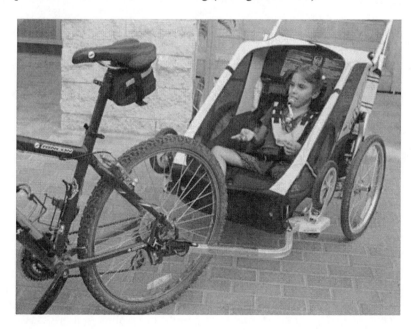

Figure XV-33. Add-on trailer.

- Cycles for self-propulsion - Practicing the act of getting on and off the cycle can serve as a functional practice helping with other tasks, such as getting in and out of bed or the bathtub. When considering self–propulsion, one should bear in mind that most individuals with RS can control either the handlebars or pedals alone, but, in most cases, will find it extremely difficult to control both simultaneously. Some users might be more successful in operating tricycles with pedals attached to the front wheel, thereby enabling the tricycle to be moved as well as steered by the legs. On the other hand, when using this type of trike, the user's posture demands movement of the thighs and knees in a manner different to regular walking (due to the flexed position) and is therefore might be found difficult to master by the apraxic person. Some of these cycles are foldable, enabling them to be easily transported from one place to the other, without the need of a special vehicle. A control bar can be attached to these tricycles so that the parent\care-giver can help propel or steer, in order to avoid obstacles. This type of tricycle is the most highly recommended since it offers the person with RS a higher level of independence, while enhancing respiratory and cardiovascular endurance and muscle activation. Individuals with RS who are usually inactive and have minor heart irregularities, shallow breathing and inactive muscles will benefit from many aspects of riding or even pedaling a cycle while it is controlled by an adult.

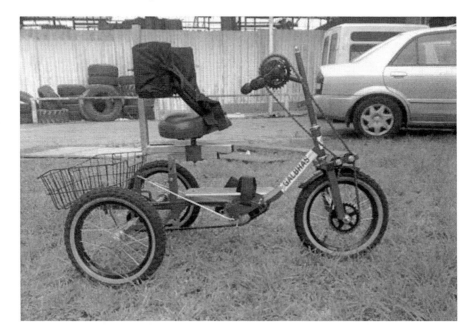

Figure XV-34. Hand-operated cycle.

- Hand-operated cycles are the least suitable type of cycle for independent riding for individuals with RS but nonetheless pose an option for using an outing as an opportunity for improving trunk and upper extremities joint range of motion (ROM). This type of cycle is designed for people who have difficulty using their legs but show functional manual abilities, such as those of individuals with spastic diplegia type cerebral palsy. They are rigorously built, are stable, and are very safe to use. Since these cycles have an elongated pedal bar at chest level, the user's hands can be attached to the pedals and can then propel the bicycle or, in the case of RS, vice versa (the cycle movement will move the hands of the user with RS). An inactive individual with RS who has high muscle tone, is occupied with stereotypic movements during most of her waking hours and maintained a kyphotic posture, is in danger of losing ROM of the trunk, shoulders, elbows and wrists. Riding this type of cycle with the user's hands attached to the pedals enables her to attain good movement of the upper limbs and trunk, which will keep her back and arms in a more flexible condition, while at the same time participating in active leisure activity (see figure XV-34).

Splints and orthopedic supports

The decision to use an orthopedic aid and the choice of which type to use must be based on an evaluation made by a physiotherapist, an orthotist and an orthopedic specialist [82]. The factors influencing this decision include: leg-joint ROM, foot position, the amount of external control required by the client to enable function, the mobility of the user, her functional level and the degree of spasticity. Since the foot and leg must also provide movement as well as stability, the influence of an orthopedic aid on these two components must be taken into consideration.

If the ankle or foot presents deviations that prevent the attainment of a neutral position when the knee is straightened without bearing weight, an orthopedic aid should not be used. Wearing an orthopedic device over a contracture at the base of the leg (the ankle or foot) will force the person to compensate in other areas and is bound to cause excessive motion and stress to other joints as well as reduced mobility at the fixated area. This is an undesirable result that might cause more damage in the long run, if not taken into consideration and supported by supplementary therapeutic intervention.

It is important to emphasize that preserving the proper length of the gastrocnemius (the calf muscle) in individuals with RS is not an impossible task. The young child should be evaluated every few months and night splints should be prepared as soon as the first spastic signs appear. This might help prevent shortening of the muscles. If shortening does develop, conventional methods such as standing on a wedge (see figureXV-17), passive stretching, serial casting, splints, active splints (see figure XV-33) or Botox injections can be used before introducing the surgical option. A daily standing program in a standing frame on a wedge has been suggested earlier in this chapter, as means by which to prevent or delay muscle shortening.

If a program for passive stretching is administered by care-givers, parents or other family members, it should be given under the guidance of a physiotherapist who will direct the manual performance of participants, supervise the administering and intensity of the program and monitor the results.

The most efficient method of serial casting involves the changing of the cast six times on a weekly basis. During the casting procedure, the physical therapist must ensure that the subtallar joint is in neutral position. The program must be continued even after the desired range in the ankle joint has been achieved in order to preserve the length of the muscle. When an intensive muscle elongation program is administered, resting splints should be made by an orthotist immediately at the end of the program in order to preserve the results and postpone or eliminate the need for more intensive/aggressive (surgical) treatment methods.

Unsuccessful serial casting is usually an indication that a more aggressive plan, such as a series of Botox injections, is needed. These injections contain a toxin known as Botulinium, which causes localized paralysis of the spastic muscles. This partial paralysis enables relaxation of the muscles for a period of 3–6 months. During this period, the care-givers of the individual with RS and her physiotherapist must employ an intensive program for the lengthening of the shortened muscle. If Botox treatment fails, surgical correction is necessary. Walking and standing can help to prevent or postpone surgical intervention. Splints and foot supports have several objectives:

- Preventing deformations — Since age-appropriate bone growth of the foot and leg is mainly achieved before 10 years of age, exerting pressure in the proper directions during those years will direct proper growth and ensure that the soft tissues are activated in the proper directions. Hypotonic children have a tendency towards deviations of the foot, such as inversion and sunken arches. The more spastic the child, on the other hand, he/she will be liable to develop an equine-type deformation in which the foot points downwards and inwards with the toes bent. An orthotic/therapeutic solution must be implemented for each of these problems.
- Controlling and preventing undesirable movement — A splint or foot support brings the foot or ankle to a neutral position and keeps the foot within a correct ROM. It also prevents the development of shortened foot muscles and keeps the foot joints, bones and tendons moving at a correct angle of motion, thereby preventing future pain and loss of function.
- Protecting and stabilizing weak muscles — Muscles that are hypotonic or weak due to tendon-lengthening surgery are not strong enough to stabilize the foot when it is moving, particularly when bearing weight. Splints can provide the necessary stability and safety. Both hypotonic and spastic individuals are liable to develop abnormal foot and ankle positions. The damage caused to the foot is increased by carrying weight. For this reason, in cases where abnormal posture of the feet is caused during weight bearing, splints are indispensable for standing.
- Controlling deviations caused by abnormal muscle tone — Muscles presenting abnormal muscle tone will function through improper direction and with improper uncontrolled amount of strength. The splint prevents incorrect movement and keeps hypertonic muscles from forcing their destructive strength on the developing foot.
- Receiving correct sensory information — If the user can walk and/or stand, she will be able to try and assume positions other than sitting. Practicing standing or walking with splints offers the brain the important opportunity to receive correct proprioceptive information based on normal foot positioning.

The following list contains the most common types of foot supports:

- Semi-stiff or stiff foot supports (SPS/MBO) — These foot supports are low and preserve the position of the calcaneus, slightly stabilize minute uncontrolled movements caused by hypotonicity, help in supporting loose tendons and prevent the drop of the medial arch, which is a common condition among young individuals with low muscle tone. Such is the case in about 60% of children and 30% of adults with RS [33]. The support that this orthotic apparatus provides is minute and only effective when used inside a high supportive leather shoe. Such foot supports can improve stability and increase function for individuals with RS who show low muscle tone, thus helping them walk and stand in an adequate foot position. This type of orthotic is ineffective if the person is extremely hypotonic, very heavy or presents high muscle tone.

- Supramaleolar orthosis (SMO) — This type of support prevents pronation and supination of the foot and maintains dorsi and plantar flexion of the ankle in natural alignment. This type of splint is a bit more stable and offers better support than SPS/MBO. It stabilizes the foot and prevents deviation of ankle movement from the center line. Overweight individuals may need to use an SMO if lesser foot supports prove insufficient.

- Ankle foot orthosis (AFO) — This type of splint prevents plantar flexion of the foot and the stretching of the Achilles tendon, neutralizes tonal reflexes, preserves the weak gastrocnemius muscle following tendons-lengthening surgery and can be used, with additional padding, as a resting/night splint. It can also be used to help stabilize the feet and ankles of individuals with RS who cannot stand independently, as well as help them to maintain a standing position and providing a natural articular alignment. These types of splints, used constantly under a daily/night program, can prevent the shortening of the Achilles tendon. Due to the efficacy of early intervention, it is important to take action before the actual shortening is noticed and apply a daily maintenance program as soon as spasticity at shin level is detected. Sometimes individuals with RS might simultaneously present several deviations of the foot. One such deviation can be the shortening of the Achilles tendon together with supination and forefoot adduction. An AFO is the only type of splint that can handle situations in which a combination of several deviations simultaneously occurs. An AFO with an ankle hinge is preferable for preserving the neutral motion of the ankle during function. Hinged AFO splints are beneficial and maintain almost natural movement when the user stands up from a sitting position, as well as when she ascends or descends stairs. It is preferable to use hinged splints for mobile individuals in order to prevent losing mobility and to avoid the weakening of the triceps-sura muscles. A hinged AFO with a stop will prevent the user from exhibiting a plantar flexion posture at the ankle as well as performing knee hyperextension [24]. Since individuals with RS have difficulty adjusting to new situations and experiences, they may have difficulty getting used to splinting and hindered movement. It is therefore advisable to initially try using an "off the shelf" modular AFO before measuring for and purchasing an individually custom-made one. In this manner, an assessment of how the person with RS moves with the splint, the way she has adjusted to the new sensory experience and whether or not there are functional improvements can be observed without excessive costs.

- Active AFO — This is a long AFO, positioned over the foot, ankle and knee joints. It is equipped with a hinge at ankle level and rubber straps in front from the top end of the splint to the anterior part of the foot. The back part of this splint straightens the knee while the Velcro straps keep the foot in place. At the same time, the rubber straps apply constant stretching over the Achilles tendon. This type of splint improves the dorsi-flexion ROM of the ankle, lengthens the triceps-sura muscles and tendons and may eliminate the need for tendo-Achilles lengthening surgery. This type of splint should be used as a resting splint in order to maintain proper length of the triceps sura, as well as to lengthen an already shortened tendon (see figure XV-35).

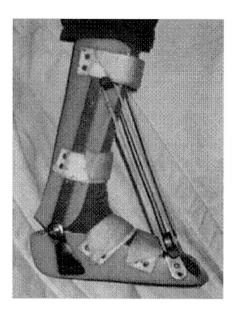

Figure XV-35. Active AFO.

Inhibitive splints or bivalved leg cast — The main objective of inhibitive splints is to decrease the influence of abnormal tonal reflexes of lower extremities. (It should be noted that extreme abnormal tonal reflexes are rare in individuals with RS.) These casts are made of plaster or fiberglass. The splint can be taken apart and has front and back sections that are joined together with Velcro straps or buckles. Splints of this type must provide the following:

- Over-straightening of the large toes
- Support and pressure application beneath the metatarsals
- Stable positioning of the ankle
- Deep pressure over the Achilles tendon

The sole of these splints is made flat in order to enable and encourage standing. The front part of these splints can be rounded at the front edge to help transfer weight forward and to encourage walking and moving. This splint helps to reduce muscle tone, straightens the big toes and their flexor tendons and assists walking for individuals who show muscle weakness under their extension hypertonic muscles, which might otherwise (without the use of such supports) cause their knees to collapse.

There is a large variety of splints and foot supports available and it is therefore important to consult with a professional before measuring for, purchasing or adapting an orthopedic aid. Individuals who are small in stature may be good candidates for devices made of relatively soft material such as Aquaplast, although it is preferable to use stiff plastic material for adults.

Conclusions

Since individuals with RS show a vast variety of functional disabilities, if the use of assistive technology can improve their function and overcome their limitations, it should be promoted. Due to the complexity of this issue, it is mandatory to introduce highly experienced clinicians in the areas of assistive technology with individuals with RS in order to enhance a process aimed at adapting special equipment for this population. Lack of professional assistance may cause the purchase of inappropriate equipment [5], later leading to its disuse and abandonment.

It is reiterated that the present chapter is a review of available scientific literature on the topic of assistive technology incorporating the clinical knowledge of the author in the field of RS; therefore scientific generalization should be limited.

Useful web sites on assistive technology:

- http://www.abledata.com — Provides a listing of over 17,000 different assistive devices
- http://www.wheelchairnet.org/ — Specifically focused on wheelchairs and other assistive technology devices
- http://www.resna.org/ — Site for the Rehabilitation Engineering and Assistive Technology Society of North America

References

[1]   Hoenig H. Assistive technology and mobility aids for the older patient with disability. Ann Long Term Care 2004;12(9):12-3,17-9.

[2]   Kerr AM. Understanding Rett disorder. A guide for professionals. An instruction DVD. Glasgow: Univ Glasgow, Section Psychol Med, 2006

[3]   Russell JN, Hendershot GE, LeClere F, Howie LJ, Adler M. Trends and differential use of assistive technology devices: United States, 1994. Adv Data 1997;292:1–9.

[4]   Yalom ID. The gift of therapy. New York: HarperCollins, 2002.

[5]   Mann WC, Hurren D, Charvat B, Tomita M. Problems with wheelchairs experienced by frail elders. Technol Disabil 1996;5: 101-11.

[6]   Edwards NI, Jones DA. Ownership and use of assistive devices amongst older people in the community. Age Ageing 1998;27:463-8.

[7]   Gitlin LN, Levine R, Geiger C. Adaptive device use by older adults with mixed disabilities. Arch Phys Med Rehabil 1993;74(2): 149-52.

[8]   Perks BA, Mackintosh R, Stewart CP, Perks BA. A survey of marginal wheelchair users. J Rehabil Res Dev 1994;31:297-302.

[9]   Baldursdottier R, Flo R, Hurnasti T, Jensen L, Sandberg K. User involvement in the development of assistive technology in the Nordic countries (USDAT). In: Marincek C, Buhler C, Cnops H, Andrich R, eds. Assistive technology. Added value to the quality of life. Amsterdam: IOS Press, 2001:95-8.

[10]   George J, Binns VE, Clayden AD. Aids and adaptations for the elderly at home: underprovided, underused, and undermaintained. BMJ 1998;296:1365-6.

[11]   Wallace JF, Flippo FK, Barcus JM, Behrmann MM. Legislative foundation of assistive technology policy in the United States. In: Flippo FK, Inge KJ, Barcus JM, eds. Assistive technology; A resource for school, work, and community. Baltimore, MD: Paul H Brooks, 1995:3-39.

[12]   Gilson BB, Huss DS. Mobility. Assistive technology for individuals with sensory impairment. In: Flippo FK, Inge KJ, Barcus JM, eds. Assistive technology; A resource for school, work, and community. Baltimore, MD: Paul H Brookes, 1995:87–103.

[13]   Hedman G. Rehabilitation technology. Binghamton, NY: Haworth Press, 1990.

[14]   Leonard S, ed. The Australian Rett Syndrome Study inaugural report. Aust: Telethon Inst Child Health Res, 2002.

[15]   Routhier F, Vincent C, Desrosiers J, Nadeau S. A new assessment tool for wheelchair users performance. In: Marincek C, Buhler C, Cnops H, Andrich R, eds. Assistive technology. Added value to the quality of life. Amsterdam: IOS Press, 2001:189–193.

[16]   Beuchel K. Physical therapy and gross motor skills in Rett syndrome. Handout, IRSA Ann Conf, Washington, DC, 2001.

[17]   Barak D. Daily accessories for the individuals with disability. In Ohry A, Shaked O, eds. Introduction to rehabilitative medicine. Tel Aviv: Min Defense, 1990:288–304. [Hebrew]

[18]   Lindberg B. Understanding Rett syndrome: A practice guide for parents, teachers and therapists. Toronto: Hognefe Huber, 1991.

[19]   Raijmakers M. Consumer survey into complaints about rollators. In: Marincek C, Buhler C, Cnops H, Andrich R, eds. Assistive technology. Added value to the quality of life. Amsterdam: IOS Press, 2001:199–203.

[20]   Brandt A, Iwarsson S. User satisfaction with wheeled walkers. In: Marincek C, Buhler C, Cnops H, Andrich R, eds. Assistive technology. Added value to the quality of life. Amsterdam: IOS Press, 2001:194-8.

[21]   International Rett Syndrome Association web site: http://www.rettsyndrome.org/content.asp?pl=147&contentid=147. Accessed 2006 Jun 21.

[22]   Hagberg B. Rett syndrome: Clinical and biological aspects. London: Mac Keith Press, 1993.

[23]   Lotan M, Elefant C. Physiotherapy and music therapy for a girl with Rett syndrome. A dual treatment approach. Fysioterapeuten 2006;2: 15-20. [Danish]

[24]   Weeks L. Rett Syndrome. Presentation, Sydney, Australia, 1997.

[25]   Tecklin JS. Pediatric physical therapy. Philadelphia, PA: Lippincott, 1994.

[26]   Hanks SB. Physical therapy strategies. Presentation, IRSA 12th Ann Conf, Boston, MA, 1996, Tape 622-08.

[27]   Hanks SB. Why physical therapy? Rett Gazette 2001;1–2:5–8.

[28]   McClure MK, Battaglia C, McClure RJ. The relationship of cumulative motor asymmetries to scoliosis in Rett Syndrome. Am J Occup Ther 1998;8(52):196–204.

[29]   Lotan M, Merrick J, Carmeli E. Scoliosis management in Rett syndrome. A case study. ScientificWorldJournal 2005;5:264–73.

[30]   Hanks SB. Motor disabilities in the Rett Syndrome and physical therapy strategies. Brain Dev 1990;12:157–61.

[31]   Budden SS. Management of Rett Syndrome: A ten-year experience. Neuropediatrics 1995;26(2):75–7.

[32]   Hoenig H, Cutson TM. Assistive and smart technologies: Improving older adults' quality of life. Durham, NC: Durham Veterans Affairs Med Center, 2002.

[33]   Kerr AM. The future for Rett syndrome girls. Int Rett Syndr Assoc Newsletter 1992;Winter:13-4.

[34]   Hunter K. The Rett syndrome handbook. Washington, DC: Int Rett Syndr Assoc, 1999.

[35]   Ellaway C, Christodoulou J. Rett syndrome: Clinical characteristics and recent genetic advances. Disabil Rehabil 2001;23:98-106.

[36]   Motil KJ, Schultz RJ, Wong WW, Glaze DG. Increased energy expenditure associated with repetitive involuntary movement does not contribute to growth failure in girls with Rett syndrome. J Pediatr 1998;132(2):228-33.

[37]   Sponseller P. Orthopaedic update in Rett syndrome. Rett Gazette 2001;1:4–5.

[38]   Personal communication: Rett syndrome with a motorized wheelchair, 2006.

[39]   Eng JJ, Levins SM, Townson AF, Mah-Jones D, Bremner J, Huston G. Use of prolonged standing for individuals with spinal cord injuries. Phys Ther 2001;81(8):1392-9.

[40]   Rubin C, Xu G, Judex S. The anabolic activity of bone tissue, suppressed by disuse, is normalized by brief exposure to extremely low magnitude mechanical stimuli. FASEB J 2001;15:2225-9.

[41]   Ward K, Alsop C, Caulton J, Rubin C, Adams J, Mughal Z. Low magnitude mechanical loading is osteogenic in children with disabling conditions. J Bone Miner Res 2004;19(3):360-9.

[42]   Haas RH, Dixon SD, Sartoris DJ, Hennessy MJ. Osteopenia in Rett syndrome. J Pediatr 1997;131(5):771–4.

[43]   Leonard H, Thomso M, Glasson E, Fyfe S, Leonard S, Ellaway C, et al. Metacarpophalangeal pattern profile and bone age in Rett Syndrome: further radiological clues to the diagnosis. Am J Med Gen 1999;12(83):88–95.

[44]   Walter JS, Sola PG, Sacks J, Lucero Y, Langbein E, Weaver F. Indications for a home standing program for individuals with spinal cord injury. J Spinal Cord Med 1999;22(3):152-8.

[45]   Dunn RB, Walter JS, Lucero Y, Weaver F, Langbein E, Fehr L, et al. Follow-up assessment of standing mobility device users. Assist Technol 1998;10(2):84-93.

[46]   Budden SS. Rett Syndrome: Habilitation and management reviewed. Eur Child Adolesc Psychiatry 1997;6(Suppl 1):103-7.

[47]   Centre for Developmental Disability Studies. Guidelines for the management of mobility and related issues for people with intellectual disability and limited mobility. Sydney: CDDS, Univ Sydney, 2003

[48]   Edlich RF, Winters KL, Woodard CR, Buschbacher RM, Long WB, Gebhart JH, et al. Pressure ulcer prevention. J Long Term Eff Med Implants 2004;14(4):285-304.

[49]   Yoshida H, Faust A, Wilckens J, Kitagawa M, Fetto J, Chao EY. Three-dimensional dynamic hip contact area and pressure distribution during activities of daily living. J Biomech 2005;39(11):1996-2004.

[50]   Stuberg WA. Considerations related to weight-bearing programs in children with developmental disabilities. Phys Ther 1992;72:35-40.

[51]   Cooper RA, Baldini FD. Prediction of pulmonary function of wheelchair users. Paraplegia 1993;31:560–70.

[52]   Solomonow M, Baratta R, D'Ambrosia R. Orthotics in spinal cord injury. Topics Spinal Cord Injury Rehabil 2000;5(4):29–53.

[53]   Lotan M, Isakov E, Merrick J. Improving functional skills and physical fitness in children with Rett Syndrome. J Intellect Disabil Res 2004;48(8):730-5.

[54]   Richards LC, Malouin F, Dumas F, Marcoux S, Lapage C, Menier C. Early and intensive treadmill locomotor training for young children with cerebral palsy: a feasibility study. Pediatr Phys Ther 1997;9:158-65.

[55]   Schindl MR, Forstner C, Kern H, Hesse S. Treadmill training with partial body weight support in non ambulatory patients with cerebral palsy. Arch Phys Rehabil 2000;8(3):301-6.

[56]   Fatouros IG, Taxildaris K, Tokmakidis SP, Kalapotharakos V, Aggelousis N, Athanasopoulos S, et al. The effects of strength training, cardiovascular training and their combination on flexibility of inactive older adults. Int J Sports Med 2002;23(2):112-9.

[57]   Pitetti KH, Boneh S. Cardiovascular fitness as related to leg strength in adults with mental retardation. Med Sci Sports Exerc 1995;27(3): 423-8.

[58]   Bauer D. Aerobic fitness for the severely and profoundly mentally retarded. Pract Pointers 1981;5(4):1-41.

[59]   Pitetti KH, Tan DM. Effects of a minimally supervised exercise program for mentally retarded adults. Med Sci Sports Exerc 1991;23(5):594-601.

[60]   Albright CL, King AC, Taylor CB, Haskell WL. Effect of a six-month aerobic exercise training program on cardiovascular responsively in healthy middle-aged adults. J Psychosom Res 1992;36(1):25-36.

[61]   Turley KR, Wilmore RH. Cardiovascular responses to treadmill and cycle erogometer exercise in children and adults. J Appl Physiol 1997;83(3):948-57.

[62]   Macko RF, Desouza CA, Tretter LD, Silver KH, Smith GV, Anderson PA, et al. Treadmill aerobic exercise training reduces the energy expenditure and cardiovascular demands of hemiparetic gait in chronic stroke patients. A preliminary report. Stroke 1997;28(2): 326-30.

[63]   Ellaway CJ, Sholler G, Leonard H, Critodoulou J. Prolonged QT interval in Rett Syndrome. Arch Dis Child 1999;80:470-2.

[64]   Sekul EA, Moak JP, Schultz RJ, Glaze DG, Dunn KJ, Percy AK. Electrocardiographic findings in Rett Syndrome: an explanation for sudden death. J Pediatr 1994;125:80-2.

[65]   Rossin L. Effectiveness of therapeutic and surgical intervention in the treatment of scoliosis in Rett syndrome. A seminar work. Pittsburgh, PA: Univ Duquesne, 1997;1-19.

[66]   Ulrich BD, Ulrich DA, Collier DH. Alternating stepping patterns: hidden abilities of eleven-month-old infants with Down Syndrome. Dev Med Child Neurol 1992;34:233-9.

[67]   Thelen E, Ulrich BD. Hidden skills. A dynamic systems analysis of treadmill stepping during the first year. Monogr Soc Res Child Dev 1991;56(1):1-104.

[68]   Witt-Engerstrom I. Autonomic monitoring in Rett syndrome at the Swedish Rett Center, Froson. Handout, Ann Conf Rett Syndr Assoc, Washington, DC, 2001.

[69]   Witt-Engerstrom I, Kerr A. Workshop on autonomic function in Rett Syndrome, Swedish Rett center, Frösön, Sweden. Brain Dev 1998;20:323-6.

[70]   Personal communication. Early differences between RS girls and their typical sisters, 1996.

[71]   Personal communication. Rehabilitation, 1997.

[72]   Personal communication. Older girls, 1997.

[73]   Larsson G, Engerstrom IW. Gross motor ability in Rett syndrome. The power of expectation, motivation and planning. Brain Dev 2001;23(Suppl 1):S77-81.

[74]   Jacobsen, K, Viken A, Von Tetchner S. Rett Syndrome and aging: a case study. Disabil Rehabil 2001;23(3/4):160-6.

[75]   Joice BU, Kirby RL. Canes, crutches and walkers. Am Fam Physician 1991;43:535-42.

[76]   Holder CG, Haskvitz EM, Weltman A. The effects of assistive devices on the oxygen cost, cardio-vascular stress, and perception of non-weight-bearing ambulation. J Orthop Sports Phys Ther 1993;18: 537-42.

[77]   Nabizadeh SA, Hardee TB, Towler MA, Chen,VT, Edlich RF. Technical considerations in the selection and performance of walkers. J Burn Care Rehabil 1993;14(2 Pt 1):182-8.

[78]   Mahoney J, Euhardy R, Carnes M. A comparison of a two-wheeled walker and a three-wheeled walker in a geriatric population. J Am Geriatr Soc 1992;40:208-12.

[79]   Personal communication I. The Hart walker, 2006.

[80]   Personal communication II. The Hart walker, 2006.

[81]   Kelley DJ, Friedman L. Go for it. San Antonio, TX: Harcourt Brace Jovanovich, 1989.

[82]   Drennan JC. The child's foot and ankle. New York: Raven Press, 1992.

ISBN: 978-1-61728-080-1
©2011 Nova Science Publishers, Inc.

Chapter XVI

Rett Syndrome: Environmental Adjustments as Fulcrum to Familial Balance

Yael Lahav-Danieli, BA Env Design, BArch[1]
and Meir Lotan, BPT, MScPT, PhD[*2,3]

[1]Department of Architecture and [2]Department of Physical Therapy, Ariel University Center of Samaria, Ariel and [3]Israel Rett Syndrome Center, National Evaluation Team, Chaim Sheba Medical Center, Tel HaShomer, Ramat Gan, Israel

In the last 50 years, many conceptual, physical and environmental changes were made in the lives of individuals with intellectual and developmental disabilities (IDD). One of the areas in which change has begun and is still constantly undergoing improvement is the quality of life and self-determination of individuals with IDD. As the different environments in which people live, learn, work and play influence many aspects of their lives, it is imperative to include such elements as self-determination, choice and autonomy when changes in the environment of the individual with IDD are planned.

Rett Syndrome (RS), the second most common multi-handicap genetic disorder after Down's syndrome, presents a special challenge in this area. Nevertheless, the literature suggests that individuals with RS have the capacity to show obvious preferences and choice-making in their lives. Therefore, the present chapter reviews the current position in environmental adaptation for individuals with IDD and suggests that the individual with RS and her family should participate in any changes to their physical environment. The chapter reviews clinical characteristics of RS that should be included when physical environmental changes for this population are in motion. This chapter presents a non traditional concept, stating that environmental changes could be suggested to the family with RS with the intent of not merely changing the physical environment, but rather the familial structure by enhancing a balance state between all members of the family. The

* Correspondence: Meir Lotan, BPT, MScPT, PhD, Department of Physical Therapy, Ariel University Center of Samaria, IL-40700 Ariel, Israel. E-mail: ml_pt_rs@netvision.net.il

chapter concludes with five case studies describing the decision-making process for this population across the life span and different settings.

Introduction

Interventions to compensate for physical impairment include adaptive techniques, assistive technologies and environmental modifications. This chapter will describe "environmental modifications" or "universal design". Environmental modifications or universal design are terms occasionally used to describe architectural designs that enable access to the widest possible range of physical abilities. Thus, generally speaking, adaptive strategies provide additional and unique ways of performing a task and assistive technologies compensate for the user's disability by increasing their functional abilities. Environmental modifications act to reduce the environmental demands on the individual and all three together help enable people with physical limitations to continue to accomplish important activities [1].

Rett Syndrome (RS), causing profound multiple disability, is a genetic disorder caused by MECP2 mutations [2,3]. Individuals with RS present a wide range of clinical severity [4,5]. The prevalence of the disorder is 1 in 10,000 of the female population [6]. The individual with RS usually has a wide array of functional difficulties that necessitates long-term nursing and environmental adaptations.

The present chapter will describe the challenges that are confronted by professionals working with individuals with intellectual and developmental disabilities (IDD) in general and with Rett Syndrome and their families specifically, when planning environmental changes. The chapter will describe the general considerations confronted when adapting the environment for individuals with IDD, describe special issues relevant for individuals with Rett Syndrome (RS), suggest actual steps to be taken when approaching this topic and give an account of five case studies.

Environment and persons
with intellectual disability

The different environments in which people live, learn, work and play influence many aspects of their lives [7]. When we address the issue of environmental adaptations we must approach it in the knowledge that this issue carries with it not only our objective professional abilities as service providers but also the assembly of a partnership with our clients. This produces change not only through their beds, doors and houses but, more importantly, within the context of their emotional capacities, their sense of loss of their personal identity and their emotional histories, attached to the labels and stereotypes that they bring into our shared interactions [8].

As professionals, we have to understand fully that the abilities of the individual with IDD will not change simply because a change in residence has accrued. A real change in abilities and attitudes will occur through guidance and teaching [9].

Today, people with IDD are seeking control over their lives. Their focus on choice and self-determination is especially directed towards those who affect their closest physical and human surroundings. People with IDD have the right to determine their personal goals and decide which support and services they want and need. For people with IDD, the focus is on living a life like every other community member and using typical community resources to accomplish their goals, whenever possible.

An important point to be considered when changes in the environment of individuals with IDD are made is to consider physical changes, together with emotional, environmental and human factors and other aspects contributing to quality of life.

When we talk about a better physical environment for the individual with IDD we have to take into consideration the complex emotional state of the individual in question [10] and his emotional well-being [11]. Since there is no point in adapting a house if little attention has been paid to the subjective quality of the individual's experience or, to them as a feeling human being [12]. Enhancing the individual's quality of life (QOL) will be promoted through allowing higher levels of personal control and choice that they have over their daily lives [13], as well as supporting their wishes and desires [14]. If individuals with IDD are supported to help make choices, participate in decisions, set goals and experience control in their lives, they will become more self-determined. As they become more self-determined, they will be more likely to assume greater control; make more choices; improve their skills in goal-setting, decision-making and problem-solving. Furthermore, they are more likely to have greater belief in their capacity to influence their lives [7]. One might also suggest that optimum environments are those in which individuals have the opportunity to express and further develop or acquire self-determination [7].

Yet at present times, for this population, it is often the case that daily routines, including work and leisure activities, are determined by service providers [15] and that these routines are, basically, denying self-determination to individuals with IDD.

Therefore, despite years of dealing with self-determination and the rights of individuals with IDD to self-determine, the notion still exists that those considered to have intellectual disabilities cannot be self-determined [7]. The underlying assumption of self-determination made by the authors of the present chapter is that all individuals with IDD\RS, at all ages, can and should have control over their lives, given the appropriate support and mediation [16,17]. Self-determination could start by establishing control over daily routines and leisure activities and include choice in the color of her/his clothes, in food items, in care-giving staff and much more. It has been found that people with disabilities, living in settings that offer more opportunities to make choices, exhibit more autonomous behavior [7]. It has been found that when greater autonomy is provided to residents with IDD, it has a positive effect on their adaptive behavior, and health [18]. Furthermore, it appears that when greater opportunities to be involved in decision-making are handed to individuals with IDD, such changes are associated with greater adaptive behavior and community integration [19] producing more successful adults and better educational outcomes for youths with disabilities [20,21].

All the above sources support the assumption that by providing opportunities for individuals with IDD to make decisions, we enable them to achieve confidence and self-efficacy, thereby gaining new skills which contribute to their ability to become integrated in to the community [22].

In order to improve the quality of life of people with IDD , the authors believe that efforts should be made to increase such individuals' experience of control over major life events and the extent to which they perceive themselves as being self-determined [23,24].

In light of the above we should always ask ourselves "what do individuals with IDD want when it comes to living accommodations?"

Needs, wishes and choice

It is presumptuous to say that we know what individuals with disabilities want when it comes to their living accommodations, especially since we can get answers to such questions from people with communication abilities, unlike most with RS. But we believe that relying on existing knowledge will give us general direction. In a study from Northern Ireland, 180 adults with intellectual disabilities were recruited to participate in 20 focus groups that dealt with the issue of present and potential living arrangements [25]. From these discussions and others [26-28], personal preferences emerged that were common to participants irrespective of where they lived:

- Single bedrooms for each person; if several people reside in one apartment [25,27,28],
- Participating in household activities [26]
- Having access to community activities [25]
- Ground floor accommodation is preferred
- Flat or small bungalow- type accommodation
- Only a few people living together; friendly with each other [27,28]
- Having a garden
- Close to family/friends
- Located in 'home town", townland or village
- Within walking distance from shops,
- Near to facilities such as doctors, pharmacies, supermarkets, public transport
- Near bus stops/public transport
- Close to a park/places to walk
- In a quiet area away from trouble (particularly loitering groups, drinking, fighting)
- Away from main roads and a lot of traffic
- Pleasant surroundings [27,28].

Some researchers have found factors relating negatively to user satisfaction such as:

- Lack of money [28,29]
- Being with incompatible co-residents [28]
- Isolation and harassment by people in local communities [28,29]
- Constraints on preferred lifestyles [30]
- Poor food [27].

The above are important issues that should be considered when engaging accommodation changes for people with IDD/RS. The general spirit of findings suggests that participants with IDD/RS value their independence, having access and choice of their support staff and the importance of relationships with co-residents and staff. Overall, the findings point to the need for greater consideration of personal preferences in home option choice-making by housing and service providers.

Physical changes in the environment

Researchers have also tried to assess the physical environment favored by those with IDD. In several studies, researchers noted that facilities with more attractive physical environments and more home-like atmospheres positively influenced adaptive behavior. The degree of variety and stimulation present in the residential environment of adults with IDD (defined by the researchers as the degree of personalization, distinctiveness and stimulation) was found to lead to higher levels of adaptive behavior [18].

Furthermore, features of the physical environment such as comfort, openness and functionality, were found to be positively related to adaptive behavior among people with IDD [31]. Further support to the previous finding was supplied by King and Raynes [32] who found that improvements in adaptive behavior were associated with environments that were individualized and stimulating. Thompson, Robinson, and associates [33] reported that people with IDD living in environments identified as having "home-like" physical features were more likely to be involved in independent household chores than were those living in "institutionalized" environments. Positive physical qualities of housing environments for older residents have also been associated with enhanced resident functioning, activity level and social contacts [34,35].

More supportive evidence as to the importance of the physical environment and to its positive influence on residents reveals that individuals who lived in more physically attractive settings (typically characterized by: interesting views from windows, distinct variation in style and décor from room to room and personalized furniture and objects in residents' rooms [19], showed evidence of higher adaptive behavior scores than did those who lived in less physically attractive settings. These findings are similar to results of studies which examined the impact of the physical design features on the behavior of older people [35,36]. An environment that is attractive, clean and well-maintained may communicate to those with IDD that they are viewed positively and as people of dignity [37].

It is probable to suppose that most of the participants in the above-mentioned discussion group and similar groups were not individuals with RS. What do we know of the choice-making abilities of this population? Are individuals with RS capable of the task of autonomy and decision-making over their own lives?

Rett syndrome

Some individuals with RS present severe multi-handicapped characteristics and it is known that some with more severe IDD tend to exercise less choice and are subject to more restrictions [38]. On the other hand we know that adults with IDD can gain knowledge and skills as they age [39,40] and they can also develop necessary skills in significant areas of their daily living [39].

Moreover, there is a strong body of evidence that demonstrates an association between the activity of the person with IDD and his adaptive behaviors and the receipt of attention, assistance or praise from care-givers, interaction between staff and residents, contact with family members, autonomy and choice [41-45].

Therefore, it is obvious that people managing individuals with RS bear the responsibility for their well-being [46]. Sometimes, the expectations from the individual with RS by their close human environment are limited, due to the underestimation of their potential [47]. Yet it is obvious now that a supportive environment can enable even a person with severe disabilities to exercise greater personal control, even if the individual has not yet been able to exercise choice independently [38].

The efforts to provide individualized support will, as suggested earlier, require that individual preferences and abilities be identified and environmental support be based upon these factors.

To date, there have been attempts to use adapted switches and toys or computer activities to motivate functional hand use of individuals with RS [48] to encourage interest in the environment and enhance awareness to give reason and effect to relationships with the environment [49-51]. Most of these attempts have proven to be favorable as they have applied to the abilities of the individual with RS.

It is customary to believe that a person's manual abilities are essential in order to operate switches that might control her/his environment, yet other responses by the participant may enable her/him to acquire control over events in the environment, thus leading to improved interest and motivation to explore toys and other objects [52].

In a case study, a child with RS participated in a research project and was taught to operate two switches, one that was placed behind her head and the other on the table in front of her at mid-line. During a year of introducing the program, the child developed increased hand-function control over a number of toys and music-playing devices and this behavior has been generalized to her home and to manual trials to manipulate toys in her vicinity. Even when the child in question was sick and the program was paused for a month, the former level of head activity and control over the switch was regained very quickly within one session from program re-initiation [52]. These experiences seemed to enhance attention to toys and to other objects in the environment and skills that apparently generalized from the class environment, to the home and ultimately to a new classroom. This case study and its results support the acknowledgement that children with Rett syndrome, despite developmental delay, severe (sometimes uncontrolled) seizure activity can learn to modify their behavior and to execute opportunities for control over some element in their environment.

A resent study verified the application of eye-tracking technology to analyze objectively the intentionality of gaze of individuals with RS. The data analysis from this project implies that intense gaze might be used by individuals with RS for communication [47], thereby enhancing environmental control. The development of new technologies that enable people to control a series of devices solely by their look is a powerful tool that will improve the quality of their lives [47]. Therefore, since evidence suggests that technological limitations are not, or in the near future will not be, a barrier for environmental control by individuals with RS, we need to look at their abilities to communicate their choices.

Choosing, choice-making and motivational factors

One of the ways to empower individuals with IDD is to enable them to make decisions for themselves [24]. Most importantly, there is evidence that people with IDD, such as those with RS, can learn to exercise choice and to make personal, independent decisions [53-55]. Not only can people with IDD learn to express preferences in a variety of situations, they can also facilitate positive behavioral outcomes when given the opportunity to choose, based on those identified preferences [56-58]. The initiation of choice-making should be executed in a meaningful arena, in situations that the individual with RS confronts daily and about which she cares, such as daily schedules (bath-time, bed-time), daily selection (clothes, types of food) and activities (listening to radio, watching television, taking a walk). If such opportunities are suggested, then the authors are certain that the possibility exists for the child with RS to gradually become an active member of her family and community.

In the light of existing literature, it is clear that the means and opportunities by which to enable those with RS to make decisions for themselves should be developed further and significant efforts should be made both to involve them in all decisions and to minimize the number of matters over which others exercise control.

Living accommodation

The relationships between the individual with RS and her family are an important part of decision-making when considering environmental changes. According to existing literature, we find that 85% of people with IDD have an excellent or good effective relationship with a sibling and that instrumental assistance is most likely to be provided by one sibling to another with disabilities when the latter has poorer functional abilities, when the siblings both live in the family home and when the person with disabilities is a sister [59]. Good relations among siblings are also apparent during adulthood when they have existed between the individual with IDD, the siblings and the mother during adolescence[60].

Another point to consider is that mothers of those with IDD experienced lesser care-giving burdens, greater care-giving satisfaction and less worry about the future care of their child with disabilities when the quality of the sibling relationship was rated highly [61]. In the light of such findings and due to the fact that relations between children with RS with their siblings are usually described as very close [62], this is a favorable aspect for the person with RS. It is therefore recommended that sibling relationships should be a consideration when planning daily routines, as well as when planning a house adaptation.

Communication challenges

On the one hand, most people with RS show considerable difficulty in verbal expression. On the other, the primary development of the child with RS leads to the belief that their communicative attunement and intentionality can be kept and used with alternative communication [63]. We also believe that individuals with RS show the emotional and social need to communicate, yet this need is cloaked by their disabilities [64], making their communicative acts hard for their human environment to interpret. Nevertheless, when their motivation is high enough and the human surroundings are attentive, the person with RS will be able to convey her needs and wants, thereby greatly improving her quality of life [65]. Communication systems such as alternative and augmentative communication (AAC) can compensate when the individual with RS has limited speech capacity. Moreover, these communication devices can function as an environmental control system (ECS) [66]. Therefore, when designing a home for the person with RS, the installation of such devices should be considered according to the child's skills and character.

Another factor that should be considered when adapting the house for the individual with RS and her family and when considering the inability of the former to verbalize, is her visibility. By creating opened-up large spaces, we enable the person with RS to be observed from other areas of the house, thereby providing a sense of independence, yet observing her and coming to her aid if the need arises.

Permanent nursing

Despite individual differences in the functional levels of individuals with RS, most with this disorder will always need close human supervision and care. In the light of this premise, it would be prudent to consider an extra living unit when adapting the family house of an RS member (if the economic burden can be tolerated). Such a unit should take account of sleeping, hygiene and other accommodation needs of the person with RS and her care-giver. Negative changes in emotional expression (crying, moody disposition) have been described in the past with regard to people with RS and have been attributed to constipation, hyperventilation, bowel pain, a noisy environment, an excess of stimuli and temperature changes [67]. Since these changes might last for periods from a few minutes to several hours, a separate unit might enable the person with RS to withdraw to her private shelter when she feels she wants to put some distance between her and the rest of the world (because of emotional outbursts that the she might experience occasionally). A separate unit will also give both the family and the care-giver a possibility of privacy and enable the family to detach itself from the person with RS and take care of the needs of other family members besides the former.

Ambulation abilities

As a group, people with IDD have been found to lead sedentary life-styles with all the later negative consequences of passivity that can arise [68-70]. Most individuals with RS are no exception in relation to this predicament. Therefore, it is recommended that the physical environment of the person with RS should enable and encourage a more active life-style. For instance, when the RS family is in the market for a home, the possibility of residing in close proximity to an accessible park or playground should be considered.

In 50-85% of children with RS [71,72] [according to the International Rett Syndrome Association, 2006] walking is achieved, yet 33-85% of the individuals who have achieved walking might later lose this ability [71,73]. Since walking abilities of those with RS should not be taken for granted, it should be obvious that an accessible, continuous pathway should lead from the family parking area to the entrance of the home.

When ambulating, the individual with RS has to confront her unreliable sensory processes (apraxia), her fear of movement, her fluctuating muscle tone and her poor muscular control attributed to ataxia. The accumulation of such challenges inflicts severe functional limitations upon the person with RS [67]. Because of her difficulty of movement, a spacious, open home is ideally recommended; since this enables her to walk with minimal interference, despite her limitations, whilst at the same time enables her care-giver to watch over her without the need to follow her around.

When designing windows for the home of the family with a Rett syndrome member, it should be considered that the individual with RS is usually of short stature, or may be ambulating in a wheelchair. Therefore it would be for the best if the windows are designed lower, closer to the ground, offering her a constant view of the outside, despite to her physical limitations.

Functional capabilities

The person with RS is usually characterized by functional deficits necessitating an adapted environment, if her control over her environment is to be maximized. It stands to reason that providing state–of-the-art medical treatment and rehabilitative equipment is essential, in order to raise quality of life (QOL) of the user [74].

One way of controlling the environment is through the use of assistive technology. In fact, in the U.S. Individuals with Disabilities Act, of 1988, Congress stated that the provision of assistive technology devices and services to individuals with IDD will enable individuals with functional difficulties to:

- have greater control over their own lives
- participate in and contribute more fully to activities in their home, school and work environments, and in their communities
- interact to a greater extent with non-disabled individuals
- otherwise benefit from opportunities that are taken for granted by individuals who do not have disabilities [75:1044]. Because of the functional limitations characteristic of

many individuals with RS, it is a probable assumption that they will gain from adapting their surroundings to become more flexible and compliant through the use of adaptive technology.

One type of assistive technology has been called an "environmental control system" (ECS). It is basically a switching device that allows disabled people to activate and control aspects of their environment that the disability otherwise prevents them from controlling [76-78]. Devices commonly controlled include domestic appliances such as television sets, radios, air condition, lights; vocational devices such as computers and telephones. ECS technology incorporates a control unit that activates these devices by means of electrical fixed wiring or remotely by infra-red or radio frequency control.

Controlling a television with their hands using a remote control device might not be possible for most individuals with RS. Therefore, using alternative means provides the switching interface assistance they need to activate the television. For instance, a person with RS may not have fine hand movement to activate a television remote control device but they usually have chin or eye movement [47]. ECS systems improve the QOL of the individual with disability, by increasing their independence in their home environment, decreasing the load placed on the care giver, increasing the self-esteem of the disabled individual [76-78] and by enhancing their ability to communicate, ameliorate their security and health, recreational capacity and control of household appliances.

Despite the facts that vast potential benefits are associated with the use of assistive technology and that many researchers have demonstrated conclusively that people with IDD can use and benefit from assistive technology devices [79-81] there is only sparse use of assistive devices by this population. The causes are lack of specific planning for this population, complexity of use of the devices in question, lack of knowledge as to the existence of such equipment and the high expenditure involved in purchasing it. However, with substantial advances in quality and quantity of ECS technology over the past 15 years, especially in the development of the interface between the user and the ECS technology [82], it is possible that such devices will soon be more available for the client with RS and her family. If the use of such technology is considered, it is desirable that ECS technology be built around the individual user [78].

Medications and alert states

Individuals with RS have been described as living under a cloud, with fluctuating levels of alertness that shift from day to day, and even within the duration of a day [83]. This phenomenon has been attributed to their medication consumption and their abnormal sleep patterns [84,85] but it is a common characteristic of RS. It is important that care-givers are acquainted with the daily waking and sleep cycles of the person with RS and introduce choice-making opportunities when the opportunity is appropriate [86]. This is true for the general population with IDD as it is for individuals with RS [87]. In one case study, the participating child with RS seemed to be in an exhausted/sleepy state most of the time. Therefore, the staff treating the child used periods of alertness to engage her in intensive periods of individual intervention. This flexibility by the staff enabled to achieve and register progress for that child [52].

Sudden death syndrome

Females with RS typically survive into adulthood, but the incidence of sudden, unexplained death is significantly higher than in non-Rett Syndrome controls of similar age [88]. This sudden death may be due, in part, to the higher incidence of longer QT intervals, T-wave abnormalities and reduced heart-rate variability in RS [89,90], but can also be relate to sudden death due to epilepsy (SUDEP) [91] or other mortality causes referred to as "complications of Rett Syndrome" [92], such as breathing abnormalities [93]. The possibility of sudden death necessitates that when preparing a separate living unit/room for the individual with RS, a monitoring device be installed to constantly relay the person's condition to the parents/care-giver.

Special room with adaptations

The bedroom

Because of the sleep disorders of individuals with RS [62,84,85], some particular attention should be paid to the beds in which they sleep. With the vast array of beds available it should be possible to find the most suitable type for a particular child with RS. When considering a bed, one should bear in mind the following factors:

- The height of the bed should fit the varied needs of each user. If the individual with RS is immobile, it is important that the bed be high enough to allow easier access when administering different treatments by the therapist and caregiver. Optimally, the bed should be height-adjustable.
- If adjustable height is not an option it may be possible to saw down the bed's legs if it is too high or alternatively to prop the bed up with a leg-elevating device, if it is too low.
- If the child is using a wheelchair, it is important to make sure that the mattress is level with the cushion on the wheelchair's seat, to provide easy transition from wheelchair to bed and back.
- If a crane is used for transporting a child to and from bed, bed height should enable access for the crane's base (11 cm. at least), and it is important to make sure that the bed's location in the room is accessible from at least two directions by the crane.
- Location of the bed is important! On the one hand, adjacent to a wall is safer, as the wall, supporting the child, will prevent her from falling off the bed. On the other, the positioning of the bed in the middle of the room will provide three points of access, which can be crucial during emergencies. One should consider bed location according to issues of security and safety and the general health and sleeping habits of the child.

- A large, double bed is recommended, because large sleeping surfaces promote movement during slumber.
- Mattresses that reduce pressure should be incorporated into beds for immobile children (there are many kinds available to consumers and it is recommended that a professional person, who is well acquainted with the various types of mattress and who knows which are suitable for the child, be consulted).
- If the bed has wheels (which makes it easier to clean the room), there has to be a brake on each wheel, for safety sake.
- A board or some other support surface may be placed under the mattress to counter any overly-soft nature of the mattress.
- Remember that mattresses that are too hard do not provide sufficient support for all the body's extremities. On the other hand, a depression is likely to form in mattresses that are too soft, causing the child to get stuck and lose the option to move.
- The right mattress is personal. Sleeping duration and relaxation levels are proof of the extent of compatibility of a mattress.
- The term "orthopedic" bed is meaningless because there is no official standard or grade of bed quality and the word "orthopedic" is used to boost sales. Therefore individual preference should be the standard for using\buying a specific mattress
- Electrically powered beds can be configured to personal settings. After personalization, the child can also alter the state of the bed (it is recommended that the manufacturer be consulted beforehand). This is an additional benefit which provides at once both independence and fun and other children just might be overjoyed to join the "voyage" on the bed, in which case the girl will be the center of attention, in her own private playground.
- If purchasing a hospital bed, it is preferable to select a three-part bed, (termed: full fowler) from which the head/leg parts move separately. This will allow the elevation of the girl's torso when she catches a cold, allowing for easy breathing.

Bathrooms

Bathroom aids typically include raised seats for the bath, shower and toilet, grab-handles and hand-held showers. A raised toilet-seat or bath-bench may be helpful to an adult who has difficulty in getting up to a standing position from sitting at normal height. A miniature toilet (as can be found in children's schools) will be more appropriate for a child who has standing and walking abilities. Many people find that a hand-held shower is helpful when using a bath-bench or shower and designs are available that can be attached to most faucets/taps and shower-heads. There are differences in the stability and sturdiness of various bath and shower chairs. It is important to ensure that the equipment provided will fit in the patient's bathroom while maintaining the user's safety and care of the back of the care-giver. A visit by a health related professional or better yet, a group of experts in the area of adaptive technology and environmental adaptations can help in making informed decisions about optimal bathroom equipment. Free-standing commodes (toilet seats) are available with fairly high seats, or raised toilet seats can be attached directly to the toilet. Free-standing commodes can be placed directly over the toilet or used in a separate room. Hydraulic lifts can be helpful for patients who have extremely limited mobility and they can be easily used even by quite frail care-givers. The use of lifts demands extensive alteration sometimes including expansion of the bathroom and passages to and from it, to allow this type of equipment to be used (ceiling lifts might be a solution that consumes much less space)

The use of grab-handles is only relevant for individuals with RS who present reliable hand grip and where the grab-handles do not endanger the child if she is left partially supervised. Nevertheless, for the person who can stand on her own and show sufficient manual ability, bars or handles may allow her to rise more safely by allowing her to compensate for weak legs using her upper extremity strength. Some raised toilet seats have bars attached to the seat itself as do most free-standing commodes. In addition, bars are available that attach easily to the back of the toilet. Appropriate statutory regulations should give guidelines for the use of bars. However; newer grab-bar technologies such as "swing-away" grab-bars may be preferred when toilet space is limited. Bars can be attached to the side of the bath or they can be attached to the wall by the bath. Special attachment techniques are available to attach bars to prefabricated baths or showers. The bars that should be planned for the individual with RS are those that present a variety of stabilizing mechanisms which might help to extend the holding ability of the person with RS and reduce the care-giver's stress in overseeing the client.

Living with family

Living with family is the dominant residential arrangement in the US for people with IDD. Recent estimates indicate that about 60% of US citizens with IDD live with their families [94,95]. Therefore this chapter will engage mainly with the analysis of the person with RS, her family and the home in which she resides.

It is in the nature of things that family relationships form a central core of the quality of life of adults with IDD/RS who live in the parental home and they figure prominently in most theoretical frameworks of quality of life [96].

Moreover, care for people with severe disability is loaded with emotional issues. It is dominated by the concern to provide an environment of care that not only meets the material needs of such people, but also fosters their development, integration and psycho-logical well-being. Western ideology currently holds that such an environment is best provided by the family of the person with the disability and numerous studies have lent support to this view [97].

Krauss and his associates [98] studied the social support networks of 418 adults with IDD, all of whom lived at home, and found that individuals with more severe disabilities had the smallest networks and were the most likely to have no friends. Such a situation calls for the professionals involved with environmental changes for the individual with RS and her family to address the issues and suggests that daily routines and physical environment will encourage social encounters (large windows to allow transparency from the world towards the individual with RS and vice-versa; daily walks in public areas to enable transient interaction with others in the community; participation of person with Rett in family/social experiences.

Person-centered planning

One of the actual ways of achieving QOL through the enhancement of self-determination of the individual with IDD is by the employment of a framework of individual planning or person-centered planning (PCP). This section will provide actual steps to go through when implementing person-centered planning in environmental changes for the individual with RS.

It is reiterated that efforts need to be made to ensure that opportunities for activity both in the home and in the community are developed and maintained by care-givers.

It is should be clear to all involved that the individual with RS must be taught how to make use of new/changed environments [40].

We (the authors) understand that by extending the capacity of users and caregivers to participate in decisions about the design, management and review of accommodation through person-centered planning, implies that more work will be passed to already hard-pressed personnel, family members, and service-users. This poses the enormous challenge of seeking the meaningful involvement of users [99] yet we believe that the efforts are worthwhile.

When forming a team of professionals to evaluate and plan accommodation changes, this team should employ the person-centered planning approach as their basic form of action.

The use of focus groups is highly recommended since such gatherings have important advantages both in reviewing present situations and assessing and defining the desired outcomes and those that can actually be achieved [100]. The dynamics generated within focus groups can:

- help participants to gain confidence
- create safe, non-threatening and non-intimidating environments for discussion
- provide for inter-member reinforcement, peer support and validation of views and experiences
- enable members to participate in activities from which they would otherwise be excluded [101].

The first step is to create a personal profile through interviews of the people who spend the most time with the individual with RS on a daily basis. The profile should contain the information such as: basic information about the person's experiences, both past and present, information about the quality of the person's life and information about personal preferences and important themes in the person's life.

When the assembly and evaluation of the above data is being forming into a more solid body of knowledge and there is an opportunity for reflection, another meeting of the team (including the individual with RS, friends, staff, family and others committed to the individual with RS) should be held. The meeting is aimed at forming a draft plan through the next stages:

- Review the data collected so far.
- Review common events (ongoing events that are likely to affect the person either in a positive or negative way) in the environment.

- Find desirable images of the future. The team begins to share their ideas about the future by brain-storming about where the person might live and possibilities and opportunities for fun and relaxation.
- Identify obstacles and opportunities. The group decides on which area of life it is most important to work first and then identifies both obstacles and opportunities that may be encountered.
- Build a support group to make these ideals happen and overcome obstacles.
- Identify strategies. The strategies are specific action steps, in which each team member is assigned a task to handle.
- Get started. The group or "circle of support" identifies up to five action steps which they will commit to completing within a short period of time.
- Identify the need for change. The meeting is concluded with two lists; a list of thing to do and one including any problem that might be "part of the system".
- During follow up meetings, the group members begin to develop strategies for making the changes happen.

Preparing the individual with RS for a change in accommodation

It is known that individuals with RS usually reject new places and situations. It is therefore crucial that, when people are considering a change in accommodation, the individual with RS should have opportunities to be prepared, through the use of early visits, to look around the new local community and experience the level of independence she might have. When considering home alterations it should be obvious that the individual with RS, besides taking part in the process, will be verbally and experientially prepared by looking, for example, at a model or at an appropriate video.

The sense of loss that one experiences when changing location or when other alterations to the existing environment occur (such as a move from one's room to another due to changes in the family) is perceived to be greater when the move is sudden. Failure to overcome such difficulties can lead to a reduced quality of life and may contribute to a poorer state of physical and mental health [102].

Home environment for the family

This part of the chapter has been written by way of an elaboration from specific cases. In this part, five case studies describing a variety of ages and living arrangements typical of individuals with RS will be described. Our aim is to suggest specific environmental designs/changes that have direct or indirect influence on interpersonal relationships within the family and on the quality of life of the person with RS and her family. We know that every family will physically adapt their home in accordance with the physical incapacity of the family member with RS and in the best way to enable direct care and ADL needs for this individual, taking into account their economic capabilities. We would like to restate our belief that such physical changes should not be implemented with the narrow objective of changing the home, but to achieve a focus for improved family functioning in a much broader sense. We hope that every reader will be able to identify some helpful hints that will aid in arranging his/her home to the benefit of family organization. All the case studies follow changes in manner in which the families behave in accordance with:

- The development and growth from childhood to adulthood of the person with Rett
- The characteristics of the family
- Cultural belonging
- Financial resources

By referring to these five cases, we shall show how physical changes in the environment (re-arrangement of furniture and rooms) can influence behavior patterns and quality of life of the family with RS. The purpose of this section of the chapter is to give examples that will enable other families to evaluate their specific situations thereby pin-pointing elements that might "disturb" the equilibrium of the household. We claim that, in many cases, physical rearrangement of the home and/or furniture can help in achieving improved quality of life for the person with RS and her family.

We would like to emphasize that any remarks made within the content of the following section are made as purely objective and non-judgmental observations. There is no good or bad mode of behavior but rather family behavior that changes according to a variety of influencers. It is for each reader to identify elements that could be changed for their situation, thereby assisting their family to achieve the best possible life-style and balance within the family structure and its habits. We have divided our observations to four main life-stages of the person with RS:

- Infancy and early childhood
- Adolescence
- Early adulthood (preparation towards leaving the home)
- Adulthood (life in a residential setting)

Each of these periods in life has its own characteristics, directly of indirectly influencing the way the home is "organized" into a balanced life constellation (with regard to individual circumstances), taking into account the needs of the family as a unit as well as a collection of autonomous individuals sharing a residential environment.

Case story 1 (infancy and early childhood)

A is a child diagnosed with RS, aged 3 at observation. She is the third in the family after two boys. She was born after an uneventful wanted pregnancy and normal delivery. She is a lively child who likes to watch television and eat. The child has the ability to stand and walk and perform transfers with considerable support and needs assistance in all life's ADL activities. The child occasionally uses Assistive Augmentative Communication (AAC) apparatus to communicate.

The home

The family resides at an apartment building with an elevator, on the third floor. The apartment can be divided into two main areas a public one and the private part. The public area includes the living room, the kitchen and a dining room, which are adjacent to a room designated as a television and study room and a small, closed balcony, mainly used as storage space. The private part includes three bedrooms (one for the parents, one for child with RS and one shared by her two elder brothers) and a bathroom. There are no open areas adjacent to the apartment (not even an open balcony).

The room of the child with RS

A long corridor leads up to the door. Immediately behind the door stands a tall baby's bed with a safety rail. This enables direct view, from the corridor and from the public area of the apartment, of the child with RS in her bed. Inside the room are a computer-desk adapted for the child's height, a television set and a closed wardrobe. Beneath the bed and along the wall we find assistive devices for the child (walkers, standing frames, etc.). The general design of the room is functional and "dry"; no apparent ornamentation or toys can be viewed.

Activity area of the child with RS – The child's waking hours, which are not devoted to developmental therapeutic intervention, personal hygiene or feeding were spent mostly in her room in front of the television or the computer screens. Therapeutic interventions were performed in the child's room. Additional therapeutic apparatus was stored on the balcony adjacent to the living room. A communication board was hung on the living room wall at a height enabling its use by the child with RS and other family members. The child was fed in the kitchen in an adapted chair (including a knee separator, side, arm and leg supports) with her back turned towards the rest of the house usually without the accompaniment of other family members aside from the feeder.

Possibilities for change in the living environment - Goals

- To reduce the present high level of anxiety and the burden of currently- invested intensive supervision given to the child by the parents.
- To integrate the child into the center of family events by establishing familiarity by family members and guests with the child's behavior/actions.

Possibile changes in the living environment

- The television was moved to the living room – thereby moving the child and her TV set in to the main public area; "the heart" of the house.
- The child's main activity center was moved to the living room – thereby enabling her to become involved in the social activity of other family members and guests

- It was suggested that the activity of her brothers (and friends) should also be carried in the living room or in its near vicinity – placing the child within the center of events.
- The child's chair was moved to a new position around the table in the kitchen, facing the center of the house – thereby enabling her to watch others and to be watched while being fed
- It was suggested that as many meals as possible should be taken in the presence of other family members, as long they do not clash with the rest of the family's schedule.
- In order to achieve some possibility for withdrawal and self-accumulation, the child's bed was moved into a more interior area of her room, were she could only be seen after her room is entered. This was done to achieve a sense of privacy, together with the aim of reducing levels of outer control and of anxiety by parents.
- The look of the child's room was changed by adding dolls, furry animals and other soft/musical toys that were visible to every visitor, combined with rescheduling a time for the child actually to play with those toys - thereby enhancing the sense of normality for the child with RS.
- It was suggested that the high bed be replaced by one with variable height- control - thereby enabling it to change from a platform designed only for functional care-giving (clothing, changing a diaper/nappy) to a low bed, enabling the normality of bedside story-telling.
- Changes in the bathroom – Due to parents' concerns about the child's weight and the difficulty in taking her in and out of the bathroom, different standard solutions (a stool at the edge and an hydraulic lift at the bottom of the bath) were suggested to help the parents in their activities of daily living (ADL)

Early childhood – generalization and discussion

Rett abruptly hits the child as well as her family. A cute, healthy breath-taking baby suddenly "turns over" and transforms before the eyes of the unbelieving family into the child with RS, with everything this implies. On the one hand, the family trying to cope with the chaotic, hectic and sudden turmoil that have unexpectedly accrued by building a supportive, yet sometimes over-protective, environment around the child. On the other, this strategy secludes her in her room both to enable autonomy and to supply proper care but, to some extant, to set apart the healthy from the ill.

In families already with children there might be an expectation of the older ones to free up more parent time and more space than they were used to before the arrival of RS. In cases in which the child with RS is the first born, the amount of energy consumed by RS is so significant that there might be no more room for other children, since every waking moment revolves around the care-giving task.

Coping with RS gives rise to different reactions. Some might start a shopping-trip, purchasing every old and new piece of apparatus that might be thought of as helpful in advancing the child's abilities. Among them one might find multi-media gadgets, a computer, a standing-frame and walkers, physical therapy equipment, etc. In the same way, helpful aids are obtained to help in ADL tasks (an elevated bed, a special chair, special bath apparatus and big pillows for support).

Usually, a home with young children and babies, looks like a well-equipped kindergarten, with a colorful abundance of clothes, toys, equipment and gear spread around, creating a constantly cheerful commotion. Yet the child with RS does not leave such tracks behind her. Sometimes, the only way to break the giant void of passivity surrounding the child with RS is by "forgetting" her equipment lying around. Eventually the house is filled with physical and occupational therapy equipment and communication devices, and the figure of the child as a disabled one is gradually built and revealed. The new appearance of the child and family is obvious to all visitors. Despite the fact that all girls with RS differ from one–another, there are some similar phenotypic commonalities that might be used to set some guidelines with regard to caring for the young child with RS. These commonalities are diverse sleep patterns, frequent changes of mood, lack of verbal communication, the need for round-the-clock supervision and the unstable character of the Rett disorder (the appearance of scoliosis, epilepsy, constipation and eating disorders). Dealing with such an array of difficulties requires enormous reserves of hope, energy and patience. Occasionally the parents may feel the need to withdraw from the energy-consuming status of being in charge of a child with RS. Undoubtedly, the child herself might need an occasional refuge from the turbulence of challenges created by Rett syndrome. The solution might be to formulate a timetable of activities for the child, yet not forgetting to establish a secluded, quiet and calming area (e.g. a form of multi-sensory environment – [105-107] enabling total relaxation for the child and her care-givers. Without planned changes in her schedule, she might gradually find herself spending time alone in front of the television set, a situation which should be avoided.

The eating difficulties presented by the child with RS [108, 109] might be resolved in well-kept meal-times which in turn might cause her to be fed separately from the rest of the household to enable the parent to be fully attentive to her needs, whilst secluding the child with RS from her family.

Summary of early childhood – what should be done?

We believe that the healthier thing to do would be to keep as normal as possible representation of the situation; i.e. the child is at that and that age, her position in the family order is as it is, she goes to school and like many her age she attends private schooling and programs in the afternoon. She has many appliances that she needs and therefore has to have her own room.

Possible recommendations for this stage:

- Enrich her toy collection - Especially adding attractive ones based on their color, texture, motion abilities, appealing sounds, etc. These should be displayed, as with those of all her peers, on shelves, around her seating space, at her side of the table at meal times – since individuals with RS enjoy touch, sound and visual stimuli, they will probably enjoy and use such objects. We highly recommend that the child be given the opportunity from a young age to obtain some control and self-monitoring over her life, for instance, with her parents by choosing the toys at the toy shop.

- Whenever there are joint family activities (dining room, living room, playground, etc.) arrange her seating position (if the child is not mobile) making sure she is seated on a seat best-adapted to her physical needs and in a position that enables her best eye and voice contact with other members of the family. If possible, arrange a communication device close to the child with RS, properly positioned to enhance the initiation of communication with other family members by the child. We are confident that with continuous practice of her communicational skills, the child will optimize her abilities, thereby, to some extent, acquiring independence and control over her life.

- Building a stable timetable – In order for the child and her family to achieve a "normative" life, responding to her physical/emotional /social needs, it is advised that the family establish regular daily habits. Outings are highly recommended since we believe that some of the stress involved in dealing with the RS disorder on a daily basis is due to confinement of the family to the home. Moreover, sensory/ social/interactive encounters with differing individuals in a rich outdoor environment can enable the child with RS to flourish as they fulfill a basic human need [110].

- Long-lasting relationships – we are sure that establishing long-lasting friendships from childhood will make a positive contribution to the child and her family, providing a source of support while dealing with the daily challenges of RS.

Moving to a residential setting at a young age

In some cases, the family might prefer to move the child into a residential setting from a young age, where she might share a room with other residents. When visiting the young child within the institute, the family has to cope with the detachment and alienation that might be encountered, as well as with their own pain of disassociating the child from the home environment. At the same time, the family has to cope with submitting their daughter to the hands of others and trust that she is well taken care of. We suggest that the room of the child with RS should be decorated in a way that will indicate a personalized identity through the use of personal belonging (toys and artifacts from home). It is recommended that the child should have a place were she can display the "presents" she gets on family visits. It would be wise to choose a residential setting geographically close to the family's residence, thereby enabling family members to "drop in" as often as possible. Another feature that should be established ahead of placing the child in the residential setting is that the residence can supply the family with a place and facilities that will enable the child and her family to spend quality time without special preparations and without the need to announce their forthcoming visit. A meeting of all family members with their child with RS in the Snoezelen environment has been found to be extremely beneficial in the past – [106], but more information on this topic can be found in the chapter regarding Snoezelen. If the child is expected to visit home occasionally, the house should be arranged to supply a familiar, comfortable accommodation, facilitating enjoyable, pleasant gatherings. When the child is absent from the house, her personal belongings represent her.

Case story 2 (adolescence)

A 16 year old person with RS who is the eldest child in the family resides at home with her two younger brothers. During daytime hours, the girl spends her time in a special education center and on her return she is taken care of by her mother. The girl is independent in transitions and ambulation and she has partial-handedness abilities, especially when strong enough motivational factors (such as communication and foodstuff) are involved.

The apartment

The apartment is located in a building in a quiet street in a small town. It is a ground floor apartment with a small, fenced garden attached. The entrance to the garden is through the living room, over a paved surface and onto a well-cultivated lawn. The public area of the house has an open kitchen, a dining corner and a living room with a T.V. area. The private area of the house includes four bedrooms and a shared bathroom for the children and a parent bedroom with an adjacent bathroom, which the girl with RS uses.

The girl's room

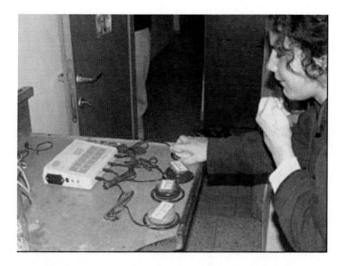

Figure XVI-1. A voice output communication device.

The girl has her own room, at the end of the corridor and it is set in a way that enables a view of the interior of the room only when standing at the entrance to it. The bed is opposite the door, under the window. The bed is at a normal height, enabling the girl to mount and dismount the bed at will. This height enables the mother to sit by her daughter's side and read her bed-time stories, which, according to the mother is much enjoyed by the girl. Above the bed there are a couple of book-shelves. In this room there is a closet used as storage room by all family members. The room also contains a big dresser with shelves hanging above it, displaying an assortment of colorful dolls and artifacts. The girl herself does not have the ability to open the dresser or take things off the shelves. On the dresser, there is a set of communication switches (see figure XVI-1), yet since the girl spends most of her waking hours in the living-room, the switches are mostly unavailable to her.

The major area of activity of the girl with RS

The girl, being sociable, likes to hang out in the public areas of the house. She usually sits on the edge of the living-room sofa "absorbing" the vigorous activity of the home. Commonly she initiates personal contacts with other family members, especially her mother. According to her mother, the girl likes to walk outside yet she usually avoids doing so since the fenced garden (as things are) is exposed to wind and sun.

Possibilities for changes in the living environment –Goals

- To enhance the privacy of the girl with RS
- To enable more freedom of movement
- To encourage shared activity of the girl and her mother
- To improve ways of communication with other family members

Possibilities for changes in the living environment

- Enjoying the outdoors on her own terms – When combining a general approach to a healthy life style, the girl's functional abilities and her love for the outdoors, we suggested that the rear garden be set up for easier access from the living room, with shaded and easily accessed resting spots created. In addition to the suggestion that independent outings by the girl are made available, we noticed that she has her own unique way of spending time in the outdoors (being out there, yet protected in some way). It was suggested that a rocking-chair be stationed in the rear garden. This chair should provide good enough support for the girl's back (due to her developing scoliosis) and enable her to get "the feel" of being out. With the intention of engulfing the girl within a relaxing, enchanted ambiance, we suggest some form of small garden gazebo with a comfortable chair, sounds of running water and colorful flowerpots. Another addition that would coincide with the girl's inclinations as well with her manual abilities would be the establishment of a pets' corner (with rabbits and hamsters). Because of the possible emotional bonding of which individuals with RS are capable, it is advised that long-lasting animals should be presented (cats, dogs, a parrot) with emphasis on warm, loving creatures.
- Enhancing communication/independence – To position around the house (or hang on the wall) some communication stations. In this case, our girl has the ability to understand and use up to about 80!! written words, including the formation of simple written sentences. It was recommended that a voice-activating device might enable

her to call out for other members of the household, thereby initiating communication at will.

- Employment – it is suggested that a work-station should be set up in her room, to include a computer, at which she could be involved in games and creative activity, including homework from school. Working regularly at her station could be a useful habit since she would be finishing school in a couple of years. It should be reiterated that her mother's (to whom the child is extremely attached) work-station is in the girl's room, so they both could sit and work together, side-by-side. Another work-station could be where the pets in question are fed and yet another possibility would be to position some elevated flowerbeds for the girl to plant and cultivate.

- Improving body image - it is suggested that a mirror be hung in the public area of the house where the girl can observe her reflection. It might be beneficial for a girl of her age and an incentive for walking around, to see herself in a mirror.

- Privacy – it is suggested that a curtain be hung at the entrance to the girl's room to allow a sense of privacy while taking care of the girl's hygiene needs.

- Enhance self-advocacy and give room for personal taste – It is suggested that the girl's room be redesigned, in a taste more becoming of a teenage girl. Meaningful artifacts and pictures might be hung on the wall opposite her bed (the girl with significant individuals/animals, photos of television/movie stars). This reorganization should be done with the girl's approval and participation in the forthcoming changes (changes of objects, colors, position of furniture, etc).

- The mother's workplace- In the light of the special bond between the girl and her mother, it seemed appropriate that the mother's work-station is located within the girl's room. If we adjoin the girl's workplace (see above) to her mother's than they could actually "work" side-by-side while the mother sets an example to her daughter.

Adolescence – generalization and discussion

When the individual with RS is entering her adolescence her "living areas" should be re-organized\refreshed.

- Privacy - It does not become adolescent girls (with or without RS) to be improperly dressed or handled in public or when privacy is due. The matter should be evaluated by the family and in some cases might necessitate change in family habits around issues of personal hygiene. When money and space are in abundance, than a separate living-unit for the person with RS might be considered. Such a unit should include a set of bedrooms for the person with RS and her care-giver, including an adjacent bathroom and rest room. When cheaper options have to be considered, than a curtain or any kind of screen might be used to delineate the girl's private area.

- Personal taste, self-care and empowerment of the self – Like others her age, the young girl with RS might take pleasure from observing her image in the mirror, from beauty-care and from up-to-date designer clothing. This might be a good time to discover and encourage expressions of personal taste, develop social behaviors (aesthetic eating, for example) and proper ways of approaching others. Nice outfits, attractive, beautifying garments, nice-looking hairstyles should be looked after and refreshed.

- Submitting to adolescent changing taste – Re-arranging the girl's room so as to make it more appropriate to the taste of an adolescent might be in order. It is, of course, advised that all changes be consulted upon with the girl, embracing her tastes in new items, colors and design of the walls, bed-covers and hung pictures. The placing of personal objects (c.d.'s, books, dolls, etc.) at accessible places might enhance the girl's sense of control.

- Addressing adolescent turmoil - By expecting and accepting hectic changes in mood and sudden outbursts and by teaching the girl to foresee such changes in advance and seek comfort, one might slightly control and/or reduce such incidences. Placing "communication stations" in proximity to the girl, enabling her to "scream" out when in times of distress.

- Outings and social life – the siblings of the girl with RS are growing along with her and suddenly they reach adolescence as well. It is expected that they will withdraw their areas of activity from the public to the private areas of the home (i.e. to their rooms) and at that point the girl with RS might find herself outside of their closed doors. Like any other human being she has a need to partake in social encounters, to live an active life-style and to be sensually stimulated. Living a full active and social life was advised from a young age and this is reiterated. Daily walks in public parks might support all the above- mentioned goals yet it is not always possible, because of logistical and mobility issues. If mobility is an issue, then the family should consult with a physical or an occupational therapist skilled in those matters, in order to overcome such limitations. Efforts should be made to enable the person with RS to have an accessible environment (routes, parks, walkways, transport, etc.) thereby keeping her and her family as mobile as possible, limited only by the girl's abilities. Time and effort spent during earlier years in constructing personal and social relationships are now paying off. Thanks to the social nature of people with RS, meeting friends could supply the girl and her care-givers with the required motivation to invest in traveling some distances.

- Education and life-skills – The rarity of RS is actually a constraint against specialization in such a disorder by health care professionals. In such a case it is common for the family to transform the home into a mini-development and support unit in an attempt to maintain and enhance the skills and education achieved by the girl over her years in school. It is advised that such a change be done through consultation with experienced professionals. Choosing familiar strategies and means for learning and advancement are also strongly recommended [111]. We recommend that individual advancement programs be directed towards enhancing activity levels and improving communication skills. Yet, we are aware that such programs can only be implemented at home if the time and availability of human resources (care-givers, parents, siblings or other family members) enables it, without harming the integrity of the household in areas that are unrelated to the person with RS.

A general remark: Adolescence is a time for disillusionment. Because of individual versatility and the frenzied nature of RS, the prognosis of the child with RS at a young age is difficult to predict and therefore there is always hope. Yet, with advancing age and through the second decade of the person's life, the care demands of the person with RS are gradually piling up and the parents now face the consequences of living with Rett syndrome. In some cases, life with the person with RS overshadows the attention to other family matters. In many cases, the difficulties of outings with the person with RS necessitate that the family becomes withdrawn indoors. This situation therefore calls for proper adaptation that will turn the home of the family with RS into a nice and pleasant place in which to be, to reflect personal taste, enable gathering of friends and to contain recreational means that will enable tension-reduction for the person with RS and for other family members. In the home there should be a place that might be turned into a safe-haven for all family members, a spot were each of them can detach themselves from the daily predicaments and replenish their energy resources with some personal quality-time. The authors claim that such an organization of the home and family does not get set up by it self. In order for the home of the family with RS to establish surroundings that support the joint, as well as the individual needs of the family and family members, a process should be initiated. It is obvious that this is a task that has to be thought out, carefully planned and implemented with openness, goodwill and patience, to accomplish finally a place that will supply all of the above qualities.

Practicalities

In order to achieve the euphoric yet necessary "entity" of a balanced household described above, we recommend that each member of the family should draw up a wish list; Writing the most important things at the top of the list, with the least important, the negligible ones, at the bottom. Then, consulting a drawing of the house, the family might agree upon public spaces and the conduct that is required in those areas, as well as upon private areas and the "ownership" of them. The person with RS should acquire, on this occasion, whatever she needs, according to what the others are willing to give up. In a similar manner, after deciding on the territorial boundaries of the living space, the design of the house will have been taken care of, first the public areas and then the private zones. Here again, the discussion should include that of the needs, wants and likes of the person with RS, with the family involving her as much possible in the debate.

We do believe that through such reorganization of the house, the family might better take care of all its members, including the person with RS, thus achieving a form of supportive equilibrium. Some families might find choosing such a route hard to establish on their own, yet we encourage them not to give up on such a process but to seek professional help (social workers, psychologists and therapists from other professions) and together, when supported by the skilled experience of others, to go ahead and establish the transformation described above.

Case story 3 (early adulthood)

An 18 year-old woman with RS with two small siblings (a brother and a sister) residing at home. During the day, the young woman is in a special education center and at her return home she is cared for by her care-giver. She has ambulatory abilities only when heavily supported. She usually communicates through mood swings and by familiar signs known to her family members.

The home

The family resides in a farmers' community settlement, in a house surrounded by a very big, open space. There are three levels to the house; the main level has a spacious open-access kitchen that includes a dining-table, a living room, a family-room with a computer and an audio-visual system, three bedrooms for the children and a shared bathroom. The young woman's bedroom is at the end of this unit, with a corridor leading to it. The parents unit (bedroom and a bathroom) is on the upper level and in the lower level there is a study. There are three exits from the house to the garden (the area closest to the house is a roofed porch). They are all situated at ground-floor level. In the garden there are two other small structures. One serves as the mother's studio and the other is the residence of the care-giver. Throughout the house there are no signs of disability, whatsoever.

The place of the young woman in the public areas of the house: The disability of the young woman does not allow her to go up to the parents' room or down a level to the study. She usually sits in a normal chair watching television. Some of her afternoon hours are spent on the porch. Since she is very strict with regard to her meal-times, she eats most of her meals alone, yet the structure of the house and her place at the table allows her to view the rest of the house and, therefore, some of the other family members.

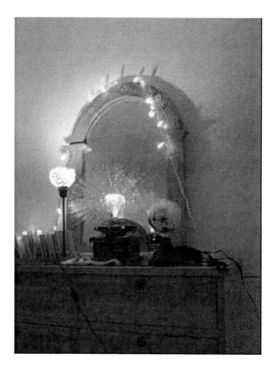

Figure XVI-2. A variety of lamps and candle holders.

The young woman's room – The room is completely devoid of any sign of disability. It is different, though, from the rooms of other women of her age. There are no posters on the walls; there is no desk; there is no computer; there are no books scattered around. Actually, the most obvious sign is the lack of nonchalant piles of cloths and the lack of order so typical of many adolescent's room. On top there other items common to people her age. There is a variety of lamps and candle holders which are placed around to room to help the young woman focus and relax to their gentle light (see figure XVI-2). The room can be easily darkened and its location in relation to the rest of the house enables sound deadening.

Communication between the young woman and her care-givers

The open and wide structure of the house and the lack of doors enable a clear view from almost every spot to the next (see figure XVI-3).

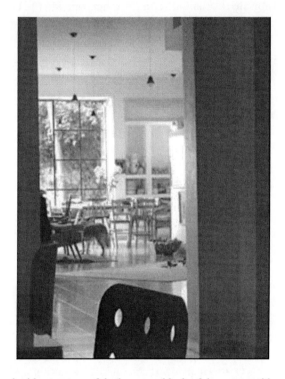

Figure XVI-3. An open and wide structure of the house and lack of doors to enable a clear view from dining sector to the recreational sector.

The parents report that when the young woman is in the house, they are constantly attuned to her every sound, finding it very difficult to draw away. On the other hand, they do feel that their daughter needs her own space and is mostly comfortable on her own in a sort of a "secluded private bubble", away from the household activities. The parents also report that, despite her severe handicap and her tendency to withdraw from accruing events, she has the ability, thanks to her love for social happenings physically and emotionally to "collect herself" and to behave in a manner that will keep her within the social life of the family (meaning that usually in social events, she will seat up, eat willingly and with grace, refrain from throwing a tantrum, etc.). The parents are also sure that she takes a lot of joy from the company of guests and is very happy to be among them. However, it should be stressed that the length of family visits is often set according to the young woman's level of interest.

Despite her lack of verbal language, the young woman has developed a wide set of gestures, enabling her to signal her wishes and therefore alerting her care-givers to assist her in avoiding "trouble" and withdraw before the "breaking of the storm".

Leaving the home

The question regarding the young woman residence was actually raised by the family, when the possibility of physical accommodations within the house was brought up. The parents at that point began wondering if the young woman should stay at home or should the family start looking for an appropriate residential setting for her, outside the house

Possibilities for changes in the living environment –Goals

- To enhance the young woman's privacy
- To ease care and management in adulthood
- To encourage and facilitate the young woman in becoming involved in activities (arts and crafts) at the termination of her educational setting (within one year).
- To maintain high levels of activity
- To prepare the young woman and other family members for the possibility of leaving the house.

Possibilities for changes in the living environment

- Enhancing privacy and easing care and management – nearing the 19th birthday of the young woman with RS's, some alterations took place. The young woman's room was widened and a direct connection between the bedroom and the adjacent bathroom was established. This new arrangement enabled full privacy for the girl and eased the work of the care-givers. Another bed was put in the young woman's room for a care-giver to sleep near her on restless nights. Colors and décor were adapted to that of a young woman preference. Some of the colors, pictures and the artifacts' positioning were chosen by the young woman her self. Another possibility that was raised and discussed was the option of installing a closed-circuit communication device that would be connected to the parents' room. The consideration in favor of the installation of such a device would be to enable door-closing and increase privacy for all family members (a demand raised by the young woman's siblings). The consideration against the installation of such a new device was that it would transmit every sound and movement from the young woman's room to the parents' room, thereby heightening their level of anxiety. Since the young woman was already manipulating her parents by using her disability to achieve attention and consideration, it seemed that the installation of such a device would only aggravate the situation and the idea was therefore, in this case, withdrawn (we do, however, suggest other families to consider the installation of such devices).
- Involvement in activities - because the young woman would be leaving school in a few months it seemed appropriate to provide her with a work-station. Since the

mother is an art therapist by profession, she found no problem in coming up with a variety of artworks that could be done by the young woman with only little assistance. A well-adapted table and chair were positioned in a small corner of the mother's studio, with good lighting, ventilation and enough space to enable room at the young woman's side for an assistant. One of her initial tasks was to prepare new decorations for her renovated room.

- Maintaining the young woman's activity levels - The young woman in question is completely dependent on a care-giver in all her ADLs. Therefore, without actively being moved, she might sit passively in her chair for long periods of time. Therefore, the house was re-arranged so that different centers of interest are scattered in various spots around the premises. In the garden there is a walkway with benches. In the kitchen, food is served but it is also a place were the young woman can sit and enjoy music from a vast audio selection. In the living room, television can be watched and the young woman's bedroom is equipped with an array of attractive lighting devices. We encouraged the family to change the young woman's position every now and then, so she might be entertained, yet at the same time enjoy the benefits of being an active person.
- First steps towards detachment – after considering the matter, the actual departure of the young woman from her parents' house, was postponed. The alterations by which the young woman's room was slightly segregated from the rest of house are, in reality, a first step enabling the parents to ponder and contemplate further on the possibility of sending her later in life to a residential facility. The implemented alterations enabled the young woman to have a small activity center at home, yet in a sense, away from home. Her new room enables taking care of her hygiene needs, acoustic separation from the rest of the house, with its noisy occupants (both siblings are very popular and the house is always storming with activity) when the young woman so prefers.
- Accessibility – It was recommended that the young woman's room be arranged with several easily-controlled items of furniture and objects (an electric, folding sofa, electronically controlled shades, etc.) to increase her control over her environment.

Early adulthood – generalization and discussion

With the end of adolescence, the young woman with RS will be terminating her education and, after many years of being used to the schedule of the education system, will be staying home for most of the hours in a day. Since the person with RS is in need of constant monitoring and care-giving, this new reality necessitates reorganization.

There are grave physiological aspects to this change yet the present chapter has dealt mainly with ways of influencing family structure and balance through the use of shaping of the physical environment.

Taking care of the young woman's needs

The young woman needs to be kept busy to prevent behavioral changes that might arise due to boredom. Therefore, a small work-station should be established at which the young woman can work. An occupational therapist or an art therapist might suggest proper activities suitable for the woman's age and functional abilities. A complete program should be planned for her, to help retain her school achievements and continue her education.

It is stressed that childhood connections and friendships might be a good source of comfort and support for the young woman with RS. Because of the complex nature of this population, it is recommended that parents of individuals with RS assemble to create a meeting group. Through regular meetings, such a group might enable recreational encounters for individuals with RS and allow the parents to brain-storm on the subject of finding proper support for themselves and for their family member with RS.

Taking care of the other family members' needs

The end of the educational period in the life of a person with RS is also a time for intensive contemplation. The parents might consider searching for alternative accommodation; consider the functional abilities of the woman with RS and her needs, their age, their strengths and their own needs. Other siblings might also be in their teens, posing their demands and needs to be filled.

Due to the rarity of RS, it is reasonable to assume that each facility that might be considered for the young woman with RS (day center or residential) will need to be appraised on the proper management of this population. The openness and the flexibility the facility shows in adapting to the specific needs of the person with RS could be considered a good measure of its appropriateness for the young woman. Because of the age of the parents and the demanding care needs of the person with RS, it stands to reason that an unfamiliar care-giver will enter the life, the house, the timetable and the habits of the family.

It is recommended that a separate room be assigned to the care-giver and if the apartment or house is short on space, than at least a separate area should be found to provide the care-giver with some privacy and prevent her/him from being unable to avoid the family. The arrival of a new person into the home might be a good time to rearrange it. If space is in abundance, it should be noted that the young person with RS has come to an age where it is appropriate to move her into her own lodgings. This could be a new experience both for the woman and her parents, preparing them for the time when the woman with RS might move to some form of residential care, a new home away from home.

Case story 4 (adulthood and residential case)

A 35 year-old woman, the eldest child in her family, resides in a small hostel were most of the residents are diagnosed with Autism. The woman is diagnosed with a Preserved Speech Variant (PSV) of RS. She is independent in terms of mobility and in transfers, in ascending and descending stairs and her manual abilities enables independence in most ADLs. She is visited by family members (mostly her mother) at least twice a week; she is taken home every other weekend.

Case story 5 (adulthood and residential case)

A 24 year-old woman, residing in a residential center within a group of severely-disabled individuals diagnosed with profound levels of IDD. She has never walked and is a constant wheelchair user. She has family visits every few weeks. She does not visit home, does not use any form of assistive communication device and is completely dependent upon care-givers to supply all her ADL needs.

Living in residential settings - generalization and discussion.

Leaving the family home is accompanied by grave concerns, usually with a long, complicated process of detaching the deep symbiotic relationship with the daughter. The acquired passivity and the challenging/demanding emotional character common to many with RS, has made the parents/care-giver ever prepared and attuned to each sign given by their child. If the parents are attuned enough and very skilled at reading their daughter's wishes, they are reworded with a peaceful home and the enormous love and affection conveyed by their child. The ability of individuals with RS to give-in emotionally and to exchange meaningful looks could become overwhelming, when sometimes the person with RS is exchanging her total dependence in return for endless attention.

Within the residential settings, the individual with RS and her family are forced to accept the outside rules enforced by the management, dealing with every piece of daily experience. The daily schedule and timetable, the living-space design, the décor; most of these issues are decided by external decision-makers. The parents and the person with RS must accept this and they are expected to adapt and obey the new rules. The parents can help their daughter to adjust by bringing household bits and pieces that will reflect their affection and everlasting love. They should insist on decorating her personal space and if necessary to install the required communication devices on the woman's wheelchair or in appropriate places in her living space.

We advise that general information regarding RS but especially the habits and behaviors of the person with RS (what makes her feel wanted and comfortable and what irritates her) should be conveyed first-hand to the her care-givers and that any piece of equipment or information that may assist the person with RS and her parents to adjust to the new situation, be delivered to the residential center. In the two case-studies in which we observed and interviewed, we saw that one person was very active, spreading her personal belonging around the public areas of the hostel yet rewarding the staff by being very friendly. The other was very dependent but her talkative eyes constantly hung on her care-givers' faces, sending messages of her ever-lasting appreciation and love for their efforts. It is quite certain that individuals with RS can enjoy living in a residential setting (as long as the human and physical environments suit their needs and personality), with the family helping by treating the place as the permanent house for their daughter by bringing loved objects and colorful items, making her place a lively, homely one through familiar shining, moving games.

It is known that individuals with RS sometimes find it hard to adjust to new places and situations and therefore may take some time to accept the new settings. Therefore, we advise doing the transition gradually, informing the person with RS, taking her for visits to get acquainted with the new place, making sure that her non-verbal communication signs are understood (a dictionary of "communication acts" [64,65] might be a good practical solution upon the transfer). More information about the construction of a personal dictionary can be found in the chapter regarding communication. After gradually lengthening visit times, taking care of her mood swings when going to and coming from her future residence, the transfer may be completed. We can only hope that, with time, she will relate to her personal room and care-givers at the residential place with the same warmth and acceptance as to her room and family members at home. The parents, for their part, should be able to let go, notwithstanding the pain and worries involved, and ensure that her room at home turns into a visiting place and the room were she lives most days of the week is turned in to her new home.

Discussion

The present chapter outlines the up-to-date knowledge on environmental adaptation for individuals with IDD, as well as that related to relevant aspects applicable to individuals with Rett syndrome, when environmental changes are considered.

The case-studies that were selected for this chapter identified changes that were suggested to families with children with RS. We also wanted to convey to the reader that it is vital to balance the child's intensive ADL and therapeutic needs with those of the whole family, including other siblings. The chapter suggested a non-traditional view of environmental changes by pointing out that environmental and physical change might be used as a fulcrum to achieve changes in the family equilibrium. This type of intervention should only be done upon the invitation of the family, because of the intrusiveness and delicateness of the process. We emphasize that such a change should only be initiated and addressed by a team of professionals, contributing in achieving a holistic change, each from his/her field of expertise. We also believe that a multi-disciplinary approach can assist the family with RS not only in moving walls and widening entrances but also in achieving a more balanced life-style, taking care of the needs of each individual in the family, as well as the whole family as a unit. The chapter points to a possible novel intervention. However, taking such a direction should be done with the outmost proficiency, bearing in mind the families' structures and strengths as the pace-makers of this process of change.

References

[1]   Hoenig H. Assistive technology and mobility aids for the older patient with disability. Ann Long Term Care 2004;12(9):12-9.
[2]   Wehmeyer ML, Bolding N. Self-determination-across living and working environments: A matched samples study of adults with mental retardation. Ment Retard 1999;37(5):353-63.
[3]   Nadirshaw Z. Expert or experience? Public or Private? A personal view of a psychologist within the health care system. J Learning Disabil 2000;4(3):187–91.

[4]   Sullivan CAC, Vitello SJ, Foster W. Adaptive behavior of adults with mental retardation in a group home: an intensive case study. Educ Training Ment Retard 1988;23:76–81.

[5]   Reed J. Understanding and assessing depression in people with learning disabilities: a cognitive-behavioral approach. In: Kroese BS, Dagnan D, Loumidis K, eds. Cognitive-behavior therapy for people with learning disabilities. London: Routledge, 1997:53–66.

[6]   Young L, Ashman AF. Deinstitutionalization for older Adults with severe mental retardation: results from Australia. Am J Ment Retard 2004;109(5):397–412.

[7]   Szivos SE, Griffiths E. Group processes involved in coming to terms with a mentally retarded identity. Ment Retard 1990;28(6):333–41.

[8]   Hughes C, Hwang B, Kim JH, Eisenman LT, Killian DJ. Quality of life in applied research: a review and analysis of empirical measures. Am J Ment Retard 1995;99(6):623-41.

[9]   Nirje B. The normalization principle and its human management implications. In: Kugel R, Wolfensberger W, eds. Changing pat-terns in residential services for the mentally retarded. Washington, DC: Gov Print Office, 1972:418–29.

[10]   Baggerman DJ, Sheldon JB, Sherman JA, Harchick AE. Balancing the right to habilitation with the right to personal liberties: The right of people with developmental disabilities to eat too many doughnuts and take a nap. J Appl Behav Anal 1990;23:79–89.

[11]   Bambera LM, Cole CL, Kroger F. Translating self-determination concepts into support for adults with severe disabilities. J Assoc Pers Severe Handicaps 1998;23:23–7.

[12]   Olney MF. Communication strategies of adults with severe disabilities: Supporting self determination. Rehabil Couns Bull 2001;44:87–94.

[13]   Heller T, Miller AB, Hsieh K. Environmental characteristics of nursing homes and community-based settings, and the well-being of adults with intellectual disability. J Intellec Disabil 1998;42:418–28.

[14]   Heller T, Miller AB, Factor A. Autonomy in residential facilities and community functioning of adults with mental retardation. Ment Retard 1999;37:449–57.

[15]   Sowers J, Powers L. Enhancing the participation and independence of students with severe physical and multiple disabilities in performing community activities. Ment Retard 1995;33:209–20.

[16]   Wehmeyer ML, Schwartz,M. Self-determination and positive adult outcomes: A follow-up study of youth with mental retardation or learning disabilities. Except Children 1997;63(2):245-56.

[17]   Heller, T. group decision-making by mentally retarded adults. Am J Ment Defic 1978;5:480-6.

[18]   Henderson KA. An interactive analysis of the teaching of decision-making in leisure to adolescents with mental retardation. Ther Recreation J 1994;28:133–46.

[19]   Stancliffe RJ, Abery BA, Springborg H, Elkin S. Substitute decision–making and personal control: Implications for self-determination. Ment Retard 2000;38:407–21.

[20]   McConkey R, Sowney M, Milligan V, Barr O. Views of people with intellectual disabilities of their present and future living arrangements. J Policy Pract Intellect Disabil 2004;1(3-4):115-25.

[21]   Holland A, Meddis R. People living in community homes: the influences on their activities. Ment Handicap Res 1993;6:333–45.

[22]   Wing L. Hospital Closure and the resettlement of residents: The case of Darenth Park Mental Handicap Hospital. Avebury: Aldershot, 1989.

[23]   Donnelly M, McGilloway S, Mays N, Perry S, Knapp M, Kavanagh S, Beecham J, Fenyo A, Astin J. Opening new doors: An evaluation of community care for people discharged from psychiatric and mental handicap hospitals. London: HMSO, 1994.

[24]   Flynn MC. Independent living for adults with mental handicap: A place of my own. London: Cassell, 1989.

[25]   Booth W, Booth T, Simons K. Return journey: The relocation of adults from long-stay hospital into hostel accommodation. Br J Ment Subnorm 1990;36:87-97.

[26]   Eyman R, Demaine G, Lei T. Relationship between community environments and resident changes in adaptive behavior: A path model. Am J Ment Defic 1979;83:330–7.

[27]   King RD, Raynes NJ. Patterns of institutional care for the severely subnormal. Am J Ment Defic 1968;72:700–9.

[28]   Thompson T, Robinson M, Farris M, Sinclair V. Interdependence of architectural features and program variables in community residences for people with mental retardation. Am J Ment Retard 1996;101:315–27.

[29]   Lawton MP. The impact of the environment on aging and behavior. In: Birren J, Shaie KW, eds. Handbook of the psychology of aging. New York: Van Nostrant Reinhold, 1977:276–301.

[30]   Moos RH, Lemke S. Assessing the physical and architectural features of sheltered care settings. J Gerontology 1980;35:571-83.

[31]   Linn MW, Gurel L, Linn BS. Patient outcome as a measure of quality of nursing home care. Am J Public Health 1977;67:337–44.

[32]   Heller T, Miller AB, Hsieh K. Eight-year follow-up of the impact of environmental characteristics on well-being of adults with developmental disabilities. Ment Retard 2002;40(5):366–78.

[33]   Amir RE, Van den Veyver IB, Wan M, Tran CQ, Francke U, Zoghbi HY. Rett syndrome is caused by mutations in X-linked MECP2, encoding methyl CpG binding protein2. Nature Genet 1999;23:185-8.

[34]   Vacca M, Filippini F, Budillon A, Rossi V, Mercadante G, et al. Mutation analysis of the MECP2 gene in British and Italian Rett Syndrome females. J Mol Med 2001;78:648-55.

[35]   Rett A. Über ein Zerebral-atrophisches Syndrom bei Hyperammonämie. Vienna: Brüder Hollinek, 1966. [German]

[36]   Hagberg B, Hagberg G. Rett syndrome: epidemiology and geographical variability. Eur Child Adolesc Psychiatry 1997;6:5-7.

[37]   Kerr AM. Rett syndrome British longitudinal study (1982-1990) and 1990 survey. In: Roosendaal JJ, ed. Ment Retard Med Care 1991;4:21-24.

[38]   Stancliffe RJ, Abery BH. Longitudinal study of deinstitutionalization and the exercise of choice. Ment Retard 1997;35(3):159-69.

[39]   Heller T, Miller AB, Hsieh K, Sterns H. Later-life planning: Promoting knowledge of options and choice making. Ment Retard 2000;38(5):395-406.

[40]   Kleinberg J, Galligan B. Effects of deinstitutionalization on adaptive behavior of mentally retarded adults. Am J Ment Defic 1983;88:21–7.

[41]   Felce D, Jones E, Lowe K, Perry J. Rational resourcing and productivity: Relationships among staff input, resident characteristics, and group home quality. Am J Ment Retard 2003;108:161–72.

[42]   Felce D, Lowe K, Beecham J, Hallam A. Exploring the relationships between costs and quality of services for adults with severe intellectual disabilities and the most severe challenging behaviors in Wales: A multivariate regression analysis. J Intellect Dev Disabil 2000;25:307–26.

[43]   Hatton C, Emerson E, Robertson J, Henderson D, Cooper J. Predictors of staff support and resident lifestyle in services for people with multiple disabilities: A path analytic approach. J Intellect Disabil Res 1996;40:466–77.

[44]   Jones E, Felce D, Lowe K, Bowle C, Pagler J, Gallagher B, Roper A, Kurlowska, K. Evaluation of the dissemination of Active Support training in staffed community residences. Am J Ment Retard 2001;106:344–58.

[45]   Jones E, Perry J, Lowe K, Felce D, Toogood S, Dunstan F, Allen D, Pagler J. Opportunity and the promotion of activity among adults with severe intellectual disability living in community residences: The impact of training staff in active support. J Intellect Disabil Res 1999;43:164–78.

[46]   Lewis JE, Wilson CD. Pathways to learning in Rett Syndrome. Teleford, Shropshire: Wozencroft, 1996.

[47]   Baptista PM, Mercadante MT, Macedo EC, Schwartzman JS. Cognitive performance in Rett syndrome girls: a pilot study using eyetracking technology. J Intellect Disabil Res 2006;50(9):662- 6.

[48]   Hanks SB. The role of therapy in Rett syndrome. Am J Med Genet 1986;Suppl 1:247-52.

[49]   Watson JU, Umansky R, Johnson C. Rett syndrome: An exploratory study. Paper presented at the international conference on infant studies, Montreal, Canada, Apr 1990.

[50]   Wesecky A. Music therapy for children with Rett syndrome. Am J Med Genet 1986;24(suppl. 1):253-7.

[51]   Zappella M. Motivational conflicts in Rett syndrome. Am J Med Genet 1986; 24(suppl.1):143-51.

[52]   Sullivan MW, Laverick DH, Lewis M. Fostering environmental control in a young child with Rett syndrome: A case study. Unpublished report, 1994:1-44.

[53]   Mahon M J. The use of self-control techniques to facilitate self-determination skills during leisure in adolescents and young adults with mild and moderate mental retardation. Ther Recreation J 1994;28:58–71.

[54]   Mahon MJ, Bullock CC. Teaching adolescents with mild mental retardation to make decisions in leisure through the use of self-control techniques. Ther Recreation J 1992;26: 9–26.

[55]   Williams R, Dattilo J. Effects of leisure education on self-determination, social inter-action, and positive affect of young adults with mental retardation. Ther Recreation J 1997;31:245–58.

[56]   Mithaug DE, Mar DK. The relation between choosing and working prevocational tasks in two severely retarded young adults. J Appl Behav Analysis 1980;13:177–82.

[57]   Parsons MB, Reid DH, Reynolds J, Bum-garner M. Effects of chosen versus as-signed jobs on the work performance of persons with severe handicaps. J Appl Behav Analysis 1990;23:253–8.

[58]   Wehmeyer ML, Metzler CA. How self-determined are people with mental retardation? The National Consumer Survey. Ment Retard 1995;33:111–9.

[59]   Pruchno RA, Patrick JH, Burant CJ. Aging women and their children with chronic disabilities: perceptions of sibling involvement and effects on well-being. Family Relat 1996;45:318–26.

[60]   Greenberg JS, Seltzer MM, Orsmond GI, et al. Siblings of adults with mental illness or mental retardation: Current involvement and expectation of future caregiving. Psychiatr Serv 1999;50:1214 – 19.

[61]   Seltzer GB, Begun A, Seltzer MM, et al. Adults with mental retardation and their aging mothers: impacts of siblings. Family Relations 1991;40:310 –17.

[62]   Hunter K. The Rett Syndrome handbook, International Rett Syndrome Association, Washington D.C. U.S., 1999.

[63]   63..   Sigafoos J, Woodyatt G. Educational implications of Rett syndrome. Eur J Ment Disabil 1996; 3(11):19-28.

[64]   Sigafoos J, Woodyatt G, Tucker M, Roberts-Pennell D, Pittendreigh N. Assessment of potential communication acts in three individuals with Rett Syndrome. J Dev Phys Disabil 1999;12(3):203-16.

[65]   Sigafoos J. Communication development and aberrant behavior in children with developmental disabilities. Edu Train Ment Retard Dev Disabil 2000;35(2) :168-76.

[66]   Pollak VA, Gallagher B. A fast communication aid for non-verbal subjects with severe motor handicaps. J Med Eng Technol 1989;13(1-2):23-7.

[67]   Lotan M, Ben-Zeev B. Rett Syndrome. A review with emphasis on clinical characteristics and intervention TheScientificWorldJournal 2006;6:1517–41.

[68]   Pitetti KH, Tan DM. Effects of a minimally supervised exercise program for mentally retarded adults. Med Sci Sports Exe 1991;23(5):594-601.

[69]   Pitetti KH, Boneh S. Cardiovascular fitness as related to leg strength in adults with mental retardation.. Med Sci Sports Exe 1995;27(3):423-8.

[70]   King D, Mace E. Acquisition and maintenance of exercise skills under normalized conditions by adults with moderate and severe mental retardation. Ment Retard 1990;28(5):311-7.

[71]   Hagberg B. Rett Syndrome: Clinical and biological aspects. London: Mac Keith, 1993.

[72]   International Rett Syndrome Association web site. Adults with Rett Syndrome http://www.rettsyndrome.org/main/adults-intro.htm Accessed January 7. 2006.

[73]   Kerr AM. The Future for Rett Syndrome girls. International Rett Syndrome Association Newsletter 1992 Winter:13-14.

[74]   Craig A, Tran Y, McIsaac P, Boord P. The efficacy and benefits of environmental control systems for the severely disabled. Med Sci Monit 2004; 11(1):RA32-9.

[75]   Technology -Related Assistance for Individuals with Disabilities Act of 1988, PL 100-407. (August 19, 1988). Title 29, U.S.C. 2201 et seq: U.S. Statutes at Large, 102, 1044-1065.

[76]   Wellings DJ, Unsworth J. Fortnightly review: Environmental control systems for people with a disability: an update. BMJ 1997;315:409–12.

[77]   Barnes MP. Switching devices and independence of disabled people. BMJ 1994;309:1181–2.

[78]   Platts R, Fraser M. Assistive technology in the rehabilitation of patients with high spinal cord lesions. Paraplegia 1993;313:280–7.

[79]   Datillo J. Computerized assessment of leisure preferences: A replication. Edu Train Ment Retard 1987;22:128-33.

[80]   Realon RE Favell JE, Phillips JF. Adapted leisure materials vs. standard leisure materials: Evaluating several aspects of programming for persons who are profoundly handicapped. Edu Train Ment Retard 1989;24:168-77.

[81]   Realon RE, Favell JE, Dayvault KA. Evaluating the use of adapted leisure materials on the engagement of persons who are profoundly, multiply handicapped. Edu Train Ment Retard 1988;23:228-37.

[82]   Thornett CEE: Designing special switches and control systems for multiply handicapped young people- a problem-led approach. J Med Eng Technol1990;14: 87–91.

[83]   Lindberg B. Understanding Rett Syndrome: A practice guide for parents, teachers and therapists. Toronto: Hognefe Huber, 1991.

[84]   Nomura Y. Sleep in relation to other behaviors in Rett syndrome. A lecture presented at the international course on Rett Syndrome, Ostersund Sweden; 2003 Jun 16-18.

[85]   Piazza CC, Fisher W, Kiesewetter BS, Bowman L, Moser H. Aberrant sleep patterns in children with Rett Syndrome. Brain Dev 1990;2:488-93.

[86]   Woodyatt G, Marinac J, Darnell R, Sigafoos J, and Halle James. Behaviour state analysis in Rett syndrome: Continuous data reliability measurement. Int J Disabil Dev Edu 2004;51(4):383-400.

[87]   Katsiyannis A, Ellenburg JS, Acton OM, Torrey G. Addressing the Needs of Students with Rett Syndrome. Teach Except Child 2001;33(5):74-8.

[88]   Kerr AM, Julu PO. Recent insights into hyperventilation from the study of Rett syndrome. Arch Dis Child 1999;80:384-7.

[89]   Sekul EA, Moak JP, Schultz RJ, Glaze DG, Dunn JK, Percy AK. Eelectrocardiographic findings in Rett syndrome: an explanation for sudden death? J Pediatr 1994;125:80-2.

[90]   Guideri F, Acampa M, Hayek G, Zappella M, Di Perri T. Reduced heart rate variability in patients affected with Rett Syndrome. A possible explanation for sudden death. Neuropediatrics 1999;30:146-8.

[91]   Annegers JF, Coan SP. SUDEP: overview of definitions and review of incidence data. Seizure 1999;8(6):347-52.

[92]   Byard RW. Forensic issues and possible mechanisms of sudden death in Rett Syndrome. J Clin Forensic Med 2006;13(2):96-9.

[93]   Julu PO, Kerr AM, Apartopoulos F, Al-Rawas S, Witt Engerström I Engerström L, Gamal AJ, Hansen S. Characterization of breathing and associated central autonomic dysfunction in the Rett disorder. Arch Dis Child 2001;85:29-37.

[94]   Fujiura GT. Demography of family households. Am J Ment Retard 1998;103: 225–35.

[95]   Braddock D. Aging and developmental disabilities: demographic and policy issues affecting American families. Ment Retard 1999;37:155– 61.

[96]   Borthwick-Duffy SA. Quality of life and quality of care in mental retardation. In: Rowitz L, ed. Mental retardation in the year 2000. New York: Springer, 1992:52–68.

[97]   Cumminns RA. The subjective well-being of people caring for a family member with a severe disability at home: a review. J Intel Dev Disabil 2001;26(1):83–100.

[98]   Krauss MW, Seltzer MM, Goodman SJ. Social support networks of adults with mental retardation who live at home. Am J Ment Retard 1992;96:432– 41.

[99]   Ramcharan P, Grant G. Views and experiences of people with intellectual disabilities and their families. (1) The user perspective. J App Res Intellect Disabil 2001;14:348–63.

[100]   Robinson N. The use of focus group methodology—with selected samples from sexual health research. J Adv Nurs 1999;29: 905–13.

[101]   Cambridge P, McCarthy M. User focus groups and Best Value in services for people with learning disabilities. Health Soc Care Commun 2001;9:476–89.

[102]   Oswin M. Am I allowed to cry? A study of bereavement amongst people who have learning disabilities. London, Souvenir Press, 1991.

[103]   Carnaby S. What do you think? A qualitative approach to evaluating individual planning services, J Intellect Disabil Res 1997;41:225–31.

[104]   Rowe D, Rudkin A. A systematic review of the qualitative evidence for the use of lifestyle planning in people with learning disabilities, J Learn Disabil Nurs Heal Soc Care 1999;3:148–58.

[105]   Lotan M. Improving staff and resident well-being using the multi-sensory treatment: Four case studies with washout periods. A poster session at the Annual International Conference of the American Association for Mental Retardation (AAMR). Philadelphia, USA, 2004.

[106]   Lotan M. Management of Rett syndrome in the controlled multisensory (Snoezelen) environment. A review with three case stories. TheScientificWorldJournal 2006 Jul 8;6:791-807.

[107]   Lotan M, Shapiro M Management of young children with Rett disorder in the controlled multi-sensory (Snoezelen) environment. Brain Dev 2005 Nov;27 Suppl 1:S88-94.

[108]   Motil KJ, Schultz RJ, Browning K, Trautwein L, Glaze DG. Oropharyngeal dysfunction and gastroesophageal dysmotility are present in individuals and women with Rett Syndrome. J Pediatr Gastroenterol Nutr 1999; 29(1):31-7.

[109]   Budden SS. Management of Rett Syndrome: a ten year experience. Neuropediatr 1995;26;75–7.

[110]   Grandin T, Johnson C, Frasier S. Animals in translation: Using the mysteries of autism to decode animal behavior. Oxford: Harcourt, 2005.

[111]   Elefant C. Emotional/musical communication of children with RS. A lecture at an annual coference on RS. Sheba hospital, Ramat-Gan, Israel. July, 2005

In: Rett Syndrome: Therapeutic Interventions
Editors: Meir Lotan and Joav Merrick

ISBN: 978-1-61728-080-1
©2011 Nova Science Publishers, Inc.

Chapter XVII

Rett syndrome: Alternative Therapeutic Interventions

Lotan Meir BPT, MScPT, PhD[*]

Israel Rett Center, National Evaluation Team, Chaim Sheba Medical Center, Tel Hashomer, Ramat Gan and Department of Physical Therapy, Ariel University Center of Samaria, Ariel, Israel

The individual with Rett syndrome (RS) experiences a range of challenging difficulties in all areas of daily living. Since there is no cure for the disorder at this point in time, parents of the individual with Rett syndrome search for different interventions that will improve the condition and quality of life of their child. In recent years, many different intervention programs have been carried out with individuals with RS. This chapter is a presentation of these methods with relevant case examples. The chapter reviews the following interventions: animal assisted therapy e.g. dolphin therapy, and dog assisted therapy; auditory integration training; hyperbaric oxygen therapy; manual therapies such as acupuncture/acupressure, aromatherapy, cranio-sacral therapy, Myo-fascial release, Traeger massage, chiropracty, and Reiki; behavior modification techniques such as the Lovaas approach, and cognitive rehabilitation; motoric interventions such as advanced biomechanical rehabilitation and the Doman-Delacato patterning approach and yoga. The present chapter is not a recommendation for any of the above mentioned techniques, but merely a review of different interventions available for the interested parent of the individual with RS.

Introduction

Rett syndrome (RS) is a neurological disorder resulting from an X-linked dominant mutation [1], affecting mainly females and found in a variety of racial and ethnic groups worldwide

---

[*] Correspondence: Meir Lotan, BPT, MScPT, PhD, Department of Physical Therapy, Ariel University Center of Samaria, IL-40700 Ariel, Israel. E-mail: ml_pt_rs@netvision.net.il

[2]. RS is a frequent cause of neurological dysfunction in females, and is the second most common cause for multiple disability among females, after Down's syndrome [3,4]. Due to the chronic nature of Rett syndrome and to the fact that the individual with RS displays an array of challenging difficulties affecting all areas of daily living [3], it is not surprising that different alleviating techniques have been suggested to this group of clients.

Since there is no cure for the disorder at this point in time, parents of the individual with Rett syndrome are constantly in search of different interventions, in order to improve the child's condition and quality of life. Research on these alternative methods is often single case study in design or conducted with small sample sizes. Such reports are difficult to interpret and generalize as the many aspects of the presented interventions may be vague or otherwise highly dubious. Such reports are not usually followed by more rigorous and controlled studies in the peer-reviewed scientific literature.

In many cases, an alternative intervention suggests "nothing but" a short, positive, and relaxing experience for the child with RS. Due to the turbulent nature of this disorder, which may be attributed to an over-active autonomic system, placing the individual with RS in a state of constant arousal [5] and a highly developed emotional state of being in individuals with RS [6], some alternative "relaxing" therapies could prove to be very beneficial for this specific group of clients.

Parents of the individual with RS should be cautious with different unconventional interventions and make well-informed decisions regarding the use of alternative treatments for their daughter. In this review a treatment approach posing some risk to the client with RS has been highlighted in text and should be carefully taken into consideration (see box XVII-1).

Box XVII-1. Wards of warning.

- o There is a vast selection of available interventions; shop for them cautiously.
- o Intervention involving termination of all other co-existing interventions for the individual with RS for the duration of treatment should be cautiously reconsidered and preferably avoided.
- o After deciding on a therapy program, a time limit for its duration with pre-excepted results should be set.
- o If by the end of a pre-determined set of intervention sessions a therapeutic result is not visible, continuation of the program should be reconsidered.
- o A quick and constant change between intervention methods should be avoided.

During the last few years, various alternative interventions have been available to individuals with RS. This review will present a short description of these methods, followed by a case study of a person with RS on whom the intervention has been carried out. When reading through the case studies, the reader should bear in mind that given the enormous phenotypic versatility presented by individuals with RS that in case of a different child, there might be dissimilar or even opposite results using the same intervention.

This review outlines the following interventions in alphabetical order:

- Animal Assisted Therapy
  o Dolphin therapy,
  o Dog assisted therapy,
- Auditory Integration Training (AIT)
- Hyperbaric oxygen therapy.
- Manual therapies
  o Acupuncture/ Acupressure,
  o Aromatherapy,
  o Chiropracty,
  o Cranio-Sacral therapy,
  o Myofascial Release,
  o Reiki
  o Traeger massage,
- Behavioral modification techniques
  o Cognitive Rehabilitation,
  o The Lovaas approach
- Motoric interventions
  o Advanced Biomechanical Rehabilitation (ABR)
  o Patterning/Doman-Delacato approach
- Yoga

It is important to emphasize that the present review is not a promotion for any of the above mentioned techniques, merely a presentation of different interventions available for the interested parent of the individual with RS.

Animal assisted therapy

Animal assisted therapy (AAT) is a goal-directed intervention in which an animal with particular characteristics is an integral part of a treatment that facilitates the healing process and rehabilitation of clients with a medical condition [7,8]. Therapeutic horseback riding is a specific type of AAT, which has been mentioned elsewhere in this book and therefore will not be addressed within the scope of the present chapter. Animal assisted therapies, available to individuals with RS include:

- Dog assisted therapy and
- Dolphin assisted therapy

Dog assisted therapy

One study has shown that children with pervasive developmental disorders (PDD) exhibited a more playful mood, were more focused and more aware of their social environments, when in the presence of a 'therapeutic' dog [8]. Individuals with RS are extremely fond of animals. Different reports have suggested that animals, mainly dogs, can be a powerful motivating factor for individuals with RS. E.g. when the family dog escorted the child with RS to physical therapy sessions, the child was found to cooperate more willingly and capable of experiencing different and far more challenging activities beyond her usual level of cooperation. It has also been reported that dogs have been used to reduce stereotypical hand movements as the girls with RS were motivated to pat the dogs [9].

Story of Claire

Claire loves dogs. The only three words she spoke in her life were: "cookie" briefly when she was six, and "dog" and "again" when she was two. "Dog" was her first word, spoken the first time she saw a friend's collie, and again later when she saw a neighbor's dog. She is attracted to large dogs and is motivated to touch their faces. Her love for dogs is strong enough to get her to actually use her hands to throw a ball to Paula's dog (see figures XVII-1, XVII-2) [10].

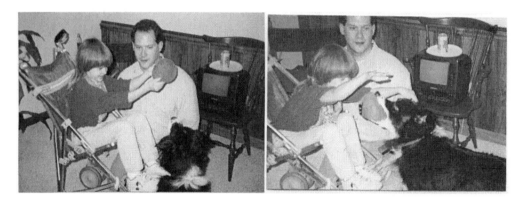

Figures XVII-1 and XVII-2. Claire with a dog.

Dolphin assisted therapy

The use of dolphin therapy for individuals with developmental disabilities is well documented [11]. Dolphins are thought to have special qualities which are believed to enhance healing potential [12]. Dolphins are also such gentle and perceptive animals that children really respond to them. They attract attention, stimulate awareness and interest, as well as provoke excitement and motivation [13], therefore they are extremely suitable for individuals with RS. Furthermore, the combination of environment, the movement of the water, the texture of the dolphin's skin, as well as the overall movement involved - is so engaging that the child's ability to interact and learn is enhanced [14]. All families who have engaged with this form of therapy have reported that it was a unique and extremely positive experience both for the child with RS as well as for themselves. One drawback was the fact that it was extremely expensive, usually involving the transporting of the whole family for a short and defined period [14-16]. Due to the costs involved in this type of intervention, it is usually a once off experience.

Story of Emily

Emily received 10 days of intensive therapy for 40 minutes a day. Emily worked with different therapists in an attempt to address her range of needs. On the first occasion she had a physiotherapist who worked with her on the dockside in the sunshine. On Emily's second trip a speech therapist massaged her mouth, face and neck to encourage Emily to talk. Sara, Emily's mom reports that "Emily had to complete a task, like pointing to 'yes' or 'no' cards in response to a question, and the reward was swimming with the dolphin (see figure XVII-3). She also sat on the dockside and the dolphin came and kissed her feet, which was lovely". "The most amazing thing was watching Emily being pushed along by the dolphin as she held on to a float. She couldn't talk but was really excited and made lots of vocal noises. I felt really emotional." *Sara, also thought it was really worth it: "Before dolphin therapy, Emily was trapped in a world of her own, crying a great deal, but since we've returned, she has been noticeably brighter, more conscious, and she's making more eye contact."* The reaction to the therapy was initially impressive, when Emily got back to school, they could not get over the difference - she just seemed so bright. Today Emily is more able to communicate and occasionally laughs and giggles. We play 'ready steady go!' where she runs from one side of the room to the other – she would never have been able to do that before. Sometimes she really looks at my husband when he is talking and we are sure she knows what he is saying. However, the benefits did not last. *"It did seem to last a while" says Sara, "but after about three months I saw her regressing"* [13,14].

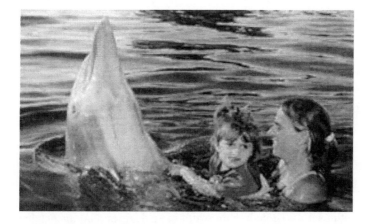

Figure XVII-3. Emily with a dolphin.

Auditory integration training (AIT)

Auditory Integration Training was first developed in France in 1982 [17] by Berard and introduced to the English speaking world in the 1990s [18]. The founder of AIT postulated that abnormal sensitivity or insensitivity to certain frequencies of sound waves, regardless of overall hearing ability, was associated with a range of behavioral and learning problems [18]. The aim of AIT was to correct poor integration between the sensory modalities. Through the presentation of special sounds and music over several sessions, it is suggested that treatment stimulates the brain in a designed manner, in order to integrate sensory functioning, thereby lessening distractibility and hyperactivity. AIT involves 10 hours of listening to electronically modified music delivered by headphones during two half-hour daily sessions over the course of 10 days. The AIT device uses filtering to dampen peak frequencies to which the individual is hypersensitive and delivers sounds modulated by random dampening of high and low frequencies and intensities [18].

This technique has been used with a variety of disorders including: autism, depression, hyperactivity and learning difficulties. Personal accounts demonstrate dramatic improvements in some individuals. Nevertheless, there is no adequate scientific research to validate AIT as a useful treatment for the majority of clients [19]. However, the treatment does show promise for some individuals. It is important that the individual with RS be assessed in advance in order to determine whether or not she has the potential to benefit from AIT.

Story of Annette

Three year old Annette from Canada, received 10 weekly sessions of Auditory Integration Therapy (AIT). According to her parents, she slept throughout the sessions. No noticeable changes were observed as result of her exposure to this intervention program [20].

Hyperbaric oxygen therapy

Hyperbaric oxygen therapy (HBOT) is the therapeutic administration of 100% oxygen at environmental pressures greater than 1 atmosphere absolute (ATA). This involves placing the patient in an airtight vessel, increasing the pressure within that vessel, and administering 100% oxygen for respiration. In this manner it is possible to deliver a greatly increased partial pressure of oxygen to the body. Typical treatments involve pressurization to between 1.5 and 3.0 ATA for periods of between 60 and 120 minutes, once or more daily. Since the 1960s there have been reports of improvement in cases of brain trauma using HBOT [21]. Hyperbaric Oxygen Therapy is based on the premise that hypoxia following closed head trauma is an integral part of the mechanism involved in secondary brain injury. Hypoxic neurons performing anaerobic metabolism result in acidosis and an unsustainable reduction in cellular metabolic reserve [22]. As the hypoxic situation persists, the neurons lose their ability to maintain ionic homeostasis, and free oxygen radicals accumulate and degrade cell membranes [23,24]. Eventually, irreversible changes result in unavoidable cell death. This gives some basis to the assertion that a form of therapy designed to increase oxygen availability may improve long-term outcome in neurological damage. The basic assumption behind the use of HBOT is its ability to compensate for decreased blood flow by increasing the oxygen content of blood plasma and body tissues and that it can even normalize oxygen levels in ischemic tissue [25].

Since HBOT has been found to improve blood flow in patients with chronic neurological conditions [26], this type of intervention has been tried during recent years with different populations, such as children with cerebral palsy [27]. In one article, it has been reported to show favorable results in 129 out of 139 (93%) pediatric patients [28]. This type of treatment was also found to improve symptoms in autistic individuals [25]. The use of HBOT may also cause negative outcomes (see box XVII-2.).

Box XVII-2. Caution

1. Since oxygen in high doses is potentially toxic to normally perfuse tissue, and the brain is a particularly at risk organ [30], it is appropriate to postulate that in some patients, HBOT may cause more harm through the action of increased free oxygen radical damage, than good through the restoration of aerobic metabolism [31].

2. Treatments using HBOT have been known to elicit epileptic seizures

3. There are anecdotal findings of the fact that HBOT intervention has caused damage to users with CP shortly after hyperbaric oxygen therapy [32].

Story of Abbey

Abbey is almost six years old. She started using the HBOT three years ago. Initially, one round of 40 "dives" was made in a big multi-places chamber at a Hyperbaric Centre. However, six months later, her family purchased a portable chamber for home use (see figure XVII-4). The portable chamber used a lower pressure than those used at HBOT centers. Her mother stated that after having the first few sessions she seemed to 'wake up' using the HBOT, and when they would stand Abbey up, instead of just flopping over, her balance was much improved. She also said that when Abbey was using the chamber regularly, she had more energy, was more alert, more communicative and had fewer illnesses and digestive problems. Her mother sums up the experience with HBOT by saying: "*it's a nice, adjunctive therapy that helps everything else we do to be more effective*" [29].

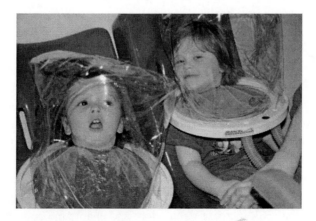

Figure XVII-4. Abbey using a portable HB chamber.

Manual therapies

The following therapies will be presented and discussed in this section:

- Acupuncture/acupressure,
- Aromatherapy
- Chiropracty,
- Cranio-sacral therapy,
- Myofascial release,
- Reiki,
- Traeger massage,

Acupuncture/acupressure

Acupuncture and acupressure are disciplines originating from a complex heritage of Chinese medicine. The original practitioners of Chinese medicine regarded the human body as a microcosmic reflection of the universe and considered the physician's role that of maintaining the body's harmonious balance, both internally and in relation to the external environment. The treatment is executed according to descriptors attached to elemental qualities (wood, fire, earth, metal, and water), and by the functional influences traditionally associated with each of the internal organs. The classical anatomy of acupuncture consists of energy channels (meridians) traversing the body. The principal energy pathways are named for organs whose realms of influence are expanded from their conventional biomedical physiology to include functional, energetic, and metaphorical qualities. Acupuncture involves the therapeutic insertion of solid needles in various combinations and patterns into the body. The adaptability of classical and hybrid acupuncture approaches in Western medical environments is the key to their clinical success and popular appeal [33].

Acupressure is an ancient healing art developed in Asia over 5,000 years ago, using the fingers to press key points on the surface of the skin to stimulate the body's natural self-curative abilities. When these acupressure points are pressed, they release muscular tension and promote the circulation of blood and the body's life force energy to aid healing. Acupuncture and acupressure use the same points and meridians, but acupuncture employs needles, while acupressure uses gentle, but firm pressure and integrates bodywork therapies, therapeutic touch, somatic work, healing imagery, energy psychology, and massage therapy techniques [34].

Research findings regarding acupuncture: There is agreement that acupuncture appears to be effective for postoperative dental pain, postoperative nausea and vomiting, and chemotherapy-related nausea and vomiting. Positive yet sometimes confusing results have been found regarding migraine, low-back pain, and temporo-mandibular disorders, fibromyalgia, osteoarthritis of the knee, and tennis elbow. For conditions such as chronic pain, neck pain, asthma, the evidence is considered inconclusive and difficult to interpret [35].

Documented benefits of acupressure include pain relief, 'balancing of the body', and the general maintenance of good health. Acupressure's healing touch has been found to reduce tension and hypertension [36], increase circulation, and enable the body to relax deeply. By relieving stress, acupressure therapy is believed to strengthen resistance to disease and promote health and wellbeing [34,37].

Story of Annette

Annette a 14 year old girl diagnosed with Rett syndrome had received a combination of acupressure, energy healing, and reflexology on a weekly basis for more than a year, at the age of 12. Her mother reported that these interventions made her relax during the session, but on the other hand made her "very upset at times, broke out in hives during some treatments". The treatments did not show any lasting changes [38].

Box XVII-3

Reviews have concluded that while not free from serious adverse events (rare they may be), acupuncture is a relatively safe procedure

Aromatherapy massage

Massage is defined as manipulation of the soft tissues of the client performed by the hands of the facilitator for the purpose of producing effects in the vascular, muscular and nervous systems of the body. Aromatherapy massage uses the non-oily pure volatile portion of aromatic plant products, normally extracted by distillation, as essential oils, for therapeutic or medical purposes. It is the chemical composition of each essential oil which gives the oil its unique therapeutic qualities. In the United Kingdom, the topical use of essential oils is now being employed by some healthcare professionals as a potential means of enhancing patients' wellbeing [39].The use of aromatherapy among the pediatric population is rapidly growing[40]. Essential oils encompass over 60 kinds of herbal oils [41], which are used to ease aching, pain and injury [42,43]. Aromatherapy is also reported to act on the central nervous system, relieving depression and anxiety, reducing stress, relaxing, acting in a sedating or stimulating manner, and restoring both physical and emotional well-being [44-46]. It has also been reported to improve night-time sleep [47] and enhance the immunological system [48].

Case study

The literature reports a single case study of a child with Rett syndrome receiving aromatherapy. The intended goal of the intervention was to reduce stereotypical hand movements and improve blood circulation to the feet. According to the report, therapy was a success and therapeutic goals were achieved [49].

Chiropracty

Chiropractors diagnose and treat patients, where health problems are associated with the body's muscular, nervous and skeletal systems, in particular the spine. Chiropractors believe that interference with these systems impairs the normal functions of the body and lowers resistance to disease. They also claim that spinal or vertebral dysfunction alters many important body functions by affecting the nervous system, and that skeletal imbalance through joint or articular dysfunction, especially in the spine, can cause pain.

The chiropractic approach to health care is holistic, stressing overall health and wellbeing. It recognizes that many factors affect health, including exercise, diet, rest, environment and heredity. In cases where difficulties can be traced to the involvement of musculoskeletal structures, chiropractors manually adjust the spinal column. Some chiropractors also use water, light, massage, ultrasound, electric acupuncture and/or heat therapy. Chiropractors counsel patients about health and wellbeing through the use of concepts such as nutrition, exercise, changes in lifestyle, and stress management. They do not prescribe drugs or perform surgery [50].

Story of Annette

Annette, a 14 year old Canadian girl with Rett syndrome, had undergone weekly therapy sessions with a chiropractor over a period of two months, at the age of four. The sessions themselves seemed to relax Annette, but no lasting changes were observed as a result of this intervention [51].

Cranio-sacral therapy

Cranio-sacral therapy (CST) is a form of touch therapy, in which the bones of the skull are adjusted along with subtle adjustments of the spine, all the way to the sacrum [52]. The basic concept behind CST is that any stresses, strains, tensions or traumas which have been "stored" in the body will restrict the cerebrospinal fluid circulation, thus harming the body's functioning and may give rise to problems over time. The effects of this stagnation may be both physical (such as back pain, migraine or digestive disorders) or emotional (such as anxiety or depression). Craniosacral therapists are trained to feel this subtle "blocks" in the body and can use their hands to provide the body with an opportunity to let go of its restrictive pattern and return to an easier mode of functioning [53].

Case studies

Allie, is a seven year old child with Rett syndrome, who had tried Cranio-Sacral therapy. According to her mother, the therapy did not appear to have much of an effect [54]. On the other hand, this type of intervention seemed to reduce teeth grinding in Lauren's case and her mother Cathy recommended it as a good technique for parents seeking some 'relaxation/recharging time' for themselves as well as for their daughter [55].

Box XVII-4. Caution

> **The theory behind cranio-sacral therapy has no anatomical or physiological basis. The intervention purportedly benefits patients with a wide range of diagnoses, and its proponents do not claim any adverse effects while published studies do not provide supporting evidence [56].**

Myofascial release

In the medical literature, the term myofascial was first used by Janet G Travell, MD in the 1940s, referring to musculoskeletal pain syndromes and trigger points. In 1976 Travell began using the term "myofascial trigger point" and published in 1983 the famous reference "Myofascial pain and dysfunction: The trigger point manual". Some practitioners use the term "myofascial therapy" or "myofascial trigger point therapy", referring to the treatment of trigger points, which is usually in a medical-clinical sense.

The term myofascial release also refers to soft tissue manipulation techniques. It has been loosely used to describe different manual therapies, applying soft tissue manipulation work (connective tissue massage, soft tissue mobilization, Rolfing, strain-counter-strain etc). Myofascial release refers to the manual massage technique of stretching the fascia and releasing bonds between fascia and ligaments, muscles and bones with the goal of eliminating pain, increasing range of motion and balancing the body. Fascia is located between the skin and the underlying structure of muscles and bones and is a seamless web of connective tissue which covers and connects the muscles, organs and skeletal structures in our body. Muscle and fascia are united, forming the myofascial system.

Injuries, stress, inflammation, trauma, and poor posture can cause restriction to fascia. Since fascia is an interconnected web, the restriction or tightness of the fascia at one place, in time, can spread to other places in the body. The goal of myofascial release is to release fascia restriction and restore its tissue health [57].

Story of Corinne

Corinne, a 10 year old child with Rett syndrome, had received myofascial release therapy from her physical therapist. As Corinne had developed some functional scoliosis and it seemed to be worsening (expressed by the fact that the muscles in her shoulders and back had become extremely tight), it was decided to implement some myofascial therapy. These techniques seemed to loosen the tightness considerably and the situation was corrected[58].

Reiki

Reiki (sometimes spelled 'Reichi') is an Asian intervention based on the theoretical assumption that 'humans are energy', and that by manipulating this energy with the hands, healing occurs [59]. It is a treatment used by individuals as an alternative or complement to Western medical treatment [60]. Several well-designed studies to date show significant positive outcomes for conditions such as wound-healing and reduction of pain and anxiety [61]. It is also suggested that Energy Healing (EH) may have positive effects on various orthopedic conditions, including muscle and connective tissue problems [61].

Story of Annette

Annette is a 14 year old Canadian girl with RS. When she was five years of age, Annette experienced a couple of sessions of Reiki. No lasting changes were documented [62].

Box XVII-5

Energy healing (such as Reiki) is an adjunctive treatment which is noninvasive and poses little downside risk to patients [61].

Traeger massage

This is a therapy developed by boxing trainer Milton Traeger, MD, which uses gentle, rhythmic movements to relieve tension, ease movement (especially in joints), and induce relaxation. Compression, elongation, and light bouncing as well as rocking motions are involved [63].

Case study

In one case study presented to the author [64], parents reported that when their child with RS received regular sessions of Traeger massage, they noticed increased relaxation and improved mobility, despite the fact that the child with RS was usually sowing extremely high muscle tone (spasticity).

Behavioral modification techniques

Cognitive rehabilitation

The goal of cognitive rehabilitation is to achieve an improved level of cognitive functioning in those where cognitive deficits interfere with their ability to live an independent life.

Treatment is based on individualized goals that take into consideration the patient's current pattern of strengths and weaknesses. Cognitive rehabilitation treatment goals include:

- Relearning of targeted mental abilities
- Strengthening of intact functions
- Relearning of social interaction skills
- Substitution of lost functions with new skills
- Optimizing control over the emotional aspects of an individual's functioning, including management of impulsivity and anger

After an initial individual diagnostic interview and discussion of the patient's goals, medical records and neuropsychological evaluation results are reviewed. A cognitive rehabilitation plan is then developed through a collaborative effort by the client and the therapist. The achievement of goals may include the use of a variety of techniques and tools:

- Auditory and/or visual attention-related tasks
- Memory compensation training, i.e. working to improve memory deficits
- Use of adaptive devices to compensate for deficits and adaptive approaches to targeted tasks
- EEG biofeedback (neuro-feedback) [65].

A systematic review of the literature from 1998 through 2002 suggested substantial evidence to support cognitive rehabilitation therapies in improving function in areas such as: attention deficits, apraxia and functional communication deficits [66]. Cognitive rehabilitation has been applied in individuals with various cognitive dysfunctions, including those with developmental disabilities [67].

Case study

A single case report was received by a therapist, who had worked with a child with atypical Rett syndrome. He claimed that through the use of cognitive rehabilitation techniques he had managed to achieve improvements in attention skills and motivation. The therapist strongly recommended the approach for individuals with RS [68].

Lovaas technique/Applied Behavioral Analysis (ABA)

Applied Behavioral Analysis (ABA) is the practice of the reinforcement of behavior, which leads to the acquisition of new skills. The essence of the technique is that for many children, the problems they experience in living with their condition result largely from difficulties in learning, which can be overcome by intensive teaching. Typically developing children learn without additional or extraordinary mediation, or the environment they are born into provides the right conditions to learn language, play, and social skills. Children with PDD (such as individuals with RS) typically have much fewer opportunities to learn from the environment. They are often capable of learning, but it takes a much more structured and adapted environment, one where conditions are optimized for acquiring the same skills that typical children learn naturally. ABA is all about setting up highly structured rules for the environment, which assist our kids to learn. Conversely, any new behavior which is not rewarded is likely to be extinguished after a while (due to a lack of motivation to repeat it). In addition, a behavior which results in something unpleasant (an aversive stimulus) is even less likely to be repeated. These are the basics of behavioral learning theory [69]. This approach is usually applied for individuals with autism spectrum disorders, and more recently there have been reports regarding the use of this approach for individuals with RS. On the surface the basic approach would not seem to fit the fragile highly emotional nature of the individual with RS. Nevertheless, a newer version of behavioral analysis, termed gentle teaching (GT) stems from the use of unconditional acceptance of the client and the disuse of avers reinforcers [70]. In this form of ABA "caregivers are encouraged to increase the level of compassion and warmth" [71]. As a response to a question posed by parents, Vicky Slonims a clinical advisor to the Rett Syndrome Association in the United Kingdom, commented that she believed "it would be necessary to make significant modifications to the teaching curriculum and teaching styles to meet the needs of a person with Rett syndrome" [72]. Some reports regarding the use of ABA with individuals with RS were extremely positive regarding the acquisition of skills and the enhancement of the individual's involvement in daily activities [73,74].

Story of Kelsey

Kelsey, a girl with Rett Syndrome, received Discrete Trial Therapy (DTT), based upon the principles of Applied Behavioral Analysis (ABA) for three years. "Although Kelsey had not progressed as quickly as some autistic children we have seen progress, she definitely made meaningful and significant progress for herself, and that is what counts."I believe all our hard work has actually managed to remediate some of the terrible effects of this disorder such as the loss of purposeful hand skills" said her mother [73].

Motoric intervention techniques

Advanced biomechanical rehabilitation (ABR)
The term ABR stands for Advanced BioMechanical Rehabilitation. ABR is a unique biomechanically-based rehabilitation approach for children and young adults with brain injury, in which it is suggested that there is recovery of musculoskeletal structures and motor functions. It is a hands-on method performed by the parents, who learn the ABR technique and receive an individual program of applications from the ABR professional staff. ABR is a method that rebuilds even the most severely distorted musculoskeletal structure. The cornerstones of the ABR philosophy are fundamental biomechanical principles of the human body's growth and development [75].

Story of Abbey

Abbey received ABR for 2.5 years (see figures XVII-5, XVII-6) and her mother reported that the (positive) changes she has achieved in her musculoskeletal structure remained, even when the program is interrupted [76].

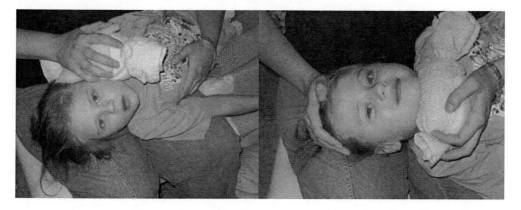

Figures XVII-5 and XVII-6. Abbey during ABR training.

Box XVII-6

> Caution: ABR is a completely new technique and the theory behind it has no anatomical or physiological proven basis. The intervention is provided to children with a wide array of brain injuries, and there are no!! Published studies to provide supporting evidence for this intervention technique.

Patterning/Doman-Delacato approach

In the 1960's, a new approach to rehabilitative intervention was initiated by Glen Doman, a physical therapist, and Carl Delacato, an educator, known as the "Doman-Delacato treatment" or "patterning". The Doman-Delacato treatment of patterning is based on theories, dating back to the 1920s-30s, of how ontogeny recapitulates phylogeny. These theories are not supported by current knowledge of the development of the central nervous system in humans [77]. The basic premise was that one can improve function by stimulating specific sensory inputs, thereby eliciting specific motor output patterns [78]. The assumption is that the accomplishment of brain development is achieved by stimulating the brain through movement of the body; for instance, if the children could not walk well, they were given the opportunity to learn crawling through many hours of therapy each day. The claim of Doman and Delacato was that mental retardation, learning problems, and behavioral disorders were caused by 'poor neurological organization' in the majority of individuals [79]. According to most researchers, studies of patterning have produced negative results and its use is not generally recommended [27]. In fact, the extreme financial and emotional burden caused by the intensive intervention program to the family of the client with developmental disabilities have caused several organizations to issue cautionary statements regarding the treatment (see box XVII-7). Despite this statement, the patterning approach has been tried by individuals with RS.

Case study

A very positive report was made by Jane George, who reported significant improvement in her daughter's functional abilities, especially crawling on all fours and independent walking. She also recommended the intellectual stimulation. She summed up the experience by saying: I think that the Doman therapy helped my daughter "get the most out of life for many years" [81].

In the case of Heather, another child with RS, her mom reported in further detail and with less enthusiasm: Heather, had undergone the Doman-Delacato intervention. According to her mother, the most useful component of the method was the overhead ladder. Training with the ladder enabled Heather to achieve independent walking for short distances. Heather enjoyed the vestibular part of the program (intended for stimulating the vestibular system). The part of the program called masking (the placing of a plastic mask over the face) dramatically increased her hyperventilation and apneas. No change was observed in relation to the patterning training in the crawl box. Neither was change observed during her participation in the intellectual stimulation program. Janet (Heather's mom) suggested that the therapy be used with caution. She also commented that when deciding on participation in such a program, careful attention needs to be paid to selecting the different parts of the program in accordance to the needs and preferences of the child [82].

Box XVII-7

Patterning has little effect on functional skills and was found inappropriate for children with motor disabilities [80].

Yoga

Yoga is a traditional Indian culture and way of life, which is intended to give the practitioner a healthy body and a sound mind. It is also believed to alleviate stress and induce relaxation [83]. The core components of the yoga technique involve breathing exercises (pranayama), postures (asanas), devotional sessions and meditation (dhyana). Many branches of yoga have been described such as hatha yoga, karma yoga, bhakti yoga and raja yoga[84].

There are several reports regarding the use of yoga in people with intellectual disability, in the rehabilitation of myocardial infarct patients, with hypertension and other medical disorders. The impact of yoga on the autonomic nervous system has been studied and effects have also been observed using the electroencephalogram [85]. Stress is considered an important precipitating factor in triggering seizures and the efficacy of yoga in stress reduction has been documented [86,87]. It is therefore suggested that Yoga could be considered as a possible therapeutic option in reducing the severity of epileptic seizures. This could be particularly beneficial in view of its non pharmacological nature, minimal adverse effects and international acceptance. Yoga has been reported as having potential as an intervention for individuals with severe disabilities [88].

Case Study

Jeanne reported that her daughter with Rett syndrome had received Yoga intervention by a trained pediatric special needs practitioner. She conveyed that the intervention was "great for relaxation and flexibility"[89].

Summary

This review has presented a small sample of alternative therapeutic approaches, which have been used in an attempt to improve function and quality of life in individuals with RS. The therapist or parent who seeks to expand the child's experience and to explore new intervention options should find some possibilities within the scope of the present chapter. The basic requirement for implementing a new and non traditional approach is of course the fact that no harm should be inflicted upon the child and her family. It must be emphasized that every new therapeutic approach should be considered and discussed with individuals proficient in the novel technique and applied only with specific, realistic and measurable goals, which are time-limited. There is a need for larger samples to be studied and detailed research to be conducted before it can be considered that a given treatment has any significant benefit for persons with Rett syndrome.

References

[1]   Amir RE, Van Den Veyver IB, Schultz R, Malicki DM, Tran CQ, Dahle EJ, et al. Influence of mutation type and X chromosome inactivation on Rett syndrome phenotypes. Ann Neurol 2000;47:670-9.

[2]   Hagberg B, Aicardi J, Dias K, Ramos O. A progressive syndrome of autism, dementia, ataxia, and loss of purposeful hand use in girls: Rett syndrome: report of 35 cases. Ann Neurol 1983;14:471-9.

[3]   Hagberg B, ed. Rett syndrome: Clinical and biological aspects. London: Mac Keith Press, 1993.

[4]   Ellaway C, Christodoulou J. Rett syndrome: Clinical characteristics and recent genetic advances. Disabil Rehabil 2001;23:98-106.

[5]   Kerr AM, Witt Engerstrom I, eds. Rett disorder and the developing brain. Oxford: Oxford Univ Press, 2001.

[6]   Elefant C. Emotional/musical communication of children with RS. A lecture at an annual coference on RS. Sheba hospital, Ramat-Gan, Israel, Jul 2005.

[7]   Rothe EQ, Vega BJ, Torres RM, Soler SMC, Pazos RMM. From kids and horses: Equine facilitated psychotherapy for children. Int J Clin Health Psychol 2005;5(2):373-83.

[8]   Martin F, Farnum J. Animal-assisted therapy for children with pervasive developmental disorders. West J Nurs Res 2002;24(6):657-70.

[9]   Levasseur KM. Pet therapy. IRSA newsletter, spring. 1996.

[10]   Personal communication (XVI) : Contact Bundlings.com. Received on July 1st 2006 from: debbie@bundlings.com

[11]   Brensing K, Linke K, Todt D. Can dolphins heal by ultrasound? J Theor Biol 2003;225(1):99-105.

[12]   Johnston L, bourne R. (2004) Is There a Dolphin in the House? http://healingtherapies,info/ dolphin.htm Assessed Jun 21, 2009.

[13]   International Dolphin Watch. Can dolphins make a difference? Assessed 2009 May 18: http://www.idw.org/html/dolphin_therapy.html

[14]   Milne T. Dolphins helped my child. BBC News Online Staff Saturday, 22 February, 2003. Assessed 2009 May 14 http://news.bbc.co.uk/1/hi/health/2736863.stm

[15]   Chess J. Stories and adventures for Zoe. A booklet made by the Chess family for Zoe's bat-mitzva, 1997.

[16]   Newman C, Newman K. Amy swims with dolphins. Rett news 2004, Spring, 17.

[17]   Berard G. Audition égale comportment. Sainte-Ruffne: Maisonneuve, 1982.

[18]   Berard G. Hearing equals behaviour. New Canaan, CT: Keats, 1993.

[19]   Sinha Y, Silove N, Wheeler D, Williams K. Auditory integration training and other sound therapies for autism spectrum disorders. Cochrane Database Syst Rev 2004;1:CD003681.

[20]   Personal communication (IX): Auditory Integration Therapy, received through the Rettnett 06 May 2006, from: annetteb@mymerit.com

[21]   Fasano VA, Nunno T, Urciolo R, Lombard G. First observation on the use of oxygen under high pressure for the treatment of traumatic coma. In: Boerema I, Brummelkamp WH, Meigne NG, eds. Clinical application of hyperbaric oxygen. Amsterdam: Elsevier, 1964:168-73.

[22]   Muizelaar JP. Cerebral blood flow, cerebral blood volume and cerebral metabolism after severe head injury. In: Becker DP, Gudeman SK, eds. Textbook of head injury. Philadelphia, PA: WB Saunders, 1989:221–40.

[23]   Ikeda Y, Long DM. The molecular basis of brain injury and brain edema: the role of oxygen free radicals. Neurosurgery 1990;27(1):1–11.

[24]   Siesjo BK, Agardh CD, Bengtsson F. Free radicals and brain damage. Cerebrovasc Brain Metab Rev 1989;1:165–211.

[25]   Rossignol DA, Rossignol LW. Hyperbaric oxygen therapy may improve symptoms in autistic children. Med Hypotheses 2005;67(2): 216-28.

[26]   Golden ZL, Neubauer R, Golden CJ, Greene L, Marsh J, Mleko A. Improvement in cerebral metabolism in chronic brain injury after hyperbaric oxygen therapy. Int J Neurosci 2002;112(2):119-31.

[27]   Liptak GS. Complementary and alternative therapies for cerebral palsy. Ment Retard Dev Disabil Res Rev 2005;11(2):156-63.

[28]   Waisman D, Shupak A, Weisz G, Melamed Y. Hyperbaric oxygen therapy in the pediatric patient: The experience of the Israel naval medical institute. Pediatrics 1998;102(5):53-63.

[29]   Personal communication (X): Hyperbaric chamber. Rettnett 2006 May 02 from thaiwillers@VERIZON.NET

[30]   Clark JM. Oxygen toxicity. In: Bennett PB, Elliott DH, eds. The physiology and medicine of diving, 3rd ed. London: Bailliere Tindall Cox, 1982:200–38.

[31]   Bennett MH, Trytko B, Jonker B. Hyperbaric oxygen therapy for the adjunctive treatment of traumatic brain injury. Cochrane Database Syst Rev 2004;4:CD004609.

[32]   Nuthall G, Seear M, Lepawsky M, Wensley D, Skippen P, Hukin J. Hyperbaric oxygen therapy for cerebral palsy: Two complications of treatment. Pediatrics 2000;106(6):80-4.

[33] Birch S, Hesselink JK, Jonkman FA, Hekker TA, Bos A. Clinical research on acupuncture. Part 1. What have reviews of the efficacy and safety of acupuncture told us so far? J Altern Complement Med 2004;10(3), 468-80.

[34] Acupressure Institute home page. http://www.acupressure.com/

[35] Berman BM. Clinical applications of acupuncture: an overview of the evidence. J Altern Complement Med 2001;7 (Suppl 1):S111-8.

[36] Kulkarni S, O'Farrell I, Erasi M, Kochar MS. Stress and hypertension. WMJ 1998;97(11):34-8.

[37] Ward SL. Caring and healing in the 21st century. MCN Am J Matern Child Nurs 1998;23(4):210-5.

[38] Personal communication (II). Acupressure/energy healing/ reflexology. Rettnett 2006 May 06 from annetteb@mymerit.com

[39] Ersser S. Touch and go. Nurs Standard 1990;4:39.

[40] Crawford NW, Cincotta DR, Lim A, Powell CVE. A cross-sectional survey of complementary and alternative medicine use by children and adolescents attending the University Hospital of Wales. BMC Complement Altern Med 2006;6:16.

[41] Price S, Price L. Aromatherapy for health professionals, 2nd ed. London: Churchill Livingston, 1999.

[42] Smith CA, Collins CT, Cyna AM, Crowther CA. Complementary and alternative therapies for pain management in labour. Cochrane Database Syst Rev 2003:CD003521.

[43] Gedney JJ, Glover TL, Fillingim RB. Sensory and affective pain discrimination after inhalation of essential oils. Psychosom Med 2004;66:599–606.

[44] Leach MJ. A critical review of natural therapies in wound management. Ostomy Wound Manage 2004;50:36–40.

[45] Buckle J. Clinical aromatherapy in nursing. London: Edward Arnold, 1997.

[46] Motomura N, Sakurai A, Yotsuya Y. Reduction of mental stress with lavender odorant. Percept Mot Skills 2001;93:713–8.

[47] Goel N, Kim H, Lao RP. An olfactory stimulus modifies nighttime sleep in young men and women. Chronobiol Int 2005;22(5):889-904.

[48] Kuriyama H, Watanabe S, Nakaya T, Shigemori I, Kita M, Yoshida N, et al. Immunological and psychological benefits of aromatherapy massage. Evid Based Complement Alternat Med 2005;2(2):179–84.

[49] Price S, Price PP. Aromatherapy for babies and children. London: Thorsous 1996.

[50] US Department of Labor. Bureau of Labor statistics occupational outlook handbook: Chiropractors. Accessed 2009 Jul 02. URL: http://www.bls.gov/oco/ocos071.htm

[51] Personal communication (VI): Chiropractor. Rettnett 2006 May 06 from: annetteb@mymerit.com

[52] Craniosacral therapy. An internet site. Accessed 2009 May 17. URL: http://www.eparent.com/welcome/alternative.htm

[53] Webhealth. Craniosacral therapy. Accessed 2009 May 18. URL: http://www.webhealth.co.uk/therapies/craniosacral_therapy.asp

[54] Personal communication (XI). Cranio-sacral therapy for Allie. Rettnett 2006 May 06 spaggis@comcast.net

[55] Personal communication (XII): Cranial-sacral therapy. Rettnett 2006 May 06 ATCath@aol.com

[56] Wirth-Pattullo V, Hayes KW. Interrater reliability of craniosacral rate measurements and their relationship with subjects' and examiners' heart and respiratory rate measurements. Phys Ther 1994;74:908-16.

[57] Wikipedia. Myofascial Release. Accessed 2009 Jun 27. URL: http://en.wikipedia.org/wiki/Myofascial_Release

[58] Personal communication (VIII). Myofascial release. Rettnett 2006 May 02 joanchris2000@optonline.net

[59] Kovalik D. Reiki as an alternative healing method. Common Factor 1995;10:9.

[60]   Nield-Anderson L, Ameling A. The empowering nature of Reiki as a complementary therapy. Holist Nurs Pract 2000;14(3):21-9.

[61]   DiNucci EM. Energy healing: a complementary treatment for orthopaedic and other conditions. Orthop Nurs 2005;24(4):259-69.

[62]   Personal communication (V). Reiki. Rettnett 2006 May 06 annetteb@mymerit.com

[63]   Spa finder. The global spa resources. Accessed 2009 May 18. URL: http://www.spafinder.com/spalifestyle/spa101/glossary_S.jsp.

[64]   Personal communication (III). Treger massage therapy. A talk with parents. IRSA Ann Conference, Las-Vegas, NV, 1999.

[65]   The center for cognitive rehabilitation and neuro-feedback. Information regarding cognitive rehabilitation. Accessed 2009 Jun 06. URL: http://www.rehabgeorgia.com/cognitive.htm

[66]   Cicerone KD, Dahlberg C, Kalmar K, Langenbahn DM, Malec JF, Bergquist TF, et al. Evidence-based cognitive rehabilitation: recommendations for clinical practice. Arch Phys Med Rehabil 2000;81(12):1596-615.

[67]   Gillette Y, DePompei R. The potential of electronic organizers as a tool in the cognitive rehabilitation of young people. NeuroRehabilitation 2004;19(3):233-43.

[68]   Personal communication (XV). Cognitive rehabilitation. Rettnet 1996 Sep 26 DentonJB@aol.com.

[69]   Autism Behavioural Intervention Association. ABA. Background information Accessed 2009 May 17. URL: http://home.vicnet.net.au/~abia/aba/whatisaba.htm

[70]   Jones RSP, McCaughey RE. Gentle teaching and applied behavioral analysis. J Appl Behv Anal 1992;25(4):853-67.

[71]   Steele D. Gentle teaching: A value based framework for helping others. A viewpoint document. Unpublished document, 2006.

[72]   Slonims V. Can you advise me whether ABA is now considered a good treatment for an individual with Rett syndrome? An answer to a question by parents. Accessed 2009 May 13. URL: http://www.rettsyndrome.org.uk/_downloads/Comm_Q5.pdf

[73]   Kelsey's story. Accessed 2009 Jun 13. URL: http://www.geocities.com/pflowerett/kelstory.html

[74]   Thomas SM. A personal profile. Personal communication, 2006.

[75]   Advanced BioMechanical Rehabilitation (ABR). Accessed 2009 May 28. URL: http://www.blyum.com/

[76]   Personal communication. Advanced Biomechanical Rehabilitation (ABR). Rettnett 2006 May 06 thaiwillers@VERIZON.NET

[77]   Holm VA. A western version of the Doman-Delacato treatment of patterning for developmental disabilities. West J Med 1983;139:553-6.

[78]   Sieben RL. Controversial medical treatments of learning disabilities. Acad Ther 1997;13:133-47.

[79]   American Academy of Pediatrics. The Doman-Delacato treatment of neurologically handicapped children. Exceptional Parent 1983;13:40-3.

[80]   American Academy of Pediatrics, Committee on Children With Disabilities. The treatment of neurologically impaired children using patterning. Pediatrics 1999;104:1149 –51.

[81]   Personal communication. Rehabilitation. 1997.

[82]   Personal communication. Rehabilitation. 2007.

[83]   Anand BK. Yoga and medical sciences. Indian J Physiol Pharmacol 1991;35(2):84-7.

[84]   Corby JC, Roth WT, Zarcone VP Jr, Kopell BS. Psychophysiologic correlates of the practice of tantric yoga meditation. Arch Gen Psychiatry 1978;35(5):571-7.

[85]   Ramaratnam S, Sridharan K. Yoga for epilepsy. Cochrane Database Syst Rev 2002;1:CD001524.

[86]   Panjwani U, Gupta HL, Singh SH, Selvamurthy W, Rai UC. Effect of Sahaja yoga practice on stress management in patients of epilepsy. Indian J Physiol Pharmacol 1995;39(2):111-6.

[87]   Schell FJ, Allolio B, Schonecke OW. Physiological and psychological effects of hatha-yoga exercise in healthy women. Int J Psychosom 1994;41(1-4):46-52.

[88] Neubert DA, Moon MS, Grigal M. Activities of students with significant disabilities receiving services in postsecondary settings. Educ Training Dev Disabil 2004;39(1):16–25.

[89] Personal communication. Yoga. 2006.

In: Rett Syndrome: Therapeutic Interventions
Editors: Meir Lotan and Joav Merrick

ISBN: 978-1-61728-080-1
©2011 Nova Science Publishers, Inc.

Chapter XVIII

Rett Syndrome: Aging

Joav Merrick, MD, MMedSci, DMSc[*,1,2],
Meir Lotan, BPT, MScPT, PhD[3,4],
Isack Kandel, MA, PhD[1] *and Mohammed Morad, MD*[1,5]

[1]National Institute of Child Health and Human Development, Office of the Medical
Director, Division for Mental Retardation, Ministry of Social Affairs, Jerusalem
[2]Kentucky Children's Hospital, University of Kentucky,
Lexington, United States of America
[3]Department of Physical Therapy, Ariel University Center of Samaria, Ariel, Israel
[4]Israeli Rett Syndrome Association, National Evaluation Team,
National Rett Syndrome Clinic, Chaim Sheba Medical Center, Ramat-Gan
[5]Department of Family Medicine, Faculty of Health Sciences,
Ben Gurion University of the Negev, Beer-Sheva, Israel

Rett syndrome (RS) is a neurological disease affecting mainly females, characterized by
an arrest of brain development caused by an X chromosome mutation. Rett syndrome is
the first human disease found to be caused by defects in a protein involved in regulating
gene expression through its interaction with methylated DNA. The disease has been
traced to a defective gene called MECP2 on the X chromosome. This review of aging
with RS revealed very few studies but the published case-studies showed that females
with RS can live even to the age of 79. The existing knowledge suggests that individuals
with RS present the therapist/physician with specific clinical challenges that require
proper, long lasting, intervention programs to be individually tailored for this population.

* Correspondence: Professor Joav Merrick, MD, MMedSci, DMSc, Medical Director, Division for Mental
Retardation, Ministry of Social Affairs, POBox 1260, IL-91012 Jerusalem, Israel. E-mail: jmerrick@
zahav.net.il

Introduction

Until recently most individuals with intellectual disability (ID) lived much shorter life spans in comparison to individuals without ID. At present adults with ID are living to advanced age due to developments in medical care and technology, which have increased life expectancy of this population [1-3]. An estimated 641,000 adults with ID at ages 60 years and up were residing in the United States in the year 2000 and official expectations are that this group will increase threefold by 2020 [4]. Not only that adults with ID are living longer and healthier lives and their life expectancy have been found to increase substantially over the last few decades, expectation are that this trend will continue in future years [5]. As persons with ID are living longer, geriatrics healthcare providers need to learn about the characteristics, healthcare needs, and common clinical issues facing this population in general as well as subgroups, such as persons with Rett syndrome.

Rett syndrome

The original observation of six girls with a peculiar disease, reported by Andreas Rett (1924-1997), from Austria, was published in German in 1966 [6], but this syndrome only gained international attention when in 1983 Bengt Hagberg from Sweden and colleagues [7] published their findings on 35 cases. This author had in fact already observed his first patient in 1960 [8].

Rett syndrome (RS) is a neurological disease [9] affecting mainly females [10] characterized by arrest of brain development [9] caused by an X chromosome mutation. RS is the first human disease found to be caused by defects in a protein involved in regulating gene expression through its interaction with methylated DNA [11] and has been traced to a defective gene on the X chromosome, called MECP2 (pronounced "meck-pea-two"). This discovery was made by Ruthie Amir, an Israeli physician who found the first mutations [11,12], working at the laboratory of Huda Zoghbi's, a neuro-geneticist at Baylor College of Medicine in Houston, Texas.

RS typically presents after the first year of life (6-18 months of age) and is one of the most common causes of multiple-disability among females. The disease incidence is one in 10,000-15,000, with a gradual reduction of speech and purposeful hand-use, seizures, autistic like behavior, ataxia, intermittent hyperventilation and stereotypic hand movements. After initial regression, the condition stabilizes and patients usually survive into adulthood [8].

Although 50% to 75% of patients achieve independent mobility in early childhood, about 75% lose the ability to walk in later years and become wheelchair-bound [13]. Some professionals recommend walking and/or other physical fitness programs as a preventive intervention that might hold back or diminish secondary regression [13-16]. The debilitating disabilities common to this syndrome are: scoliosis, appearing in up to 85% of affected individuals [14], constipation and osteoporosis at a young age. All the above medical conditions have been known to be affected positively by physical therapy and other intervention programs suggesting physical activity for this population.

Rett syndrome stages

The stages of RS have been described as, onset or pre-regression (or stage 1); destructive, motor deterioration or regression (or stage 2); essentially stable or plateau (or stage 3) and in some cases the term fourth stage (late motor deterioration) has been used in circumstances in which an individual who achieved walking abilities at a young age becomes very handicapped and loses ambulation [17, 18]. Development in females with RS proceeds in an apparently normal fashion in-utero and during the first 6-18 months of life, at which point their development comes to a halt with regression and loss of many of their acquired skills [19]. Thereafter, a rapid deterioration, with loss of acquired speech and purposeful hand use, ensues. A deceleration of head growth and jerky body movements of the trunk and limbs accompany the developmental deterioration in individuals with RS. Typically, they present with a broad-based gait and swaying movements of the shoulders when walking [20]. Other physical problems, such as seizures, scoliosis and breathing abnormalities may appear [21], which require constant care for the rest of the person's life [22]. The scoliosis is a prominent feature in females with RS, but can vary from mild to severe [23]. Apraxia (Developmental dyspraxia), the inability to program the body to perform motor tasks, is the most fundamental and severely handicapping aspect of the syndrome. Apraxia can interfere with all body movement, including eye gaze and speech, making it difficult for individuals with RS to execute what they want to do. To sum up, the child adolescent and adult with RS is in need of an intensive and comprehensive management program throughout their life span (estimated life expectancy of individuals with RS in the past was around 50 years) [24].

Longitudinal follow-up of adults with Rett syndrome

Studies conducted about aging and RS are scarce, with only a few case studies available. The present paragraph describes longitudinal follow-up of adults with RS, thereby emphasizing the importance of such documentation. One case-study [25] described a woman with RS from Norway, who lived to the age of 60 years. That paper provides no information about any genetic test, only a clinical diagnosis. The study was based on medical records, older and more recent videotapes and interviews with her sister and care-giving staff. After 21 years without being able to walk, following intensive physiotherapy, the woman regained that ability, walking without support. A few years before she died, she also showed improvement in hand use. During the early regression, she appeared to lose social interest. The interest improved after some time but she remained wary of people whom she did not know.

Another case study was published from Denmark of a 77-year-old woman [26], born in 1923 after a normal pregnancy and delivery, who walked unsupported at the age of about one. She deviated from normal development at two years of age. At 38 years of age, she had lost all purposeful hand use and performed the hand mannerisms typical of RS constantly. She developed severe kyphosis and at 41 years of age, ambulation was lost. At age 66, she was diagnosed as RS with the following mutation in her MECP2 alleles: a C to P transition in exon 4 leading to a substitution of threonine by methionine at position 158, T158M in the conserved methyl binding domain (MBD), of the corresponding gene product. The XCI showed a non-random pattern with an inactivation ratio of 10:90. This T158 mutation is a common mutation in RS and her skewed XCI may have resulted in her long survival. She died, at the age of 79 from peritonitis, caused by an abscess after the removal of a large spleen.

Hagberg [27] described three cases to illustrate long-term clinical follow-up in RS. The first case-study was of a girl born in 1957, who had developmental delay and was referred at 3½ years of age but not diagnosed with RS until 19 years of age. At that time, the main problems were her apraxia, her general developmental retardation and her aggressive behavior. In addition, she was considerably growth retarded, had developed a severe kyphosis and a more modest left convex C scoliosis. Her epileptiform symptomatology, which started at age 6 months, was under full control and no longer a problem. At the last follow-up (age 47 years), she was a very small woman, 134 cm. tall, weighing 50 kg., with an occipitofrontal head circumference (OFC) of 54 cm. She had short, thin, slightly distorted feet (only 34 cm. long). She was still able to walk unsupported but showed some balance problems. She was less active in motor-terms and had signs of excessively early gross motor-muscle aging of the legs. She had hand-finger stereotypes more or less continuously but a more subtle form of the regular hand stereotypic wringing and twisting performed by females with RS. Her neurology was characterized by a complex gross motor dysfunction of the RS type, not only a complete grasp apraxia but also some sort of dyspraxia in her whole-body movement pattern. She had a complex MECP2 rearrangement with deletions both of exon 3 and exon 4.

The second case-study was of a female born in 1960, the second of three siblings, in a healthy family. Her pre- and perinatal history was uneventful with birth at full term (weight 3,720 g., length 50 cm., OFC 34.5 cm.). Her first 1¼years of life were reported to have been uneventful. At that age, she was able to walk with support, pincer-grasp and manipulated toys as expected. She had, however, never learned to crawl on all-fours. At that point a general stagnation occurred, followed rapidly by marked developmental regression. At the age of 1¾ years, she had stopped walking completely, had lost contact with her parents, had developed intense "hand-clapping" stereotypes (film documented) and showed "autistic-like" behaviors. In parallel, her head growth curve indicated a marked deceleration. At 23 years of age, she was diagnosed as a classic Rett Syndrome patient. At the last visit (44 years of age), she was extremely handicapped, very small and thin, with a small head (height 130 cm., weight 24 kg, OFC 48.5 cm.). She had a complex S-curved RS kyphoscoliosis and a markedly distended abdomen of the RS bloating type. Her feet were cold and sweaty, bluish in color, and extremely thin and small (length only 22 cm.). Her examination was characterized by a dystonic-rigid syndrome of the advanced RS type with a right-sided dominance. She was reported to have repeated, unmotivated, long laughing attacks, as well as paroxysmal night screaming. She had never had any epileptic seizures. She had a commonly found MECP2 mutation inaxon 4 (R270X).

The third case, born in 1965, was one of two siblings in a healthy family. Her peri- and neonatal histories were uneventful, as were her developmental abilities when she was born at full term (weight 3,590 g, length 50 cm., OFC 34 cm.). She developed normally but at a health check-up at one year old, she was considered to be "late" but able to creep on her knees and sit up and walk with support and play with toys. She could say many single words. After 1½ years of age, she slowly regressed, did not use her hands as before, was found socially detached from her parents and was more or less in her "own world". At the same time, she stopped crawling and talking and repeatedly had unmotivated screaming attacks. At the age of 2½, her skull growth had stagnated significantly. She was slightly hypotonic and had some sort of ataxic movement patterns of the truncal ataxia type, as well as intention-tremor in her hands and stereotypic movement patterns. She did not develop seizures. Throughout the following three decades, she successively deteriorated neurologically into a generalized most severe dystonic-atrophic syndrome, with side-asymmetric secondary deformities, contractures and a collapsed scoliosis. She died at the age of 36 in a deformed, growth-retarded, emaciated state.

Resent findings

A large North American cohort (N=1,928) examined the longevity of individual with RS and found that about 80% of individuals diagnosed with atypical RS and 60% of individuals with typical RS survive to the age of 50 years [28]. Nevertheless, the authors themselves suggest that given that clinical management has improved considerably from the time when RS was first recognized, improved survival among each successive cohort might be expected. Moreover, we believe that since the research was done only on people currently diagnosed with RS, institutionalized undiagnosed adults might change the data, suggesting even greater longevity in this population.

In another project conducted by researchers from Maastricht University in Holland in association with the Dutch Rett syndrome association, questionnaires were sent to families and caregivers of individuals with RS aged 16 years and older [29]. It was found that concerned living conditions and use of care facilities that about third (36%) of the research population resided with their parents and the rest (71%) in residential facilities.

Health of the individuals was assessed on a 5-point scale ranging from very good (1) to very bad (5). In general, the respondents valued the health of individuals with RS as good (mean 2.15), but A significant relationship was found between health and apnea, breath holding spells, mood changes, spasticity and joint deformities. In regards to weight status 49% of the participants were underweight, 40% had a normal weight and 11% were overweight. In regards to communication a third of the participants with RS were able to express themselves sometimes by spoken language and/or signals. Communication was found considerably better in the older age groups. These findings support previous knowledge regarding adults with RS [30-32].

Cold feet were notified in 96% of participants with RS and pressure sores and vesicles occurred in 46%. Half of the participants with RS showed sleeping problems on a nightly occurrence and the prevalence of sleeping problems was higher in the older age groups. Daytime sleeping was reported in 85% of the research population. Apnea (38%), hyperventilation (39%), breath holding spells (73%) and air swallowing (41%) were reported with a much lower prevalence in the oldest age group (in regards to apnea).

Night screaming was reported in 39%, prevalence of mood changes in 66% and abnormal agitation reported in 54%. Two thirds of the research population showed anxiety. The prevalence of scoliosis in the study was 90%, of those 36% had undergone surgery, while the prevalence of kyphosis was found in 16%,

In contrast to other areas gross motor in the research population was found to slowly but continuously decline over the years, which has also been found by other researchers [17,33-35]. Ambulation and mobility were very limited in all age-groups and no relationship with age was found. The prevalence of spasticity was 52%, mainly affecting the arms and legs. Joint deformities, mostly of the feet were found in 60% of the research population. A history of epilepsy was present in 74%, of whom 95% used anticonvulsive treatment.

In general, in both research projects better communication and autonomic function in the oldest age group was found compared to the younger age groups, which is in line with previous findings [35-37]. The research demonstrate the potential for prolonged survival in this population and suggest the need for careful planning for long-term care, as well as continued observation of the effects of improved clinical management on longevity.

Clinical manifestations of the aging person with Rett syndrome

The person with RS presents some clinical manifestations that are common for this syndrome and therefore require specific acknowledgement, proper evaluation and specific intervention:

- Scoliosis – 80%-85% of individuals with RS [30,38] are diagnosed with scoliosis. It has been found that intensive therapeutic intervention with adequate sensory [21] and physical [15] support can regress the deterioration of the scoliosis [15] and might even prevent the child from the need to undergo corrective surgery [21].
- Epilepsy – according to differing studies, 30%-90% of individuals with RS will be diagnosed with epilepsy [30,36, 39-41]. Individuals with RS show acute reactions to anti-epileptic medication and therefore the diagnostic procedure and medication prescription should be performed by physicians acquainted with this specific disorder [30]. Moreover, since many individuals with RS tend to have irregular night sleep [42] and excessive amounts of daytime sleep [43] anti-epileptic medication should be introduced only if the seizures disturb the child's daily routine or functions. Since it has been found that 82% of individuals with RS show breathing abnormalities that might sometimes appear as epileptic-like attacks, telemetry or electro-encephalogram (video EEG) should be performed to avoid anti-epileptic over-medication. Another aspect of epilepsy typical of this population is the fact that many of them show reduction in the severity and frequency of epileptic attacks in adulthood. Therefore, a slow reduction of anti-convulsive medication should be performed under the supervision of a neurologist knowledgeable with adults with RS [30]. Phenobarbitone and, to a lesser extent, benzodiazepines display a severe effect on the level of alertness and responsiveness of the client with RS, to a point of sudden pseudo-motor deterioration Therefore their use should be avoided as much as possible [31].

- Cranitine - Cranitine is a biological enhancer that is needed for cell- fat metabolism. Reduction in cranitine level might cause muscle weakness, liver-insufficiency, neurological problems and hypotonia. All these behaviors might damage the functional ability of the individual with RS, yet they are masked by the fluctuating nature of the RS manifestation. Since individuals with RS have been found in the past to show low levels of Cranitine, and since the supply of cranitine has been found to contribute positively to the height, weight and motor function of these individuals [44,45], cranitine level should be evaluated and supplied in cases of deficiency. Moreover, the combination of anti-convulsive medication, especially depakot, with cranitine has been found to be beneficial for this population.
- Constipation - Constipation is common in individuals with RS [43]. It is estimated that 85% of individuals with RS will experience severe constipation at least once in their life [46]. Constipation in this population is derived from a lack of physical activity, low muscle tone, improper diet, medication, scoliosis and reduced liquid intake [47]. Since all the above aspects contributing to constipation are treatable, their use should be examined prior to the use of laxatives and enemas [48].
- Nutrition - intestinal problems are present in 74% of individuals with RS [41] and are a significant component of this syndrome. There is evidence that these symptoms worsen with age in connection to their functional/orthopedic situation [23,32] and therefore, constant and proper evaluation should be a part of the follow-up procedure of the adult with RS. Moreover, moderate to severe malnutrition is present in 85% of individuals with RS [49] and is aggravating with age [36, 47]. Yet many of the nutritional problems of this population are treatable [48] when properly diagnosed.
- Osteoporosis - Osteoporosis occurs frequently in females with RS and has been reported in very young girls [50-52]. Patients with RS have been found with decreased bone mineral density compared to controls [53]. These findings support the need for routine checking from childhood of bone density of individuals with RS and to commence physical (such as intensive standing and walking programs [16,54], nutritional [48] and medical intervention [50] as preventive intervention when the situation necessitates such courses of action [31].
- Dental treatment – specific dental disorder-related problems have been identified in individuals with RS [55,56]. These problems include gum problems, teeth closure [56], bruxism, high risk of falling and facial trauma [32], teeth damage due to prolonged use of anti-convulsive medication and reflux [21]. These accumulating problems require the dentist's acknowledged attention and care [57,58].
- Functional improvements – a few studies have demonstrated that proper intervention can improve function of children [16] and adults with RS, up to a point were walking was restored for a woman with RS who had stopped walking 20 years previously [25]. Because of the possible life-spans of individuals with RS, it is suggested that proper and intensive care should be provided to clients with this syndrome at all ages in the hope of preventing or at least reducing the age-related deterioration that is typical of this population [59].

All the above symptoms are typical of people with RS and can be treated with conventional intervention, thereby contributing to the longevity and quality of life of this population. Therefore longitudinal follow-up for proper evaluational procedures and intervention implementation is needed for this population as it ages.

Identifying adults with Rett syndrome

Due to the fact that RS has been acknowledged by Western medicine only in the past 23 years, after the publication of the first English article on Rett syndrome by Hagberg and his colleagues [7], the majority of adults with RS are misdiagnosed and might therefore lack proper intervention.

In the attached figures the prevalence of RS in Israel is presented. It is evident from the graph that many RS adults over the age of 15 years have not been located and diagnosed and older adults (25 years and up) have been scarcely detected.

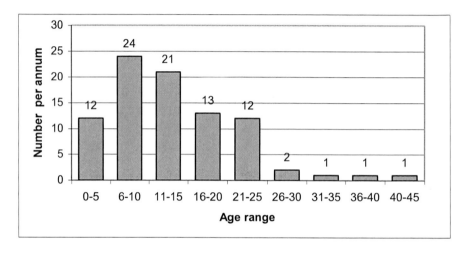

Figure XVIII-1. Prevalence of individuals diagnosed with RS in Israel, according to age.

Due to the specific medical challenges presented by adults with RS, the authors call for a widespread organized search for this population to detect, diagnose and implement proper intervention programs adapted for the specific needs of individuals with RS. Initial findings from an ongoing survey to detect undiagnosed adults with RS in residential care centers in Israel, suggest that about 3% of females in residential settings might be diagnosed with RS. Moreover, some of the typical characteristics of RS such as bruxism, bloating, sleep disorders, breathing abnormalities and sometimes even hand-mannerisms (reduced to subtle finger movements as described by Hagberg [30]) are less frequent in adulthood than in childhood within this population. Therefore, detection of these individuals requires a person, who is experienced in working with RS.

Mortality in Rett syndrome

People with RS can survive into middle and old age, but life expectancy is reduced and the occurrence of sudden death is greater than in the general population. Longitudinal records of people with RS began in the United Kingdom in 1982 and developed into the British Survey in 1993. From this British Survey, the mortality rate for RS has been estimated at 1.2% per annum [59], with 48% of deaths occurring in debilitated people, 13% from natural causes, 13% with prior severe seizures and 26% sudden and unexpected [59-62]. Respiratory dysrhythmias were usually present. Neuropathological studies confirmed reductions in cortical dendrites and in one case, immaturity of cardiac conducting tissues [59]. The possible causes of sudden death can include brain-stem autonomic failure (respiratory failure, apnoea, cardiac arrhythmias) [59-62].

Discussion

This review of aging individuals with Rett Syndrome (RS) revealed very few studies and we have still to wait for additional, larger follow-up studies and large cohort studies in the future.

The five case-studies from Norway, Denmark and Sweden showed deceleration of head growth appearing at an early stage, that was associated with increased motor disability and with the appearance of epilepsy [27]. The hand stereotypes, which are the trade mark of RS from early childhood, usually change in adult middle-age toward frozen and stiff mal-positions or remain as finger movement. From childhood to young adulthood, some gross motor-functions appear to improve slightly with a temporary recovery and compensation, in contrast to the loss of fine motor-abilities. In the long term, middle-aged women with RS lose a great deal of muscle volume, strength and power and present with generally premature neuromuscular aging, necessitating the introduction of physical fitness intervention programs. The early general growth deceleration not only affects body and skull growth but also involves the overly thin, small, cold and sweaty feet and the insufficient, compressed, and curved spine [15,27].

Epilepsy occurs in more than 90% of cases with onset of clinical seizures at around 3-5 years of age, with a peak frequency in adolescence, into young adulthood and successively decreases in early middle-age, with only rare and minor problems occurring after the age of 40 years [27,63]. Therefore, after 40 years of age, an attempt should be made to gradually withdraw anti-epileptic drugs [27,63].

Many common characteristics of adults with RS are known. These include constipation, osteoporosis, functional abilities, dental problems, nutritional needs, orthopedic problems, as well as medicational needs. All the above aspects necessitate special evaluation, which should lead to improved, more focused intervention for this population. Nevertheless the novelty of this syndrome requires a search for undiagnosed adults with RS to enable the implementation of proper care.

The case stories presented here and resent findings showed that females with RS can live even to the age of 79 years and suggest significant longevity for this population. Due to the observed longevity of individuals with RS, it is suggested that proper, long term and intensive care should be provided at all ages in the hope of preventing or at least reducing the age-related deterioration that is typical of this population.

References

[1]   Patja K, Iivanainen M, Vesala H, Oksanen H, Ruoppila I. Life expectancy of people with intellectual disabilities: A 35-year follow-up study. J Intellect Disabil Res 2000;44:591-9.

[2]   Maaskant MA, Gevers JPM, Wierda H. Mortality and live expectancy in Dutch residential centres for individuals with intellectual disabilities, 1991–1995. J Appl Res Int Dis 2002;15:200–12.

[3]   Fisher K, Kettl P. Aging with mental retardation: Increasing population of older adults with MR require health interventions and prevention strategies. Geriatrics 2005;60:26–9.

[4]   Heller T, Janicki MP, Hammel J, et al. Promoting healthy aging, family support, and age-friendly communities for persons aging with developmental disabilities: Report of the 2001 Invitational Research Symposium on Aging with Developmental Disabilities. Chicago, IL. University of Illinois at Chicago Website. Accessed 2009 Apr 17. URL: http://www.uic.edu/orgs.rrtcamr/gsa.pdf.

[5]   Tyler CVJr, Noritz G. Healthcare issues in aging adults with intellectual and other developmental disabilities. Clinical geriatrics 2009;17(8).

[6]   Rett A. Uber ein eigenartiges hirnatrophisches Syndrom bei Hyperammonamie im Kindesalter. Wiener Medi-zinische Wochenschrift 1966;116:723-38. [German].

[7]   Hagberg B, Aicardi J, Dias K, Ramos O. A progressive syndrome of autism, dementia, ataxia and loss of purposeful hand use in girls: Rett's syndrome. Report of 35 cases. Ann Neurol 1983; 14:471-9.

[8]   Hagberg B. Rett Syndrome: Swedish approach to analysis of prevalence and cause. Brain Dev 1985;7:277-80.

[9]   Armstrong DD. The neuropathology of Rett syndrome overview 1994. Neuropediatrics 1995;26:100-4.

[10]   Amir RE, Van den Veyver IB, Schultz R, Malicki DM, Tran CQ, Dahle EJ, et al. Influence of mutation type and X chrom-osome inactivation on Rett syndrome phenotypes. Ann Neurol 2000;47:670-9.

[11]   Amir RE, Van den Veyer IB, Wan M, Tran CQ, Francke U, Zoghbi HY. Rett syndrome is caused by mutations in X-linked MECP2, encoding methyl-CpG-binding protein 2. Nature Genetics 1999;23:185-8.

[12]   Amir RE, Zoghbi HY. Rett syndrome: Methyl-CpG-binding protein 2 mutations and phenotype-genotype correlations. Am J Med Genetics 2000;97:147-52.

[13]   Lotan M, Hadar-Frumer M. Hydrotherapy for Rett syndrome. Physiother Bull 2002; 4:23-8. [Hebrew]

[14]   McClure MK, Battaglia C, McClure RJ. The relationship of cumulative motor asymmetries to scoliosis in Rett syndrome. Am J Occup Ther 1998;52(3):488-93.

[15]   Lotan M, Merrick J, Carmeli E. Managing scoliosis in a young child with Rett syndrome: a case study. ScientificWorldJournal 2005;5:264-73.

[16]   Lotan M, Isakov E, Merrick J. Improving functional skills and physical fitness in children with Rett syndrome. J Intellect Disabil Res 2004;48(8):730-5.

[17]   Kerr AM. Annotation: Rett syndrome: recent progress and implications for research and clinical practice. J Child Psychol Child Psychiatry 2002;43(3):277-87.

[18]   Lotan M, Merrick J. Rett syndrome management with Snoezelen or controlled multi-sensory stimulation. A review. Int J Adolesc Med Health 2004;16(1):5-12.

[19]   Graham JM. Rett syndrome. Information packet. Los Angeles, CA: Cedars-Sinai Med Center, 1995.

[20]   Kerr AM, Stephenson JBP. Rett syndrome in the West of Scotland. BMJ 1985;291(6495):579-82.

[21]   Budden SS. Management of Rett syndrome: A ten years experience. Neuropediatrics 1995;26(2):75-7.

[22]   Leonard H, Fyfe S, Leonard S, Msall M. Functional status, medical impairments, and rehabilitation re-sources in 84 females with Rett syndrome: a snapshot across the world from the parental perspective. Disabil Rehabil 2001;23(3-4):107-17.

[23]   Sponseller P. Orthopedic update in Rett syndrome. IRSA-Int `Rett Syndr Ass Inf Resources. www.rettsyndrome.org/main/orthopaedic-update.htm

[24]   Percy AK. International research review. IRSA-Int Rett Syndr Ass 12th Ann Conf, Boston, MA, 1996 May 24-27.

[25]   Jacobsen K, Viken A, von Tetzchner S. Rett syndrome and Ageing: A case study. Disabil Rehabil 2001;23(3-4):160-6.

[26]   Nielsen JB, Ravn K, Schwartz M. A 77-year-old woman and a preserved speech variant among Danish Rett patients with mutations in MECP2. Brain Dev 2001;23:S230-2.

[27]   Hagberg B. Rett syndrome. Long-term clinical follow- up experiences over four decades. J Child Neurol 2005;20(9):722-6.

[28]   Kirby RS, Lane JB, Childers J, Skinner SA, Annese F, Barrish JO, Glaze DG, MacLeod P, Percy AK. Longevity in Rett syndrome: Analysis of the North American database. J Pediatr 2010;156:135-8.

[29]   Halbach NSJ, Smeets EEJ, Schrander-stumpel CTRM, Van Schrojensein Lantman De Valk HHJ, Maaskant MA, Curfs LM. Aging in People With Specific Genetic Syndromes:Rett Syndrome. Am J Med Genet A 2008;146A:1925–32.

[30]   Hagberg B. Rett syndrome: Clinical and biological aspects. London: Mac Keith, 1993.

[31]   Lotan M, Ben-Zeev B. Rett syndrome. A review with emphasis on clinical characteristics and intervention ScientificWorldJournal 2006;6:1517–41.

[32]   Lotan M. Angels of silence: Caring for Rett syndrome. Tel Aviv: Rotem, 2006. [Hebrew]

[33]   Steffenburg U, Hagberg G, Hagberg B. Epilepsy in a representative series of Rett syndrome. Acta Paediatr 2001;90:34–9.

[34]   Hagberg B. Clinical manifestations and stages of Rett syndrome. Ment Retard Dev Disabil Res Rev 2002;8:61–5.

[35]   Williamson SL, Christodoulou J. Rett syndrome: New clinical and molecular insights. Eur J Hum Genet 2006;14:896-903.

[36]   Ellaway C, Christodoulou J. Rett syndrome: Clinical characteristics and recent genetic advances. Disabil Rehabil 2001;23:98-106.

[37]   Julu PO, Kerr AM, Apartopoulos F, Al Rawas S, Engerstrom IW, Engerstrom L, Jamal GA, Hansen S. Characterization of breathing and associated central autonomic dysfunction in the Rett disorder. Arch Dis Child 2001;85:29–37.

[38]   Rossin L. Effectiveness of therapeutic and surgical intervention in the treatment of scoliosis in Rett syndrome. A seminar work. Pittsburgh, PA: Univ Duquesne, 1997:1-19.

[39]   Nieto MA, Candau RS, Prieto P. Contribution to studies of seizures in Rett syndrome analysis of critical forms of four cases. Rev Neurol 1995; 23:1185-89.

[40]   Glaze D. Epilepsy. Presentation, IRSA 12th Ann Conf, Boston, MA, 1996 May 24-27, tape 622-18.

[41]   Leonard S. The Australian Rett Syndrome study inaugural report. Aust: Telethon Inst Child Health Res, 2002.

[42]   Nomura Y. Early behavior characteristics and sleep disturbance in Rett syndrome. Brain Dev 2005;27(Suppl 1): S35-42.

[43]   Piazza CC, Fisher W, Kiesewetter BS, Bowman L, Moser H. Aberrant sleep patterns in children with Rett syndrome. Brain Dev 1990;2:488-93.

[44]   Plioplys AV, Kasnicka I. L-Carnitine as treatment for Rett syndrome. South Afr Med J 1993;86:1411-2.

[45]   Glaze D. Research updates from Baylor College. IRSA Ann Conf, Las Vegas, NV, 2000 May 18-21, Tape RS 10.

[46]   Saavedra JM. Gastrointestinal crises in Rett syndrome. Int Rett Syndr Assoc Newsletter 1997; Winter:3-5.

[47]   Reilly S, Cass H. Growth and nutrition in Rett syndrome. Disabil Rehabil 2001;23:118-28.

[48]   Lotan M, Zysman L. The digestive system and nutritional considerations for individuals with Rett syndrome. ScientificWorldJournal 2006;6:1737–49.

[49]   Hunter K. The Rett syndrome handbook. Washington, DC: Int Rett Syndr Assoc, 1999.

[50]   Zysman L, Lotan M, Ben-Zeev B. Osteoporosis in Rett syndrome: A study on normal values. ScientificWorldJournal 2006;6:1619–30.

[51]   Budden SS, Gunness ME. Possible mechanisms of osteopenia in Rett syndrome: bone histomorphometric studies. J Child Neurol 2003;18(10):698-702.

[52]   Leonard H, Thomson M, Glasson E, Fyfe S, Leonard S, Ellaway C, Christodouloon J, Bower C. Metacarpophalangeal pattern profile and bone age in Rett syndrome: Further radiological clues to the diagnosis. Am J Med Genetics 1999;12(83):88-95.

[53]   Haas RH, Dixon SD, Sartoris DJ, Hennessy MJ. Osteopenia in Rett syndrome. J Pediatr 1997;131(5):771-4.

[54]   Weeks L. Rett syndrome. Presentation, Sydney, 1997.

[55]   Tesini DA, Fenton-Sanford J. Oral health needs of persons with physical or mental disabilities. Dent Clin North Am 1994;38:483-98.

[56]   Ribeiro RA, Romano AR, Birman-Goldenberg E, Mayer MP. Oral manifestations in Rett syndrome: A study of 17 cases. Pediatr Dent 1997;19:349-52.

[57]   Tenisi DA. Developing dental health education programs for persons with special needs. A training guide and reference text. Amherst, MA: Massachusetts Res Inst, Massachusetts Dept Dental Health, 1988.

[58]   Tenisi DA. Providing dental services for citizens with handicaps: a prototype community program. Ment Retard 1987;25:219-22.

[59]   Kerr AM, Armstrong DD, Prescott RJ, Doyle D, Kearney DL. Rett syndrome: analysis of deaths in the British Survey. Eur Child Adolesc Psychiatry 1997;6(Suppl 1):71-4.

[60]   Acampa M, Guideri. Cardiac disease and Rett syndrome. Arch Dis Child 2006;91:440-3.

[61]   Ohya T, Yamashita Y, Matsuishi T. [Sudden death in Rett syndrome]. Nippon Rinsho 2005;63(7):1178-82. [Japanese]

[62]   Byard RW. Forensic issues and possible mechanisms of sudden death in Rett syndrome. J Clin Forensic Med 2006;13(2):96-9.

[63]   Steffenburg U, Hagberg G, Hagberg B. Epilepsy in a representative series of Rett syndrome. Acta Paediatr 2000;89:198-202.

In: Rett Syndrome: Therapeutic Interventions
Editors: Meir Lotan and Joav Merrick

ISBN: 978-1-61728-080-1
©2011 Nova Science Publishers, Inc.

Chapter XIX

About the editors

Meir Lotan, BPT, MScPT, PhD is a physiotherapist working as lecturer at the School of Health Sciences, Department of Physical Therapy, Ariel University Center of Samaria, Ariel. He is affiliated with the Israeli National Rett Syndrome evaluation team. He has a special interest in physiotherapy and persons with intellectual disability, Snoezelen and physical activity for children and adults with intellectual disability with an emphasis on individuals with Rett syndrome. His work with individuals with RS has been continuous since 1992, including research, daily physical therapy sessions and evaluations of over 300 individuals with RS both in Israel and abroad and in the year 2000 awarded by the IRSA (Int Rett Syndr Assoc) for his service to individuals with Rett syndrome. Numerous publications in international peer-reviewed journals in his areas of interest. E-mail: ml_pt_rs@ netvision.net.il

Joav Merrick, MD, MMedSci, DMSc, is professor of pediatrics, child health and human development affiliated with Kentucky Children's Hospital, University of Kentucky, Lexington, United States and the Zusman Child Development Center, Division of Pediatrics, Soroka University Medical Center, Ben Gurion University, Beer-Sheva, Israel, the medical director of the Health Services, Division for Mental Retardation, Ministry of Social Affairs, Jerusalem, the founder and director of the National Institute of Child Health and Human Development. Numerous publications in the field of pediatrics, child health and human development, rehabilitation, intellectual disability, disability, health, welfare, abuse, advocacy, quality of life and prevention. Received the Peter Sabroe Child Award for outstanding work on behalf of Danish Children in 1985 and the International LEGO-Prize ("The Children's Nobel Prize") for an extraordinary contribution towards improvement in child welfare and well-being in 1987. E-Mail: jmerrick@internet-zahav.net; Home-page: http://jmerrick50.googlepages.com/home

In: Rett Syndrome: Therapeutic Interventions
Editors: Meir Lotan and Joav Merrick

ISBN: 978-1-61728-080-1
©2011 Nova Science Publishers, Inc.

Chapter XX

About the Israel Rett Syndrome Center

In 2003 the association known as the Israel Rett Syndrome Center (IRSC) was established by families of individuals with RS. It is also managed by the families. The main goal of the Rett Syndrome Center was to improve the quality of life for individuals with RS and their families. This goal is attained through several routes:

- By promoting awareness of RS among the general public and among the medical and health related professional community, in view of the fact that it is a rare disorder
- By providing support and counseling for parents of individuals with RS
- By assessing of individuals with RS by a team of experts
- By providing guidance for educators and therapists working with individuals with RS
- By promoting and funding research on RS.

Two structures were established for this purpose:

- The Rett Syndrome Medical Clinic at the Safra Children's Hospital, Sheba Medical Center, Tel-Hashomer
- The Rehabilitation/Education Assessment and Counseling Center of the Israel Rett Syndrome Center.

The aim of the RS clinic is to provide comprehensive medical services for individuals with RS and their families in an effort to meet their medical and therapeutic needs, while taking the unique characteristics and requirements of each child and her family into consideration. These services are aimed at helping the child to attain optimal function. Diagnosis and assessment at the facility will enable guidance in areas such as:

- Counseling for the family and other supportive frameworks
- Recommendations and guidance for a holistic treatment program within the community framework
- Regular follow-up and a comprehensive treatment program

Description of activities

The Rett Syndrome Medical Clinic treats all girls in Israel who have been diagnosed with Rett syndrome (as of today there are approximately 130 known individuals with RS in Israel). The director of the clinic is a senior pediatric neurologist, Dr. Bruria Ben-Zeev. The team includes an orthopedic surgeon, a gastroenterologist, an endocrinologist, a geneticist and a dietician. The Rett syndrome clinic continues to follow each individual's progress on an annual or semiannual basis, depending on the age of the client and the severity of her phenotypic expression.

The Rehabilitation/Education Assessment and Counseling Center - The evaluation and guidance team was established with the objective to assess individuals with RS and to counsel the therapeutic, educational and rehabilitation staff, who supports the individual with RS on a daily basis.

The Rett Center Assessment Team (RS team) is a transdisciplinary team consisting of a special education teacher/advisor, a music therapist, a speech therapist, an occupational therapist and a physiotherapist. The aim of this team is to conduct assessment and advice on services for each child within her special education facility/residence in the presence of the local educational/habilitation staff and the family. In certain cases, such as when the child is too small to be integrated into a kindergarten or is in transition between special education facilities, assessment and guidance are conducted at the Tel Hashomer clinic. All of the assessments are fully funded by the Israel Rett Syndrome Center. The RS team has developed a unique assessment model that provides answers to the comprehensive needs of individuals with RS.

Contact
Sigal Hertz-Tirosh, Director
Israel Rett Syndrome Center
Rehov Leve Eskol 110/15
IL-69361 Tel Aviv
Israel
E-mail: info@rett.org.il

In: Rett Syndrome: Therapeutic Interventions
Editors: Meir Lotan and Joav Merrick

ISBN: 978-1-61728-080-1
©2011 Nova Science Publishers, Inc.

Chapter XXI

About the National Institute of Child Health and Human Development in Israel

The National Institute of Child Health and Human Development (NICHD) in Israel was established in 1998 as a virtual institute under the auspicies of the Medical Director, Ministry of Social Affairs and Social Services in order to function as the research arm for the Office of the Medical Director. In 1998 the National Council for Child Health and Pediatrics, Ministry of Health and in 1999 the Director General and Deputy Director General of the Ministry of Health endorsed the establishment of the NICHD.

Mission

The mission of a National Institute for Child Health and Human Development in Israel is to provide an academic focal point for the scholarly interdisciplinary study of child life, health, public health, welfare, disability, rehabilitation, intellectual disability and related aspects of human development. This mission includes research, teaching, clinical work, information and public service activities in the field of child health and human development.

Service and academic activities

Over the years many activities became focused in the south of Israel due to collaboration with various professionals at the Faculty of Health Sciences (FOHS) at the Ben Gurion University of the Negev (BGU). Since 2000 an affiliation with the Zusman Child Development Center at the Pediatric Division of Soroka University Medical Center has resulted in collaboration around the establishment of the Down Syndrome Clinic at that center. In 2002 a full course on "Disability" was established at the Recanati School for Allied Professions in the Community, FOHS, BGU and in 2005 collaboration was started with the Primary Care Unit of the faculty and disability became part of the master of public health course on "Children and society". In the academic year 2005-2006 a one semester course on "Aging with disability" was started as part of the Master of Science program in gerontology in our collaboration with the Center for Multidisciplinary Research in Aging.

Research activities

The affiliated staff has over the years published work from projects and research activities in this national and international collaboration. In the year 2000 the International Journal of Adolescent Medicine and Health and in 2005 the International Journal on Disability and Human development of Freund Publishing House (London and Tel Aviv), in the year 2003 the TSW-Child Health and Human Development and in 2006 the TSW-Holistic Health and Medicine of the Scientific World Journal (New York and Kirkkonummi, Finland), all peer-reviewed international journals were affiliated with the National Institute of Child Health and Human Development. From 2008 also the International Journal of Child Health and Human Development (Nova Science, New York), the International Journal of Child and Adolescent Health (Nova Science) and the Journal of Pain Management (Nova Science) affiliated and from 2009 the International Public Health Journal (Nova Science) and Journal of Alternative Medicine Research (Nova Science).

National collaborations

Nationally the NICHD works in collaboration with the Faculty of Health Sciences, Ben Gurion University of the Negev; Department of Physical Therapy, Sackler School of Medicine, Tel Aviv University; Autism Center, Assaf HaRofeh Medical Center; National Rett and PKU Centers at Chaim Sheba Medical Center, Tel HaShomer; Department of Physiotherapy, Haifa University; Department of Education, Bar Ilan University, Ramat Gan, Faculty of Social Sciences and Health Sciences; College of Judea and Samaria in Ariel and recently also collaborations has been established with the Division of Pediatrics at Hadassah, Center for Pediatric Chronic Illness, Har HaZofim in Jerusalem.

International collaborations

Internationally with the Department of Disability and Human Development, College of Applied Health Sciences, University of Illinois at Chicago; Strong Center for Developmental Disabilities, Golisano Children's Hospital at Strong, University of Rochester School of Medicine and Dentistry, New York; Centre on Intellectual Disabilities, University of Albany, New York; Centre for Chronic Disease Prevention and Control, Health Canada, Ottawa; Chandler Medical Center and Children's Hospital, Kentucky Children's Hospital, Section of Adolescent Medicine, University of Kentucky, Lexington; Chronic Disease Prevention and

Control Research Center, Baylor College of Medicine, Houston, Texas; Division of Neuroscience, Department of Psychiatry, Columbia University, New York; Institute for the Study of Disadvantage and Disability, Atlanta; Center for Autism and Related Disorders, Department Psychiatry, Children's Hospital Boston, Boston; Department of Paediatrics, Child Health and Adolescent Medicine, Children's Hospital at Westmead, Westmead, Australia; International Centre for the Study of Occupational and Mental Health, Düsseldorf, Germany; Centre for Advanced Studies in Nursing, Department of General Practice and Primary Care, University of Aberdeen, Aberdeen, United Kingdom; Quality of Life Research Center, Copenhagen, Denmark; Nordic School of Public Health, Gottenburg, Sweden, Scandinavian Institute of Quality of Working Life, Oslo, Norway; Centre for Quality of Life of the Hong Kong Institute of Asia-Pacific Studies and School of Social Work, Chinese University, Hong Kong.

Targets

Our focus is on research, international collaborations, clinical work, teaching and policy in health, disability and human development and to establish the NICHD as a permanent institute at one of the residential care centers for persons with intellectual disability in Israel in order to conduct model research and together with the four university schools of public health/medicine in Israel establish a national master and doctoral program in disability and human development at the institute to secure the next generation of professionals working in this often non-prestigious/low-status field of work.

Contact

Joav Merrick, MD, DMSc
Professor of Pediatrics, Child Health and Human Development
Medical Director, Health Services, Division for Mental Retardation, Ministry of Social Affairs and Social Services, POB 1260, IL-91012 Jerusalem, Israel.
E-mail: jmerrick@inter.net.il

In: Rett Syndrome: Therapeutic Interventions
Editors: Meir Lotan and Joav Merrick

ISBN: 978-1-61728-080-1
©2011 Nova Science Publishers, Inc.

Chapter XXII

About the Book Series
on Disability Studies

Disability studies is a book series with publications from a multidisciplinary group of researchers, practitioners and clinicians for an international professional forum interested in the broad spectrum of disability, intellectual disability, health and human development.

- Reiter S. Disability from a humanistic perspective: Towards a better quality of life. New York: Nova Science, 2008
- Knotkova H, Cruciani R, Merrick J, eds. Pain. Brain stimulation in the treatment of pain. New York: Nova Science, 2010.
- Prasher VP, ed. Contemporary issues in intelletual disabilities. New York: Nova Science, 2010.
- Lotan M, Merrick J, eds. Rett syndrome. Therapeutic interventions. New York: Nova Science, 2010.

Contact

Professor Joav Merrick, MD, MMedSci, DMSc
Medical Director, Division for Mental Retardation
Ministry of Social Affairs, POBox 1260
IL-91012 Jerusalem, Israel
E-mail: jmerrick@internet-zahav.net

Index

B

C

G

H

M

N

O

Q

R

S